YOU'VE HEARD THE HYPE.
NOW IT'S TIME TO SEPARATE FACT FROM FICTION.

FACT: Many medications can cause vitamin deficiencies. *Find out how vitamin absorption can be jeopardized by laxatives, painkillers, contraceptives, and common prescription drugs.*

FACT: Most herbal drug products lack quality control. *Learn how to tell if you are getting the dosages you need.*

FACT: It is crucial that minerals are kept in careful balance. *Discover how taking one mineral supplement can cause a serious deficiency of another—and how to avoid the health risks that accompany this common pitfall.*

FACT: RDAs or DRIs may be too low to ensure optimal health. *Discover what recommended doses will offer maximum benefits.*

FACT: Even those on healthy diets often lack many essential vitamins and minerals. *Find out why—and what you can do about it.*

FACT: A particular food's nutritional content can vary drastically depending on where it is grown and how it is cooked. *Discover how to buy and cook food to get optimal nutritional value.*

FACT: Alcohol, cigarettes, surgery, aging, and depression can change your nutritional needs. *Learn how to supplement wisely according to your individual conditions.*

THE
VITAMIN BOOK

REVISED EDITION

Harold Silverman, Pharm.D.

Joseph Romano, Pharm.D.

Gary Elmer, Ph.D.

NEW YORK • TORONTO • LONDON • SYDNEY • AUCKLAND

To Judi (HMS)

To my heroes—Linda, my wife and Anthony, my father. (JAR)

To my mother, Julia Ann Elmer, and father, Harrel Denison Elmer, in gratitude for providing many opportunities (GE)

ACKNOWLEDGMENTS

The authors would like to thank Judith I. Brown, and Nancy Monson for their invaluable assistance in updating *The Vitamin Book*.

THE VITAMIN BOOK

A Bantam Book

PUBLISHING HISTORY

Bantam paperback edition / August 1985

Revised paperback edition / July 1999

ISBN 0-553-57957-6

PRINTED IN THE UNITED STATES OF AMERICA

OPM   10   9   8   7   6   5   4

Contents

Part 5
DIETARY SUPPLEMENT PROFILES

Part 6
VITAMIN, MINERAL, AND HERBAL DRUG
INTERACTIONS

Appendix
VITAMIN AND MINERAL CONTENT
OF FOODS

TABLES

Introduction

Vitamins, minerals, and herbals are a big part of nearly everyone's life, as Americans spend billions of dollars on these products every year. Supplements continue to be a hot news topic; practically every day we read or hear about a new cancer cure, a miracle diet, a new approach to maintaining or improving health, or an amazing new vitamin, mineral, or herbal combination that will provide special benefits. What are these miracle remedies that are the source of eternal youth, beauty, and sexual prowess, these cures for the diseases that plague and endanger our lives? Do they really help?

Experts agree that vitamins and minerals are needed for everyday functions of the human body as well as to prevent deficiency conditions that occur when they are not present in the diet. But when you venture beyond the scientifically proven uses for vitamins and minerals, you enter a world of controversy and disagreement about how much of each vitamin and mineral you should take every day, what benefits these supplements can be expected to provide, and how to get these nutrients into your body. Some experts believe that you can, and should, get all the nutrition you need by eating a sensible balanced diet. Others feel that our calorie-counting, fast-paced lifestyles make it virtually impossible to eat enough of the right foods. Still others believe that doses of vitamins and minerals higher than the daily recommended amount can provide specific medical benefits, while others counter that there is no merit to the notion of treating disease with mega-doses of nutrients. Yet others see the mounting evidence for vitamin C, vitamin E, calcium, zinc, and other nutrients as the tip of a "nutriceutical" iceberg. The problem is, they say, we don't know enough about the important role played by these nutrients and how they can help us.

And the controversy continues to mount if you consider herbals, which, unlike vitamins, are not necessary for basic body function. Herbs have long been used as the sole source of medicine in many cultures, uses that pre-date the development of modern medicine. Millions of people around the world use herbs to supplement or replace "modern" medicines. How do they work? How do we know they work? How have the most popular herbals earned their reputations? Have modern herbal products been subjected to the same level of scrutiny and research as modern medicines? Are all herbal products the same? How can you know which herbal product to buy? Even though we now know more about herbal supplements than ever before, few of the products you can buy today could meet stringent federal criteria for approval as a drug product.

So how can you decide which vitamins, minerals, and herbals are right for you? Unfortunately, there are still few places for you to go for straightforward and scientifically based answers to the questions we most want answered about vitamins, minerals, and herbals. Most consumer-oriented books on the subject are written by vitamin or herbal advocates who hard-sell their product or program. These works are often based on scanty data and anecdotal evidence and may offer nonscientific advice on how to select the vitamins, minerals, and herbals you need to maintain your health.

Information in *The Vitamin Book,* however, comes from hundreds of scientific publications, and this revised and completely updated edition incorporates the most up-to-date research and information available. We have tried to dispel the myths, mysteries, and untruths commonly associated with these products. Here you will learn what vitamins, minerals, and herbals are, where and how they work in your body, when you need them, what they can do for you, how much to take, and how to select a vitamin, mineral, herbal, or combination preparation from the dizzying variety that are available in health food stores, pharmacies, and vitamin shops, as well as on the internet.

We believe that most—but not all—people can benefit by taking vitamins and minerals. In general, these supplements are not harmful, except perhaps when large doses are taken to modify the course of a disease. At these doses, vitamins and minerals are not being used as nutrients. They are being used as *drugs,* with the potential for drug-like side effects. Even in those cases where research has shown that vitamins may be beneficial (vitamin E to prevent heart disease, for example), some experts still feel that more research is needed to establish the true nature of their value. In *The Vitamin Book* we tell you how to use vitamins and minerals, and our recommendations are based on current knowledge of the safety and effectiveness of larger doses of selected vitamins and minerals.

Future research may show new ways in which vitamins can become an integral part of the prevention and treatment of diseases such as cancer, heart disease, and arthritis. Until then, your choice to take large doses of vitamins and minerals should be based on objective information about the benefits and risks of those nutrients, information that you will find in this book.

The same holds true for many herbals, some of which may also prove to be important in treating and preventing certain diseases. Unfortunately, many studies of herbal products do not meet modern scientific standards. Thus, we cannot recommend many herbal products for all of their currently popular uses. Ongoing research, especially research into the active medicinal components of herbs, will provide us with the information needed to develop them into important medicinal agents. Hopefully, this will lead to the creation of a specially regulated new class of medicines based on natural ingredients, as is already the case in many other countries. Until then, consumers will have to spend considerable time and effort to educate themselves on how to find and use quality herb products. We believe that this book will be useful in this effort.

In the final analysis, only you can determine how to make the best use of the information in this book. The information on the pages that follow will help you make reasonable decisions about the vitamins and other dietary supplements you and your family use as part of your plan to achieve and maintain good health.

Harold M. Silverman, Pharm.D.
Joseph A. Romano, Pharm.D.
Gary W. Elmer, Ph.D.

Part 1

SHOULD YOU TAKE VITAMINS AND MINERALS?

1

WHAT ARE VITAMINS AND MINERALS AND HOW DO THEY WORK?

There are some forty different substances known to be essential elements of human nutrition. Of these, thirteen are recognized as vitamins, and fifteen are recognized as either essential minerals (which are needed in large amounts), trace minerals (which are needed only in small amounts), or electrolytes. The remaining twelve are amino acids.

VITAMINS

The scientific discovery of vitamins as separate nutrients was launched in the late nineteenth century, when scientists and nutritionists began to examine specific foods already known for centuries to prevent the occurrence of certain diseases: oranges for scurvy and unpolished rice for beriberi and pellagra. Then, in the early twentieth century, Casimir Funk, a Polish biochemist working in London, isolated a crystalline substance from rice polishings and coined the word *vitamine* to describe this "amine" (a kind of chemical structure) that is essential for life. Later it was shown that not all vitamins share the amine structure and the final *e* was dropped, giving us the modern spelling, *vitamin*.

Research continued through the 1930s and 1940s, when many of the basic facts about vitamins were discovered. This history of vitamins offers some interesting scientific stories and is associated with several Nobel prizes.

The most recent vitamin and mineral research has been directed toward learning more about their effects on the body and newer uses for them. Much of this work was spurred by accidental discoveries about possible new uses for vitamins and minerals and others were based on theoretical but unproven roles for them. However, many of these studies have yielded little useful information or results that could not be reproduced by other investigators, rendering their conclusions questionable. Rumors of secret benefits to be reaped by taking certain vitamins and minerals have led to millions of health conscious baby boomers adopting inappropriate nutritional supplement products.

What Is a Vitamin?

Vitamins are essentially substances made by plants with the help of sunlight or by lower forms of life such as bacteria; in a few cases, vitamins can also be created by animals or the human body. They are always combinations of several chemical elements.

Most of our vitamins come from plants, and interestingly, the amount of a vitamin found in a given plant is always the same because the plant always makes just the right amount it needs to stay alive. For example, the average-size orange usually has about 85 mg of vitamin C. Vitamins found in animal products, such as eggs, are by-products of the plants ingested by the animal or were created by bacteria.

Over the years, scientists have developed three criteria by which a substance can be defined as a vitamin. If one of the three criteria is not satisfied, the substance in question is not considered a vitamin in the strictest scientific sense:

1. A vitamin is a nutrient required in small amounts for normal body function. With few exceptions, vitamins are not made in the body and must be supplied from an outside source. Even in those few circumstances where vitamins are made in the body, the process generally involves an important ingredient from outside the body, such as the bacteria normally found in our intestines. These bacteria are part of the normal flora that find their way into our body and reside within each of us.
2. A vitamin must be an organic chemical; that is, every vitamin has at least one carbon atom in its molecular structure. This automatically excludes minerals and other non-carbon-containing substances.
3. There is a specific set of symptoms or a specific disease associated with a deficiency of each vitamin, and it can be corrected by taking the appropriate amount of that vitamin.

It is unfortunate that advocates of vitamin treatments for illness have used the word *vitamin* improperly. Many of the proposed treatments involve doses of vitamins so far beyond the amounts required for normal nutrition that they are, in fact, no longer vitamins but drugs. Also, many treatments involve substances that do not meet the established criteria for vitamins: pseudovitamins. These include PABA, choline, inositol, and other substances that have been labeled vitamins to simply lend them public credibility.

Pressure from the United States Food and Drug Administration has forced the elimination of most pseudovitamins from multivitamin products. Despite the fact that these substances are either abundant in the food we eat or are not needed for daily function, they are still available for purchase in any health food store or vitamin center.

How Vitamins Work

Vitamins are chemical components in the complex machine that we call the human body. Each vitamin fits into a different part of the machine, and all of them are necessary for normal body function.

Chemists would call most vitamins cofactors (or catalysts). A cofactor is a substance that helps chemical reactions occur (usually more rapidly) but is not a primary ingredient in the reaction. A rough analogy is the oil in your car's crankcase: Although it is an essential ingredient to your automobile engine, it is not a major ingredient in the chemical reaction that makes the engine work. The major ingredients are gasoline, oxygen, and electrical spark. The oil helps this chemical reaction reach maximum efficiency by keeping all of the moving parts of your engine running as smoothly and friction free as possible.

Vitamins perform the same function in the body. For example:

- Vitamin B_1 (thiamin) is a cofactor in the series of chemical reactions that burn carbohydrates (sugars) in the body. Without thiamin, you would not be able to provide sufficient energy for body functions.
- Vitamin B_2 (riboflavin) serves as a cofactor in many chemical reactions involving the release of energy from body

proteins. For this reason, your riboflavin needs are directly related to the amount of energy you use each day.

• Folic acid serves as a cofactor in one of the chemical reactions that are basic to normal cell division in your body. Cell division is essential to many basic functions, including the replacement of worn-out body cells with new ones, providing new cells needed for growth and development, and healing wounds by making new cells.

Is There More than One Category of Vitamin?

Vitamins fall into two basic categories: those that dissolve in water, and those that dissolve in fat.

Water-Soluble Vitamins

The water-soluble vitamins are B_1 (thiamin), B_2 (riboflavin), B_3 (niacin or nicotinic acid), B_5 (pantothenic acid), B_6 (pyridoxine), B_{12} (cyanocobalamin), C (ascorbic acid), biotin, and folic acid.

These vitamins can be easily absorbed directly through the gastrointestinal tract into the bloodstream and don't require bile acids or other special substances to assist in this process. Once absorbed, they circulate in body fluids and are available when needed for body function.

Most water-soluble vitamins are not stored in large quantities for long periods of time. Once a certain reserve level (the threshold or saturation level) is reached, much of the excess water-soluble vitamin is eliminated from the body via the urine. Your urine may actually discolor (turn bright yellow). Therefore, taking more of these vitamins than you need—according to the recommendations discussed in the next chapter—is literally flushing money down the drain and can lead to toxic side effects.

Fat-Soluble Vitamins

The major fat-soluble vitamins are A, D, E, and K.

These vitamins are oily substances that require the addition of bile acids, your body's natural emulsifying agents, to be dissolved in intestinal contents and then absorbed into the bloodstream. The process can be compared to how we use soaps and detergents as emulsifying agents when washing out oily dirt from clothing. Since oil and water don't mix, oily dirt cannot be removed by water alone. The detergent allows the oil in the dirt to emulsify in the wash water, making it easier to remove.

Some fat-soluble vitamins, however, can be purchased in a "water-soluble" form. These products, such as the prescription vitamin Aquasol A, consist of vitamin that has been mixed with an emulsifying agent and can be absorbed without the assistance of bile acids.

Once absorbed, the fat-soluble vitamins migrate to their storage sites in body fat. When they are needed in the body, special carrier proteins take the vitamins from their storage areas to where they are needed.

You need to use good judgment because of this storage capability, since excessive amounts of some of these vitamins can be retained by the body and result in unpleasant or even hazardous symptoms. Therefore, taking more of this category of vitamin than you need can be not merely a waste of money, as in the case of water-soluble vitamins, but uncomfortable and even dangerous to your health.

Each vitamin has a specific action. Some are used more widely than others and are required in larger quantities. The specific functions of each vitamin and its role in human metabolism and function can be found in the individual profiles in Part 2 of this book.

MINERALS

Unlike vitamin research, serious study of the roles of the various minerals in the human body has been carried out mostly during the last two decades. Some minerals have been extensively studied, but many others are not well understood. Minerals such as chromium, magnesium, manganese, molybdenum, nickel, selenium, and zinc are now the subject of research projects all over the world. We believe that the next few decades will shed a vast amount of light not only on how these minerals function but also on how they can be used as possible therapeutic agents.

What Is a Mineral?

Minerals are basic elements that have their origin in the earth and, unlike vitamins, cannot be made by living systems. Those that have been found to be essential to body function are calcium, phosphorous, magnesium, iodine, iron, and zinc. Very small amounts of the important trace minerals copper, chromium, fluoride, manganese, molybdenum, and selenium are also needed by your body. Little scientific information is known about the other trace elements—arsenic, cadmium, cobalt, nickel, silicon, tin, and vanadium. The best guess is that they are required in very small amounts and that even the most nutritionally inadequate diet contains sufficient quantities.

As in the case of vitamins, we get most of our minerals from plants and from animal products that contain minerals as a result of the animal's consumption of mineral-rich plant life. However, whereas the vitamin content of a plant is stable, the mineral content is not. In fact, the amount of any particular mineral in a plant varies dramatically from region to region because of variations in the mineral content of the soil. For instance, iodine is found in much higher concentrations in seaside soils than in those inland. Accordingly, dietary sources of iodine that originate in the sea or areas near the sea are much higher in iodine than those that do not. Plant sources of the mineral usually provide about one-twentieth as much iodine as animal sources that have originated in the sea, such as shrimp, crab, halibut, perch, and other seafoods. Plants from the sea such as kelp and seaweed provide more than forty thousand times as much iodine per ounce as plants grown inland.

How Minerals Work

In the body, minerals work through a variety of mechanisms. One of the most important roles involves building basic body structure: Calcium, phosphorous, magnesium, and fluoride, for example, are major elements in forming bones and teeth. Some minerals are involved with enzyme activity, or they may combine with other chemicals to perform functions that are essential to life. Iron, for example, is a basic component of hemoglobin, the chemical contained in red blood cells that carries oxygen throughout our bodies. Copper plays a role in the process of building red blood cells and is also found in several different body enzymes, and chromium is involved in the metabolism of glucose.

Unlike vitamins, minerals are neither manufactured nor broken down within the body because they are basic elements. Minerals must combine with vitamins, enzymes, or other body substances to produce their effects. These combinations can be broken down, used up, or eliminated from the body and therefore must be recycled or remade.

Many minerals can cause definite adverse effects if you take too much of them, in contrast to vitamins, which are not as often associated with severe adverse effects. This potential for toxicity has been a natural barrier to the inappropriate use of minerals in the same way as vitamins have been misused.

Since there is so much we don't know about the specific functions of minerals in the body, there is considerable speculation as to their possible roles. Some people have even promoted minerals as a tool for life extension and a treatment for disease, but although every possibility must be examined, we believe that it is premature to conclude that any of these claims is valid. The specific functions of each mineral and its role in human metabolism and function can be found in the individual profiles in Part 3 of this book.

Electrolytes

Electrolytes are minerals that serve very specific functions. The most important of these is related to the maintenance of the balance of water within the body. Electrolytes regulate the flow of water across cell membranes by osmosis, a process wherein water shifts from areas of high electrolyte concentration to areas of low concentration in a natural effort to establish a balance. When electrolytes move, water moves with them! Electrolytes also have a role in certain enzyme and chemical reactions and are responsible for transmission of electric impulses across cell membranes. The specific functions of the major biological electrolytes, sodium and potassium, can be found in Part 3 of this book. Others are not discussed because only sodium and potassium are widely supplemented.

2

HOW MANY VITAMINS AND MINERALS DO I NEED?

There are four official sources of information on the average requirements of vitamins and minerals for good nutrition:

- RDA (Recommended Dietary Allowances) tables, prepared by the National Academy of Sciences.
- Dietary Reference Intake (DRIs) tables that replace the RDAs for certain nutrients. These are also prepared by the National Academy of Sciences, and are designed for use by both Americans and Canadians. The DRIs for calcium, phosphorus, magnesium, vitamin D, and fluoride, which were released in 1997, include and update the RDAs for these nutrients. Eventually the DRIs will replace all of the RDAs, since they are more comprehensive and specific.
- Daily Value (DV) tables prepared by the United States Food and Drug Administration (FDA). DVs, which are used for product-labeling purposes, are composed of two nutrient reference sets: Daily Reference Values (DRVs) and Reference Daily Intakes (RDIs). (The RDIs replace the U.S. RDAs that were once listed on vitamin labels.)
- Foreign and international nutrient standards, prepared by individual governments or the United Nations Food and Agriculture Organization (FAO) and the World Health Organization (WHO).

Of these, the RDAs and the DRIs will be the most helpful to you. Historically, the RDAs have been used as the basis for data on vitamin and mineral requirements. DRIs include the RDAs for many nutrients and are more appropriate for diet and meal planning. Both are cited throughout this book.

RDA TABLES

The RDAs are used as the basis for many U.S. governmental policy decisions relating to food and nutrition. They were first published in 1941 and are revised every few years to incorporate new knowledge. The last update was published in 1989 (and some of the recommendations in that report have been supplanted by the DRIs released in 1997). Two committees within the Food and Nutrition Board were charged with compiling these RDAs. The first, called the Dietary Allowances Committee, was specifically created to prepare all of the RDA tables from one incarnation to the next; the second, a subcommittee of the Food and Nutrition Board itself, was formed for the express purpose of composing *this* edition of the RDAs.

Basically, the RDAs are recommendations for average, safe, and adequate amounts of daily nutrient intake by 97 percent to 98 percent of healthy men, women, boys, and girls in different age groups. The RDAs also reflect the minimal amounts of vitamins and minerals that the body needs to ward off nutrient deficiencies. RDAs are intended to be met by consuming a broad variety of foods. Specific recommendations are given for infants, children, teenagers, pregnant and breast-feeding women, and adults through age fifty. Everyone over age fifty is grouped into the fifty-one-plus category. (The DRIs represent an advance over the RDAs because they contain a separate category for older adults age seventy and up.)

There is no way of knowing each person's specific nutrient needs, as the actual need for many nutrients is based on personal factors, diet, and exercise. So, the RDAs estimate the average requirement for a male or female of a certain age and then add on a little more to account for variations in need within a particular group of people.

How the RDAs Are Determined

There are four basic steps to the establishment of an RDA for each nutrient.

First, scientific studies are undertaken and existing information is reviewed to determine the approximate amount of each vitamin and mineral needed to maintain the health of an average person. The daily needs of healthy young males (except for iron, where women's needs are considered more essential) are used as a criterion and the results are then extrapolated to other age groups.

Second, the average amounts arrived at from the studies are increased by an additional arbitrary value that the experts feel will meet the requirements of nearly all people in the age/sex group under consideration. This is done in an attempt to ensure that everybody in the specific group receives all the nutrients they need.

The third step involves the addition of another increment to each RDA. This increment is meant to take into account natural differences in the amounts of nutrients absorbed and utilized by different people.

In the case of some nutrients, this difference is directly related to the amount of energy expended each day. Since the B-complex vitamins are involved in the process of generating energy, the more active you are, the more B vitamins you need. Some minerals may be needed in larger amounts by the young and growing (iron and calcium), by older people (calcium), or by pregnant women (calcium and iron). Others who might need more of a specific vitamin are smokers (vitamin C) and people who don't get outdoors (vitamin D). Specific information on why different people need different amounts of certain vitamins and/or minerals is provided in each of the vitamin and mineral profiles.

The fourth step involves the application of professional judgment. When data are limited or of poor quality, the experts take it upon themselves to interpret what little information they do have and come up with an allowance for a specific vitamin or mineral. If the available data are considered of good quality, no additional interpretation is needed.

Does the RDA Really Mean Daily?

No. The human body is a highly evolved and complex organism with many backup or secondary systems. In the case of vitamins and minerals, the body is able to store limited quantities of excess supplies of some nutrients for use on those days when the supplies are short. Thus the daily needs specified in the RDAs do not have to be taken in every day. They can be averaged out over a period of several days or weeks without causing you any adverse effect.

The RDAs as a Scientific Standard

The RDAs are standards arrived at by scientists. Nutritionists and others interested in studying human needs for various vitamins and minerals have used them as a guide but they will be replaced by DRIs for this purpose. The RDAs have no legal status, but are used by the Food and Drug Administration to set the legal standards, known as the DRVs (Daily Reference Values).

DRIs

The DRIs expand and update the RDAs in regard to certain nutrients—in fact, they will eventually replace the periodic revisions of the RDAs (although the term *RDA* will remain and the RDAs will be included in the more complex DRI recommendations). The DRIs are more specific in terms of age groups than are the RDAs. (They include a seventy-plus age group for nutrient intake, whereas the RDAs have only a fifty-one-plus age group). They were developed by the Standing Committee on the Scientific Evaluation of Dietary Reference Intakes (DRI Committee) of the Food and Nutrition Board, which is part of the Institute of Medicine, which is part of the National Academy of Sciences. Health Canada was also involved in the development of the DRIs, which are applicable to Canadians as well as Americans.

The DRIs came about as a result of cutting-edge research about the role vitamins and minerals play in promoting long-term good health and in reducing the risk of chronic diseases such as high blood pressure, diabetes, osteoporosis, heart disease, and even cancer.

TABLE 1
Recommended Dietary Allowances (RDAs)[a]
Food and Nutrition Board, National Academy of Sciences—National Research Council
Revised 1989

Designed for the maintenance of good nutrition of practically all healthy people in the United States

	Age (years)	Weight (kg)	Weight (lb)	Height (cm)	Height (in)	Protein (g)	Vitamin A (mcg RE)[c]	Vitamin D[d] (mcg)	Vitamin E (mg α-TE)[e]	Vitamin K (mcg)	Vitamin C (mg)	Thiamin (mg)	Riboflavin (mg)	Niacin (mg NE)[f]	Vitamin B6 (mg)	Folate (mcg)	Vitamin B12 (mcg)	Calcium[*] (mg)	Phosphorus[*] (mg)	Magnesium[*] (mg)	Iron (mg)	Zinc (mg)	Iodine (mcg)	Selenium (mcg)
Infants	0.0–0.5	6	13	60	24	13	375	7.5	3	5	30	0.3	0.4	5	0.3	25	0.3	400	300	40	6	5	40	10
	0.5–1.0	9	20	71	28	14	375	10	4	10	35	0.4	0.5	6	0.6	35	0.5	600	500	60	10	5	50	15
Children	1–3	13	29	90	35	16	400	10	6	15	40	0.7	0.8	9	1.0	50	0.7	800	800	80	10	10	70	20
	4–6	20	44	112	44	24	500	10	7	20	45	0.9	1.1	12	1.1	75	1.0	800	800	120	10	10	90	20
	7–10	28	62	132	52	28	700	10	7	30	45	1.0	1.2	13	1.4	100	1.4	800	800	170	10	10	120	30
Males	11–14	45	99	157	62	45	1,000	10	10	45	50	1.3	1.5	17	1.7	150	2.0	1,200	1,200	270	12	15	150	40
	15–18	66	145	176	69	59	1,000	10	10	65	60	1.5	1.8	20	2.0	200	2.0	1,200	1,200	400	12	15	150	50
	19–24	72	160	177	70	58	1,000	10	10	70	60	1.5	1.7	19	2.0	200	2.0	1,200	1,200	350	10	15	150	70
	25–50	79	174	176	70	63	1,000	5	10	80	60	1.5	1.7	19	2.0	200	2.0	800	800	350	10	15	150	70
	51+	77	170	173	68	63	1,000	5	10	80	60	1.2	1.4	15	2.0	200	2.0	800	800	350	10	15	150	70
Females	11–14	46	101	157	62	46	800	10	8	45	50	1.1	1.3	15	1.4	150	2.0	1,200	1,200	280	15	12	150	45
	15–18	55	120	163	64	44	800	10	8	55	60	1.1	1.3	15	1.5	180	2.0	1,200	1,200	300	15	12	150	50
	19–24	58	128	164	65	46	800	10	8	60	60	1.1	1.3	15	1.6	180	2.0	1,200	1,200	280	15	12	150	55

Age (years)	Weight (kg)	Weight (lb)	Height (cm)	Height (in)	Protein (g)	Fat-Soluble Vitamins				Water-Soluble Vitamins							Minerals						
						Vitamin A (mcg RE)[c]	Vitamin D[d] (mcg)	Vitamin E (mg α-TE)[e]	Vitamin K (mcg)	Vitamin C (mg)	Thiamin (mg)	Riboflavin (mg)	Niacin (mg NE)[f]	Vitamin B6 (mg)	Folate (mcg)	Vitamin B12 (mcg)	Calcium* (mg)	Phosphorus* (mg)	Magnesium* (mg)	Iron (mg)	Zinc (mg)	Iodine (mcg)	Selenium (mcg)
25–50	63	138	163	64	50	800	5	8	65	60	1.1	1.3	15	1.6	180	2.0	800	800	280	15	12	150	55
51+	65	143	160	63	50	800	5	8	65	60	1.0	1.2	13	1.6	180	2.0	800	800	280	10	12	150	55
Pregnant					60	800	10	10	65	70	1.5	1.6	17	2.2	400	2.2	1,200	1,200	300	30	15	175	65
Lactating 1st 6 months					65	1,300	10	12	65	95	1.6	1.8	20	2.1	280	2.6	1,200	1,200	355	15	19	200	75
Lactating 2nd 6 months					62	1,200	10	11	65	90	1.6	1.7	20	2.1	260	2.6	1,200	1,200	340	15	16	200	75

[a] The allowances, expressed as average daily intakes over time, are intended to provide for individual variations among most normal persons as they live in the United States under usual environmental stresses. Diets should be based on a variety of common foods in order to provide other nutrients for which human requirements have been less well defined.

[b] Weights and heights of reference adults are actual medians for the U.S. population of the designated age. The use of these figures does not imply the height-weight ratios are ideal.

[c] Vitamin A concentration is expressed as retinol equivalents. 1 retinol equivalent = 1 μg retinol or 6 μg of beta carotene.

[d] Vitamin D is expressed as cholecalciferol (a form of vitamin D). 10 μg cholecalciferol = 400 IU of vitamin D.

[e] Vitamin E potency is expressed as α-tocopherol equivalents (a form of vitamin E). 1 mg d-α tocopherol = 1 α-TE.

[f] 1 NE(niacin equivalent) is equal to 1 mg of niacin or 60 mg of dietary tryptophan.

* NOTE: The RDAs for calcium, phosphorus, magnesium, and vitamin D have been changed per the Dietary Reference Intakes (DRIs) of 1997. A recommendation for intake of the mineral fluoride has also been added. See following section and Tables 2 and 3 for more information. In addition, other DRIs are due to be created by the year 2000 for folate and other B vitamins, antioxidants such as vitamins C and E, and selenium.

The first DRI report was released in the summer of 1997 and focused on minerals and vitamins that contribute to bone health: calcium, phosphorus, magnesium, vitamin D, and fluoride. Another DRI report, released in April 1998, concerns folate and other B vitamins. Additional topics that will be explored over the next few years are antioxidants (vitamins C and E, and selenium); macronutrients (protein, fat, and carbohydrates); iron and zinc; electrolytes (sodium and potassium) and water; and other food components (fiber and phytoestrogens).

The DRIs consist of three types of recommendations that are relevant to you as a consumer:

• *Recommended Dietary Allowances (RDAs):* If an RDA has been established, the DRIs use the RDA as the basis for the recommendation for a specific nutrient. However, the DRIs may also increase or decrease some of the RDAs over the 1989 recommended levels. For instance, the RDA for calcium has been raised for many age groups in the DRIs to reflect current knowledge about the role of this mineral in preventing the bone-thinning disorder osteoporosis.

• *Adequate Intakes (AIs):* Where no RDA exists because of a paucity of scientific data, the DRIs set an adequate intake level that experts believe is sufficient to preserve health.

• *Tolerable Upper Intakes (ULs):* The most groundbreaking aspect of the DRIs is the establishment of a Tolerable Upper Intake Level for each nutrient. These ULs cap the recommended intakes of certain nutrients from foods, fortified foods, and nutrient supplements. Since food is no longer our sole source of nutrition and many of us take supplements or eat fortified foods, the potential for adverse health effects related to overconsumption of certain nutrients has become a concern. Hence, the ULs were established as a guide to help decrease the risk of side effects resulting from the ingestion of excess amounts of a particular vitamin or mineral. The UL of a nutrient is not meant to be a goal or recommended level of intake, however.

As you can see from Table 2, the DRIs have increased the calcium requirement for most adults from 800 mg to 1,000 mg. Children ages nine to eighteen should get 1,300 mg of calcium daily, and adults over the age of fifty should consume 1,200 mg. Pregnant and nursing women should actually receive just the amount recommended for their age group—1,000 mg to 1,300 mg—rather than the 1,200 mg recommended in the 1989 RDA. The DRIs also change and make more specific the recommendations for phosphorus, magnesium, and vitamin D, and, for the first time, tell consumers how much fluoride they should be ingesting.

Admittedly, the new DRI system is confusing—especially in light of all the other nutritional acronyms the government has thrown at us of late (RDA, U.S. RDA, RDI, DV, and so on; see next section). Yet it is worth understanding the recommendations, because they go beyond the scope of the RDAs and relate to current consumer habits, including supplementing various nutrients and eating enriched products. In short, while the RDAs still offer a guide for minimal intakes, the DRIs give very specific information about maximal intakes for good health.

Some bottom-line guidance: For the nutrients calcium, magnesium, phosphorus, vitamin D, and fluoride, try to achieve either the RDA or the AI level as described in Table 2. Don't consume more nutrients than the Tolerable Upper Intake Levels (UL) shown in Table 3. The Tolerable Upper Intake Levels should not be considered a goal to be achieved through dietary or other means. For all other nutrients, use the RDAs as your guide (see Table 1).

TABLE 2
Dietary Reference Intakes (DRIs) for Calcium, Phosphorus, Magnesium, Vitamin D, Fluoride, Thiamin, Riboflavin, Niacin, Vitamin B$_6$, Folate, Vitamin B$_{12}$, Pantothenic Acid, Biotin, and Choline

Established 1997 and 1998 by the Institute of Medicine—National Research Council

AGE	NUTRIENTS (MEASURE)													
	Calcium (mg/day)	Phosphorus (mg/day)	Magnesium (mg/day)	Vitamin D* (mcg/day)	Fluoride (mg/day)	Thiamin (mg/day)	Riboflavin (mg/day)	Niacin (mg/day)	B$_6$ (mg/day)	Folate (µg/day)	B$_{12}$ (µg/day)	Pantothenic Acid (mg/day)	Biotin (µg/day)	Choline (mg/day)
0–5 months														
Males	210 (AI)	100 (AI)	30 (AI)	5 (AI)	0.01 (AI)	0.2 (AI)	0.3 (AI)	2 (AI)	0.1 (AI)	65 (AI)	0.4 (AI)	1.7 (AI)	5 (AI)	125 (AI)
Females	210 (AI)	100 (AI)	30 (AI)	5 (AI)	0.0 (AI)	0.2 (AI)	0.3 (AI)	2 (AI)	0.1 (AI)	65 (AI)	0.4 (AI)	1.7 (AI)	5 (AI)	125 (AI)
6–11 months														
Males	270 (AI)	275 (AI)	75 (AI)	5 (AI)	0.5 (AI)	0.3 (AI)	0.4 (AI)	3 (AI)	0.3 (AI)	80 (AI)	0.5 (AI)	1.8 (AI)	6 (AI)	150 (AI)
Females	270 (AI)	275 (AI)	75 (AI)	5 (AI)	0.5 (AI)	0.3 (AI)	0.4 (AI)	3 (AI)	0.3 (AI)	80 (AI)	0.5 (AI)	1.8 (AI)	6 (AI)	150 (AI)
1–3 years														
Males	500 (AI)	460 (RDA)	80 (RDA)	5 (AI)	0.7 (AI)	0.5 (RDA)	0.5 (RDA)	6 (RDA)	0.5 (RDA)	150 (RDA)	0.9 (RDA)	2 (AI)	8 (AI)	200 (AI)
Females	500 (AI)	460 (RDA)	80 (RDA)	5 (AI)	0.7 (AI)	0.5 (RDA)	0.5 (RDA)	6 (RDA)	0.5 (RDA)	150 (RDA)	0.9 (RDA)	2 (AI)	8 (AI)	200 (AI)
4–8 years														
Males	800 (AI)	500 (RDA)	130 (RDA)	5 (AI)	1.1 (AI)	0.6 (RDA)	0.6 (RDA)	8 (RDA)	0.6 (RDA)	200 (RDA)	1.2 (RDA)	3 (AI)	12 (AI)	250 (AI)
Females	800 (AI)	500 (RDA)	130 (RDA)	5 (AI)	1.1 (AI)	0.6 (RDA)	0.6 (RDA)	8 (RDA)	0.6 (RDA)	200 (RDA)	1.2 (RDA)	3 (AI)	12 (AI)	250 (AI)
9–13 years														
Males	1,300 (AI)	1,250 (RDA)	240 (RDA)	5 (AI)	2.0 (AI)	0.9 (RDA)	1.3 (RDA)	12 (RDA)	1.0 (RDA)	300 (RDA)	1.8 (RDA)	4 (AI)	20 (AI)	375 (AI)
Females	1,300 (AI)	1,250 (RDA)	240 (RDA)	5 (AI)	2.9 (AI)	0.9 (RDA)	0.9 (RDA)	12 (RDA)	1.0 (RDA)	300 (RDA)	1.8 (RDA)	4 (AI)	20 (AI)	375 (AI)

14–18 years													
Males	1,300 (AI)	1,250 (RDA)	410 (RDA)	5 (AI)	3.2 (AI)	1.2 (RDA)	1.3 (RDA)	16 (RDA)	1.3 (RDA)	400 (RDA)	2.4 (RDA)	5 (AI)	25 (AI)	550 (AI)
Females	1,300 (AI)	1,250 (RDA)	360 (RDA)	5 (AI)	2.9 (AI)	1.0 (RDA)	1.0 (RDA)	14 (RDA)	1.2 (RDA)	400 (RDA)	2.4 (RDA)	5 (AI)	25 (AI)	400 (AI)
19–30 years													
Males	1,000 (AI)	700 (RDA)	400 (RDA)	5 (AI)	3.8 (AI)	1.2 (RDA)	1.3 (RDA)	16 (RDA)	1.3 (RDA)	400 (RDA)	2.4 (RDA)	5 (AI)	30 (AI)	550 (AI)
Females	1,000 (AI)	700 (RDA)	310 (RDA)	5 (AI)	3.1 (AI)	1.1 (RDA)	1.1 (RDA)	14 (RDA)	1.3 (RDA)	400 (RDA)	2.4 (RDA)	5 (AI)	30 (AI)	425 (AI)
31–50 years													
Males	1,000 (AI)	700 (RDA)	420 (RDA)	5 (AI)	3.8 (AI)	1.2 (RDA)	1.3 (RDA)	16 (RDA)	1.3 (RDA)	400 (RDA)	2.4 (RDA)	5 (AI)	30 (AI)	550 (AI)
Females	1,000 (AI)	700 (RDA)	320 (RDA)	5 (AI)	3.1 (AI)	1.1 (RDA)	1.1 (RDA)	14 (RDA)	1.3 (RDA)	400 (RDA)	2.4 (RDA)	5 (AI)	30 (AI)	425 (AI)
51–70 years													
Males	1,200 (AI)	700 (RDA)	420 (RDA)	10 (AI)	3.8 (AI)	1.2 (RDA)	1.3 (RDA)	16 (RDA)	1.7 (RDA)	400 (RDA)	2.4 (RDA)	5 (AI)	30 (AI)	550 (AI)
Females	1,200 (AI)	700 (RDA)	320 (RDA)	10 (AI)	3.1 (AI)	1.1 (RDA)	1.1 (RDA)	14 (RDA)	1.5 (RDA)	400 (RDA)	2.4 (RDA)	5 (AI)	30 (AI)	425 (AI)
>70 years													
Males	1,200 (AI)	700 (RDA)	420 (RDA)	15 (AI)	3.8 (AI)	1.2 (RDA)	1.3 (RDA)	16 (RDA)	1.7 (RDA)	400 (RDA)	2.4 (RDA)	5 (AI)	30 (AI)	550 (AI)
Females	1,200 (AI)	700 (RDA)	320 (RDA)	15 (AI)	3.1 (AI)	1.1 (RDA)	1.1 (RDA)	14 (RDA)	1.5 (RDA)	400 (RDA)	2.4 (RDA)	5 (AI)	30 (AI)	425 (AI)
Pregnancy													
≤18 years	1,300 (AI)	1,250 (RDA)	400 (RDA)	5 (AI)	2.9 (AI)	1.4 (RDA)	1.4 (RDA)	18 (RDA)	1.9 (RDA)	600 (RDA)	2.6 (RDA)	6 (AI)	30 (AI)	450 (AI)
19–50 years	1,000 (AI)	700 (RDA)	350–360 (RDA)**	5 (AI)	3.1 (AI)	1.4 (RDA)	1.4 (RDA)	18 (RDA)	1.9 (RDA)	600 (RDA)	2.6 (RDA)	6 (AI)	30 (AI)	450 (AI)
Lactation													
≤18 years	1,300 (AI)	1,250 (RDA)	360 (RDA)	5 (AI)	2.9 (AI)	1.5 (RDA)	1.6 (RDA)	17 (RDA)	2.0 (RDA)	500 (RDA)	2.8 (RDA)	7 (AI)	35 (AI)	550 (AI)
19–50 years	1,000 (AI)	700 (RDA)	310–320 (RDA)***	5 (AI)	3.1 (AI)	1.5 (RDA)	1.6 (RDA)	17 (RDA)	2.0 (RDA)	500 (RDA)	2.8 (RDA)	7 (AI)	35 (AI)	550 (AI)

* Vitamin D is expressed as cholecalciferol (one form of vitamin D). 10 mcg of cholecalciferol = 400 IU of vitamin D. Please note that amounts are recommended in the absence of sufficient exposure to sunlight.

**350 mg is for women ages 19–50; 360 mg is for women ages 31–50.

***310 mg is for women ages 19–30; 320 mg is for women ages 31–50.

AI = Adequate Intake, the intake that has been established as a goal level in the absence of the scientific data needed to establish an RDA.

RDA = Recommended Dietary Allowance, the intake that meets the needs of most healthy people in a specific age and sex group.

> = greater than

≤ = less than or equal to

Niacin equivalents: 1 mg niacin = 60 mg tryptophan

Folate listed as 1 µg food folate = 0.6 µg folate from fortified food supplement consumed as food = 0.5 µg of synthetic (supplemental) folic acid taken on an empty stomach.

Although AIs have been set for choline, it may be that the choline requirement can be met by endogenous synthesis at some ages.

Since 10% to 30% of older people may malabsorb food-bound B_{12}, it is advisable for those older than 50 years to meet their RDA mainly by eating fortified foods or a B_{12} supplement.

In view of the evidence linking folic acid with neural tube defects in the fetus, it is recommended that all women capable of becoming pregnant consume 400 µg of synthetic folic acid from fortified foods and/or supplements in addition to consuming folate from a varied diet.

It is assumed that women will be taking 400 µg of folic acid until their pregnancy is consumed and they enter pre-natal care, which ordinarily occurs after the critical time for the formation of the neural tube.

TABLE 3
Tolerable Upper Intake Levels for Calcium, Phosphorus, Magnesium, Vitamin D, Fluoride, Thiamin, Riboflavin, Niacin, Vitamin B₆, Folate, Vitamin B₁₂, Pantothenic Acid, Biotin, and Choline

Established 1997 and 1998 by the Institute of Medicine—National Research Council

AGE	NUTRIENTS (MEASURE)													
	Calcium (g/day)	Phosphorus (g/day)	Magnesium* (mg/day)	Vitamin D+ (mcg/day)	Fluoride (mg/day)	Thiamin (mg/day)	Riboflavin (mg/day)	Niacin (mg/day)	B_6 (mg/day)	Synthetic Folate (μg/day)	B_{12} (μg/day)	Pantothenic Acid (mg/day)	Biotin (μg/day)	Choline (mg/day)
0–5 months	-	-	-	25	0.7	-	-	-	-	-	-	-	-	-
6–11 months	-	-	-	25	0.9	-	-	-	-	-	-	-	-	-
1–3 years	2.5	3	65	50	1.3	-	-	10	30	300	-	-	-	1.0
4–8 years	2.5	3	110	50	2.2	-	-	15	40	400	-	-	-	1.0
9–13 years	2.5	4	350	50	10	-	-	20	60	600	-	-	-	2.0
14–18 years	2.5	4	350	50	10	-	-	30	80	800	-	-	-	3.0
19–70 years	2.5	4	350	50	10	-	-	35	100	1,000	-	-	-	3.5
>70 years	2.5	3	350	50	10	-	-	35	100	1,000	-	-	-	3.5
Pregnancy	2.5	3.5	350	50	10	-	-	35	100	1,000	-	-	-	3.5
Lactation	2.5	4	350	50	10	-	-	35	100	1,000	-	-	-	3.5

Note: A Tolerable Upper Intake Level represents the maximum intake that is unlikely to cause adverse health effects in most healthy individuals in a specific age group.

* The figure for magnesium represents amounts from supplements only and does not include ingestion of magnesium in food and water.

+ Vitamin D is expressed as cholecalciferol (a form of vitamin D). 10 μg cholecalciferol = 400 IU of vitamin D.

> = greater than

≤ = less than or equal to

ULs were established to protect the most sensitive members of the general public. Tolerable limits have not been established for thiamin, riboflavin, B_{12}, pantothenic acid, or biotin because of insufficient data. However, this does not mean that people can tolerate the intake of these nutrients at levels that exceed the RDA or AI over a long period.

RDIs, DRVs, AND DAILY VALUES AND PRODUCT LABELING

Early attempts by the federal government to regulate the safety and effectiveness of vitamins and minerals in our foods and in supplements resulted in the establishment of a minimal daily requirement for six vitamins and four minerals. These were re- placed in 1973 when the United States Food and Drug Adminis- tration published the first U.S. RDAs. The U.S. RDA values were derived from the RDA values and were meant to be a sim- plification of the RDA—to make it easier for manufacturers and food packagers to label their products with nutrient content. However, many people were confused by the terms *RDA* and *U.S. RDA,* so in the early 1990s the government replaced the U.S. RDAs with the RDIs. The RDIs, along with daily reference values (DRVs) for various food components such as fat, satu- rated fatty acids, cholestrol, fiber, sodium, and protein, comprise the Daily Values (DVs) (see Table 4).

If you're confused—and who wouldn't be by the alphabet soup of abbreviations—simply remember that *the DVs are simi- lar to the RDAs and in addition provide vitamin, mineral, and other food component information to guide you in making food choices.* The DVs are used as the standard for labeling all con- sumer products with nutritional value in America, including packaged foods and vitamin supplements.

Information on vitamin and mineral content is always given as a percentage of the DV and is based on a 2,000-calorie adult diet. However, when calculating your daily vitamin intake from labeled foods, we recommend that you use the actual content and the RDA/DRIs rather than the DV percentages listed on the package. Why? Because those percentages may not apply to your age and sex on the RDA/DRI tables, and the RDA/DRIs are far more comprehensive.

TABLE 4
Daily Values (DVs)

Reference Daily Intakes (RDIs)

Nutrient	Amount
Vitamin A	5,000 IU (1,000 mcg)
Vitamin C	60 mg
Thiamin	1.5 mg
Riboflavin	1.7 mg
Niacin	20 mg
Calcium	1,000 mg
Iron	18 mg
Vitamin D	400 IU (10 mcg)
Vitamin E	30 IU (20 mg)
Vitamin B_6	2.0 mg
Folic acid	400 mcg
Vitamin B_{12}	6 mcg
Vitamin K	80 mcg
Phosphorus	1,000 mg
Iodine	150 mcg
Magnesium	400 mg
Manganese	2 mg
Zinc	15 mg
Copper	2 mg
Biotin	300 mcg
Pantothenic acid	10 mg
Selenium	70 mcg
Chromium	120 mcg
Molybdenum	75 mcg
Chloride	3,400 mg

Daily Reference Values (DRVs)*

Food Component	DRV
Fat	65 g
Saturated fatty acids	20 g
Cholesterol	300 mg
Total carbohydrate	300 g
Fiber	25 g
Sodium	2,400 mg
Potassium	3,500 mg
Protein**	50 g

*Based on 2,000 calories a day for adults and children over 4 only.

**The DRV for protein does not apply to certain people; instead RDIs have been established for children ages 1–4 (16 g), infants under 1 year of age (14 g), pregnant women (60 g), and nursing mothers (65 g).

RDA/DRI VERSUS DV

The RDA/DRIs represent the most detailed and logical approach to daily vitamin requirements available to the American public. But they are far from perfect and because a number of adjustments must be made in deciding on any given value in order to cover variations among human beings, they are subject to a great deal of comment and criticism. Nevertheless, they are the best guidelines we have. Hence, we have designated the RDA/DRIs as the "gold standard" of *The Vitamin Book* for all of the vitamins and minerals covered.

We are not using the DVs as our standard because of the extremely general nature of their listings. They contain no age classifications (the RDAs and the DRIs have ten), do not differentiate between the sexes (the RDA/DRIs have separate listings for males and females at many ages), and they differ from the RDA/DRIs for several nutrients. They also don't offer the groundbreaking Tolerable Upper Intake Levels of the DRIs.

NEW FOOD LABELS

The Nutrition Labeling and Education Act of 1990 mandated that the United States Food and Drug Administration revamp food labels on all packaged foods. After much debate and consideration, labels were changed in 1994. Now every food product has a "Nutrition Facts" box that lists its nutrient content (see Figure 1). The new labels are much easier to read than the old ones, and they help you to better see how your food selections fit into a balanced diet and how well they meet your requirements for various nutrients.

Each label contains information about serving size, calories, and the percent of DVs the product contains for fat, cholesterol, sodium, total carbohydrates, dietary fiber, sugars, protein, vitamins, and minerals. In addition, food claims are now strictly defined and standardized for all products, so you don't have to spend your time figuring out what terms like "fat free," "low sodium," and "extra lean" really mean.

**FIGURE 1
A Sample Food Label: Spaghetti Sauce**

Nutrition Facts	
Serving Size ¹/₂ cup (120 mL)	
Servings Per Container about 6	
Amount Per Serving	
Calories 150 Calories from Fat 45	
	% Daily Value*
Total Fat 5 g	8%
Saturated Fat 1.5 g	8%
Cholesterol 0 mg	0%
Sodium 670 mg	28%
Total Carbohydrate 23 g	8%
Dietary Fiber 3 g	12%
Sugars 14 g	
Protein 2 g	

Vitamin A	25%	•	Vitamin C	25%
Calcium	4%	•	Iron	6%

* Percent Daily Values are based on a 2,000 calorie diet.
Your daily values may be higher or lower depending on
your calorie needs.

	Calories	2,000	2,500
Total Fat	Less than	65 g	80 g
Sat Fat	Less than	20 g	25 g
Cholesterol	Less than	300 mg	300 mg
Sodium	Less than	2,400 mg	2,400 mg
Total Carbohydrate		300 g	375 g
Dietary Fiber		25 g	30 g

FOREIGN AND INTERNATIONAL STANDARDS

Some countries simply adopt the FAO/WHO recommendations as their own or use the American RDAs. In other countries, agencies concerned with nutrition utilize a number of different studies and surveys. Logically, one would think that human nutrient needs are identical for all people, regardless of the country they live in, and that daily requirements should therefore be the same for everyone. While it's true that the research data on vitamins and minerals are the same, it is also true that the data are subject to slight differences in interpretation.

Table 5 presents some of the U.S. and non-U.S. nutrient standards.

TABLE 5
Foreign and International Nutrient Standards (Adults)

	World Health Organization	United States	Canada
Vitamin			
A	800–1,000 mcg RE	800–1,000 mcg RE	2,500 IU
C	50–60 mg	25–40 mg	30 mg
D	5–10 mcg	2.5–5 mcg	—
E	8–10 mg α-TE	5–10 mg α-TE	—
B_{12}	2 mcg	1–2 mcg	2 mcg
Folate	150–200 mcg	145–220 mcg	200 mcg
Niacin	13–19 mg	14–23 mg	19.8 mg
B_5	—	—	—
B_6	1.4–2 mg	1.4–2 mg	—
B_2	1–1.5 mg	1–1.6 mg	1.8 mg
B_1	1–1.5 mg	0.8–1.3 mg	1.2 mg
Mineral			
Calcium	800–1,200 mg	700–1,100 mg	400 mg
Iron	10–15 mg	8–13 mg	5 mg
Magnesium	280–350 mg	130–200 mg	—
Zinc	12–15 mg	9–12 mg	—

WHAT IF YOU TAKE IN MORE OR LESS THAN THE RDA/DRI FOR A VITAMIN OR MINERAL?

What happens if you don't take in as much of a given vitamin or mineral as called for by its RDA/DRI? What happens if you take in much more than is recommended? Unfortunately, these simple questions require a complicated answer, but here are some important points to remember in considering the RDA/DRI for each vitamin and mineral:

1. The RDA/DRI value for each nutrient is not an absolute measure of what your daily intake should be. It is only a guide to the amount of a nutrient appropriate for good health; specific needs can vary from one person to the next.
2. It is possible to maintain good health even if you don't reach the RDA/DRIs for some vitamins. Remember, the RDAs have been adjusted upward *twice,* to allow for differences in how individuals process the nutrients they take in and in how much of any given nutrient they need.

3. If you are planning to satisfy all of your vitamin and mineral requirements through a varied diet, you will inevitably take in more than the minimum amounts of some vitamins. Not only do foods contain more than one vitamin and/or mineral, but the vitamin content of foods is uneven and, in some cases, not even completely known.
4. If your regular diet provides more than the RDA/DRIs of certain nutrients, be careful about the vitamin supplements you use; it is possible to consume excessive amounts of some vitamins and minerals. Don't go over the Tolerable Upper Intake Levels (see Table 3).

Each vitamin and mineral must be considered individually when it comes to symptoms of deficiency or the possibility of toxicity. These potential problems are discussed in detail in the individual vitamin and mineral profiles in Parts 2 and 3. However, some generalizations can be made by category.

Water-soluble vitamin deficiencies, except for vitamin B_{12}, usually make themselves known sooner than those of the fat-soluble vitamins because the body retains much smaller amounts as backup storage. The actual appearance of deficiency symptoms, however, may take a month or more, depending on personal circumstances. For example, active people will show deficiency symptoms of the B-complex group (involved in body reactions that generate and use energy) sooner than sedentary individuals because they are using these vitamins at a more rapid pace.

As a ground rule, most water-soluble vitamins are not toxic, even when you take more of them than you can possibly use, because the excess is eliminated through the urine. As a result, there tends to be a general lack of concern on the part of most health professionals about severe adverse effects from self-medication with very large doses (megadoses) of this category of vitamin.

However, as you might expect, there are exceptions, and these are vitamins B_{12}, B_6, and, to some extent, vitamin C. Vitamin B_{12} is stored in the liver and can accumulate in the body to a toxic level. Vitamin B_6 also is stored in the liver and has been observed to be toxic in doses over 2 g; in addition, even as little as 50 mg a day has been shown to cause temporary nerve damage in women who use this vitamin to fight symptoms of premenstru syndrome. As for vitamin C, the body normally stores about 1,500 mg (1.5 g) of vitamin C in body tissues. After using its daily requirement of the vitamin at about 60 mg, the body will ordinarily discard, through the urine, anything in excess of the 1,500 mg it already has stored. But when the backup, or inventory, is partially depleted, perhaps because of reduced intake or unusually high use to fight infection, the body will replenish its inventory from either food or vitamin supplements, until the limit of 1,500 mg has been reached. After that, the body will return to using its 60 mg a day and discard any additional vitamin C in the urine.

Deficiencies of most fat-soluble vitamins will reveal themselves only after extensive body stores are used up, a process that can take months. On one hand, this is bad because a nutritionally deficient diet is masked for quite a long time. Once the deficiency makes itself known through the development of a deficiency disease, very large amounts of the vitamin are required to replace the depleted stores and return you to a healthy state. On the other hand, huge stores of fat-soluble vitamins can offer some protection if you find yourself in an unusual circumstance where you are unable to supplement your intake of fat-soluble vitamins.

Deficiency in fat-soluble vitamins can be caused by some drugs. For instance, taking these vitamins together with mineral oil—a widely used laxative—can cause a deficiency because the vitamins may dissolve in the mineral oil. If this happens, the vitamins will be eliminated from the body with the mineral oil, instead of being emulsified and absorbed into the bloodstream.

Among the fat-soluble vitamins, only relatively small amounts of vitamins E and K are stored in the body, even when large doses of these vitamins are taken. However, these vitamins, too, can be toxic. And if you take more of vitamins A and D than you need, the excess will accumulate in your liver and body fat, where it will remain. Health professionals are rightly alarmed by people who self-medicate with high doses of vitamins A and D because the accumulation can lead to symptoms of toxicity.

Minerals present somewhat different problems in terms of inadequate or excessive intake. Relatively small amounts of minerals are needed by the average person, and deficiencies in most minerals are therefore rare. The only major exceptions are the high incidence of iron deficiency in women during the childbearing years and calcium depletion in the postmenopausal years that may be aggravated by a lifelong calcium deficiency.

Several of the minerals are conveniently stored in large quantities in the form in which they can best serve the body. Calcium, for example, is stored in the structure of the bones and teeth. Zinc and other minerals are stored as enzyme or protein complexes; magnesium also makes up a part of bones and teeth. This storage potential, although beneficial, can lead to toxicity. The body's metabolic machinery is not very efficient in rapidly eliminating an excess of an inorganic element such as a mineral. Hence, taking more than the required amount can be toxic for some minerals. For example, copper, which is recommended for adults in daily amounts of 1.5 mg to 3 mg, becomes toxic if it is taken in doses of 10 mg or more a day. Likewise for fluoride, which is recommended in a daily dose of 3.1 mg for adults to prevent the formation of tooth cavities. People taking 10 mg to 20 mg of this element per day can develop a toxic condition in which their tooth enamel paradoxically becomes weakened, discolored, and *more* susceptible to decay.

Another consideration determining correct intake is the fact that interactions between vitamins and minerals may impede the absorption of one or both nutrients. When one is ingested in excess, it may inhibit the availability of one or more of the others. These interactions take place mainly between minerals with similar electronic structures. They have been discovered in studies on farm animals and in some cases in laboratory animals. The best-known example is the interaction between copper and molybdenum, which was discovered in cattle who developed a disease called scours when grazing on pasture where the herbage contained high levels of molybdenum. The copper deficiency occurred even when copper levels in the plants were considered to be in the normal range. The mechanism by which molybdenum causes a copper deficiency is not well understood, but there appears to be both decreased copper absorption and decreased copper utilization. Those interactions considered important to humans are discussed in the section on Vitamin, Mineral, and Herbal Drug interactions on page 385.

ARE THE RDA/DRIs TOO LOW?

There is controversy today over whether the RDA/DRI levels are actually sufficient to meet the needs of the American population. Many experts stand by the RDA/DRIs, just as they stand by the idea that we can get all of the nutrients we need from a well-balanced diet. Others feel the RDA/DRIs are too low and that supplements are the only way to provide the body with the nutrition it needs. For instance, a government-funded study suggests that the adult RDA for vitamin C needs to be tripled, to around 200 mg. The existing guideline of 60 mg was basically devised to provide minimal protection against the disease called scurvy. But the recent focus on the immunity-boosting and antioxidant properties of vitamin C spurred researchers to find a dose that would perform a greater service. This study showed that while 1,000 mg caused no apparent harm, a dose of 200 mg best satisfied the RDA criteria to meet the body's needs without causing problems.

The study had several drawbacks, however: Only seven healthy young men participated, and it did not look at women. However, it was very strictly controlled—the men actually lived in a hospital environment—and it lasted for four to six months.

Until planned follow-up studies are performed on women and other populations, the researchers suggest extrapolating the 200 mg recommendation to all adults. In addition, they say that it is possible to obtain 200 mg of vitamin C from your diet if you eat the government-recommended five servings of fruits and vegetables a day.

It is likely that as more studies are conducted on the effects of vitamins and minerals in preventing disease, some of the RDAs will be adjusted upward for many groups of people. Indeed, one of the goals of the DRIs is to offer more specific and extensive guidance for the use of nutrients to promote good health than do the RDAs.

FOOD VERSUS SUPPLEMENTS

Traditionally, the government, the American Dietetic Association, and the medical community have believed it is best to obtain the vitamins and minerals the body needs by eating a variety of foods. In recent years, however, given the explosion of interest in supplements and the vast amount of research showing that vitamins and minerals can protect against and treat many illnesses, they are beginning to soften their stance. We believe that vitamins and minerals are absolutely essential for some people, not all. See Chapter 4 "Who Needs Supplemental Vitamins and Minerals?" for specific recommendations.

Here, then, are summaries of the official statements on this topic from important nutrition groups.

The 1989 RDA Committee: "RDAs are neither minimal requirements nor necessarily optimal levels of intake. They are amounts intended to be consumed as part of a normal diet. If the RDAs are met through diets composed of a variety of foods derived from diverse food groups rather than by supplementation or fortification, such diets will likely be adequate in all other nutrients for which RDAs cannot currently be established."

The 1997 DRI Committee: The 1997 DRI report does not take a position on whether the recommended levels should be met through food, supplements, or a combination of the two. However, the report does recognize that it may be difficult to obtain the sometimes higher DRI levels from foods—especially since many of us have trouble reaching the 1989 RDA levels. Hence, the report states that "eating fortified food products represents one method by which to increase or maintain intakes without major changes in food habits. For some individuals at higher risk of chronic disease, use of nutrient supplements for some nutrients may be desirable in order to meet RDAs or AIs."

The United States Department of Health and Human Services (from the Dietary Guidelines for Americans): "Supplements of vitamins, minerals, or fiber . . . may help to meet special nutritional needs. However, supplements do not supply all of the nutrients and other substances present in food that are important to health. Supplements of some nutrients taken regularly in large amounts are harmful. Daily vitamin and mineral supplements at or below the Recommended Dietary Allowances are considered safe, but are not usually needed by people who eat the variety of foods depicted in the *Food Guide Pyramid*."

The American Dietetic Association: "It is the position of The American Dietetic Association that the best nutritional strategy for promoting optimal health and reducing the risk of chronic disease is to obtain adequate nutrients from a wide variety of foods. Vitamin and mineral supplementation is appropriate when well-accepted, peer-reviewed, scientific evidence shows safety and effectiveness."

THE MEGADOSE ISSUE

Using Vitamins to Prevent Disease

Many vitamin enthusiasts today are recommending that we take very large quantities, or megadoses, of vitamins to prevent disease. This is not always a bad idea, although available data and government policies, as well as much of the nutrition and medical establishment, say this form of supplementation can be dangerous and is ill-advised.

There's no doubt that megadoses of certain vitamins (A and D come to mind) *can* be harmful. But when it comes to the antioxidant vitamins C and E and to folic acid, which clinical studies linked to decreasing the risks of cancer and heart disease, we part ways with the establishment.

While we applaud the skepticism of these groups, we feel they are mistaken in taking such a conservative and closed-minded stance in demanding incontrovertible scientific evidence of the benefits claimed for megadoses of antioxidants and folic acid before saying yes to supplementation. At this point in time, we believe the evidence for benefit is there, though the precise benefits and risks remain to be defined by further research. We don't believe it is wise or necessary to take a wait-and-see approach until studies bear fruit. Such a delay could take years off your life.

It is our contention that the evidence about the value and safety of larger doses of vitamins C and E and folic acid than recommended by the current RDAs has been proven to a great enough degree to warrant taking such products in or along with a multivitamin. DRIs, including Tolerable Upper Intake Levels, have not yet been established for the antioxidants, so we're not sure where the government will go with this issue, but the 1998 DRIs include an acknowledgment of the key role played by folate and an important increase in the intake levels for everyone. However, we advocate early and consistent antioxidant and multivitamin/mineral use starting in childhood and continuing for your whole life. Supplementation is not just for the young or old. Today, the data clearly indicate that it has benefits for all of us.

A forward-thinking group that agrees with our position is the Alliance for Aging Research, a nonprofit, national public health organization. In 1994 this group took the bold step of advocating that consumers take large amounts of antioxidant vitamins to fight age-associated damage to the body's cells. They recommended taking vitamin C in a daily dose of 250 mg to 1,000 mg and vitamin E in a dose of 100 IU to 400 IU per day. (The alliance also recommended beta carotene supplementation, which we do not.)

The alliance based its recommendations on over two hundred clinical and epidemiological studies conducted over the past two decades that suggest these vitamins can reduce the risk of developing cancer, heart disease, and cataracts as you age. In addition, their analysis found that these vitamins are safe and effective for most individuals to take, and that it is difficult to get the high doses needed from foods alone. (Besides which, most Americans are already falling short in consuming the more conservative number of servings of various foods—especially fruits and vegetables—the government recommends for good health.)

Using Vitamins to Treat Disease

In contrast, the trend toward people taking massive doses of vitamins and minerals to treat disease (not just prevent it) without guidance from a physician is troubling to us. Such people are using these substances as drugs, not as food supplements. We strongly encourage you to seek the advice of a physician if you wish to use megadoses of vitamins to treat disease.

More information on this controversial topic will be found in Chapter 5, "Vitamins and Minerals as Drugs," and in each of the individual vitamin and mineral profiles in Parts 2 and 3.

FUTURE TRENDS

The future will likely see an expansion of research into the disease-preventive and treatment properties of vitamins and minerals. New forms of vitamin and mineral applications will become a reality. We'll increasingly see our food fortified with necessary nutrients, just as folic acid was recently added to grain products to supplement the diet of reproductive-age women so they receive an adequate amount of the vitamin in case of pregnancy. (Folic acid can prevent birth defects such as spina bifida and may also protect against cervical cancer, heart disease, and stroke.)

Genetically engineered foods designed to enhance nutrient content, taste, and shelf life can also be expected. Three such products are currently on the market. The Flavr Savr tomato was developed to maintain its vine-ripened freshness during shipping. The second is chymosin, an agent that is used in cheese production because it makes milk curdle. The third is recombinant bovine somatotropin (rbST), a growth hormone given to cows to increase their milk production.

A variety of new nutrients will surely be discovered in foods. These will include phytochemicals—the hundreds or thousands of hidden compounds in plant foods. Currently recognized phytochemicals include limonene in citrus fruits, isoflavones in soybeans, phytic acid in grains, and indoles in cruciferous vegetables. As more and more of these phytochemicals are discovered and studied, we suspect they may become the vitamins of the future.

3

GETTING VITAMINS AND MINERALS FROM THE FOODS YOU EAT

Most nutrition experts agree that the foodstuffs available in the United States and other industrialized nations have the capacity to provide all the nutrients we need. And surveys clearly show that Americans are more nutrition- and health-conscious than ever before. Yet the fact remains that many of us are deficient in one or more nutrients, or would be if we did not take supplemental vitamins and minerals.

The vitamin inadequacy of the average diet can be verified by information gathered from the most recent national health survey. According to the What We Eat in America survey of ten thousand individuals, conducted by the United States Department of Agriculture (USDA), our population is vitamin-deficient in some key areas. Between 1994 and 1995, most adult women did not meet the RDAs for six nutrients—iron, zinc, vitamin B_6, calcium, magnesium, and vitamin E—and adult men failed to meet the RDAs for zinc and magnesium. In addition, although children and teenage boys did meet the RDAs for most nutrients, the survey found that teenage girls were averaging 85 percent or less of the RDAs for calcium, magnesium, zinc, and vitamin E.

The 1991 to 1995 Framingham Nutrition Studies of 1,375 women and 1,145 men found similar deficiencies in Americans' diets. By analyzing three days' worth of food diaries, the investigators reported that more than half of the women surveyed fell short of the RDAs for beta carotene, vitamin E, vitamin B_6, and calcium. More than half of the men did not meet RDAs for beta carotene, vitamin E, calcium, and sodium.

If we couple this information with the fact that vitamin deficiencies are more likely to occur in certain groups of people—as discussed in the next chapter—the picture of a society deficient in vitamins and minerals begins to emerge.

Why is this? Is modern agriculture destroying the quality of our food? Are our diets inadequate to our needs? Are the RDAs too high? Are we storing and processing our foods improperly? This chapter attempts to shed some light on these important and controversial questions.

THE CONTROVERSY OVER AGRICULTURAL METHODS

Some people are concerned that our soil is becoming depleted of trace minerals by continuous farming on the same fields. They fear that the foods we eat are becoming depleted of vital minerals. This is a complex issue about which not a great deal is known, but the lack of evidence of mineral deficiencies in our population speaks to the adequacy of our soil. (Indeed, plants simply wouldn't grow if the soil didn't contain enough minerals to nourish them.) Furthermore, trace minerals are replenished in soil in rainwater and especially by irrigation water that is obtained from rivers or wells, which draw from other soil or rock formations far away from farms.

On the other hand, agricultural practices that remove the total crop from the field year after year with no replenishment of trace minerals can, over time, result in a crop poor in these minerals. Of course, the farmer could apply fertilizer to the fields, but with most fertilizers this practice would replenish only potassium, phosphates, and nitrogen. Rotating a "green manure" crop such as clover, which is plowed under after the end of the growing season, would renew only nitrogen in the soil, not trace elements. There is a growing realization, therefore, that so-called organic farming makes good commercial sense and would help to minimize depletion. In organic farming there is no reliance on chemical fertilizers; rather, soil is invigorated by the application of manure and by the plowing in of compost and crop wastes such as corn stalks and bean vines. These techniques return organic material and trace minerals back to the soil and are to be commended. However, for maximum yields, a chemical fertilizer may be required in addition to manure and plant waste.

Some critics of modern farming methods fear that the hardier species of fruits and vegetables that have been developed to make shipment easier have resulted in a loss of vitamin content.

This concern is unfounded because the creation of vitamins by plants is an automatic biological process. Any variety of plant will make the full complement of vitamins it needs.

Conversely, several popular writers have advanced the notion that extensive vitamin and mineral supplementation of animals' feed has resulted in excess nutrients finding their way into our diets. In fact, most of the nutrients fed to animals are used up within their own bodies to carry out normal metabolic activities. A portion of the remaining vitamins are stored just as they would be in the human body, but most of them are simply passed out of the animal's body via the urine.

In our opinion, critics of American agricultural methods—insofar as they reflect on nutrition—have not made a case for their point of view. Our soil and the produce it grows are not deficient. We must look elsewhere to find out why we do not get all of the vitamins and minerals we need from the foods we eat.

CAN YOU EAT ENOUGH TO SATISFY YOUR VITAMIN AND MINERAL NEEDS?

In theory, yes, according to the government guidelines outlined in the Food Guide Pyramid (page 43). (See below for more information on the Pyramid.) In practice, probably not.

Surveys have shown that few of us are able to meet the established RDAs for all vitamins and minerals through dietary means. We either can't eat the volume of food that would be required to provide the nutrients, don't want the calories found in the foods required to obtain the necessary vitamins, or simply won't devote the time needed to select the proper foods. And many of us won't give up the junk foods and new low-fat, high-calorie substitutes that clutter our diets.

In addition, large amounts of some vitamins are lost from foods that have been subjected to the processing techniques normally used in the food industry. These include the treatment of foods by heat or irradiation prior to canning or freezing, and other processes to which our foods are subjected before we actually eat them.

Since it is difficult for most of us to meet normal vitamin and mineral requirements through dietary measures, it follows that achieving higher individual levels of vitamin and mineral intake by dietary means is almost impossible. For example, if you

wanted to get an additional 500 mg of vitamin C from your
diet every day, you would have to eat an *extra* 2½ cantaloupes
(400 calories), 7¾ pounds of blueberries (2,200 calories), or
6½ cups of grapefruit sections (550 calories). You could mix
your fruits with other vitamin C sources for variety, but
you would still have to eat an awful lot of extra food. If you
wanted an additional 400 units of vitamin E from everyday foods, you would have to eat twenty-one cups of sunflower seeds (17,100 calories), four pounds of English walnuts
(11,812 calories), or twenty cups of black raspberries (2,000
calories).

Nutritional needs at higher levels than the RDA/DRIs are
discussed in the individual vitamin and mineral profiles (see
Parts 2 and 3), and supplements to a daily diet would clearly be
needed in such cases. For the average person, some supplements
may also be necessary to bring daily intake up to the RDA/DRI
levels, even when serious attention is paid to food intake.

THE "AVERAGE DIET" THEORY

It would be nice to offer a solution to the problem of good nutrition
by drawing up diets that would be right for everyone. Unfortunately, this is not as easy as it sounds, for several reasons.

First, foods that are commonly found in one area of the country
or in the diet of one ethnic or economic group may be uncommon in another. People's eating habits also vary widely, even
within ethnic groups and regions of the country.

Second, a diet evaluation must include only food that is actually eaten. If considerations are based only on what is bought or
prepared, the resulting nutritional picture will be distorted.

Third, the way you prepare and cook raw and processed
foods at home may affect their vitamin content. For example,
paring certain vegetables before cooking often results in the loss
of most of their water-soluble vitamins. Baking and other cooking methods can also lead to vitamin loss.

When estimating the vitamin losses from your food during
preparation, remember that it is unreasonable to expect that the
preparation conditions of test foods will be identical to those being prepared in your home. Therefore, individual diets can be
evaluated only by analyzing the final food product.

Fourth, your dietary or body level of one vitamin or mineral may influence your requirement for another. For example, many of the water-soluble vitamins' functions are interrelated because they all participate in the series of chemical reactions known as the Krebs cycle, which is involved in energy generation. Thus, a deficiency in one vitamin may affect the ability of the other vitamins to function. The nutrients that are interrelated in this way are niacin, thiamin, pyridoxine, riboflavin, biotin, pantothenic acid, choline, and cyanocobalamin.

Vitamin needs can also be related to the nature of your dietary intake. More thiamin, niacin, riboflavin, and other water-soluble vitamin requirements are needed in a high-carbohydrate diet. In contrast, a high-protein diet calls for increased pyridoxine and has an effect on the amount of riboflavin the body stores. Zinc seems to play a role in the action of vitamin A, so that vitamin A deficiencies can be more easily corrected if there is a sufficient amount of zinc in the diet. And vitamin C (ascorbic acid) is a factor in the efficient absorption of iron from the gastrointestinal tract. Thus it is possible that you are taking enough iron but don't have enough ascorbic acid in the diet to get the full value of that iron. Usually, however, the situation is reversed, with more than enough C and too little iron in the diet.

Fifth, it is difficult and time consuming to translate information from nutrition value tables to our daily diet. For example, to determine the vitamin content of a simple ham sandwich on white bread, we must find the listing for "Ham: piece, approx. 4⅛ in. long, 2¼ in. wide, ¼ in. thick; wt. 1½ oz." Assuming that three such slices are used in our sandwich, we can determine that, from the ham alone, we will gain no vitamin A, 7.2 mg of niacin, 0.37 mg of riboflavin, 0.81 mg of thiamin, and no vitamin C. Similar steps must be followed for every part of the sandwich, and then for total food intake.

Interestingly, the technology explosion has led to the introduction of a number of programs and services that will analyze your diet for vitamin and mineral content—as well as for fat, cholesterol, sodium, and other nutritive components—using a computerized listing of the information contained in the United States Department of Agriculture (USDA) tables on the nutritive value of American foods.

These computer programs can help you find an optimal diet

by pointing out where your diet is lacking and making suggestions as to how to improve your eating patterns.

Below we've provided a list of some of the programs available as computer software or via the Internet. Please note that we are not endorsing any one product. Nor is this a complete list; there are many, many programs out there—enough so that you can surely find one that suits your needs and pocketbook.

Software:

Balance Your Diet, Diet Analysis, Eating Machine
Queue, Inc.
800-232-2224
Apple-compatible

Executive Diet Helper/Menu Planner/Weight Loss Planner (set)
Food Label Analyzer
Ohio Distinctive Software
614-459-0453
Windows- and Macintosh-compatible

The Diet Balancer
Nutridata Software Corporation
800-922-2988
Windows- and Macintosh-compatible

Diet Wise–Energy Wise
Dine Healthy
Nutritional Data Resources
800-NDR-DIET
Diet Wise–Energy Wise is Windows-compatible
Dine Healthy is Macintosh-compatible

FoodWorks
The Nutrition Company
888-65WORKS
Written for registered dietitians, but sophisticated consumers may also benefit from its use.
Windows

Nutribase
Cybersoft
800-959-4849
www.nutribase.com
Windows, Macintosh

Idaho Diet Analysis
University of Idaho, Agriculture Communication Center
208-885-7982
Windows-compatible

Nutritionist Five
First Data Bank
800-633-3453
www.firstdatabank.com

NutriGenie Zone Diet Meal Planners
NutriGenie
800-242-4775
www.pslweb.com
Windows

Nutristar CD-ROM
Hopkins Technology
612-931-9376
Windows-compatible

What Did You Eat Yesterday? The Pyramid Version
Learning Seed
800-634-4941
Windows-compatible

Internet:

Food Finder (Fast Food)
Olen Publishing
http://www.olen.com/food

Nutrient Data Laboratory
USDA/Center for Nutrition Policy and Promotion
http://www.nal.usda.gov/fnic/foodcomp/

Nutrition Analysis Tool
University of Illinois
http://www.ag.uiuc.edu/~food-lab/nat/

Nutrition Software Finder
http://nutrition.miningco.com

THE DIETARY GUIDELINES FOR AMERICANS

Over the years, nutrition and food researchers have developed a set of standard recommendations for the kinds of foods we should eat to maintain a healthy nutritional state.The Dietary Guidelines for Americans are the official policy of the United States Department of Agriculture and are updated every five years. The guidelines describe food choices that will help you meet the RDA/DRIs. They also intersect with the nutrition labeling that now appears on all packaged food products.

Here are the basic recommendations contained in the latest edition of the Dietary Guidelines for Americans:

• *Eat a variety of foods.* No one food can supply all of the vitamins, minerals, and other nutrients your body needs. By varying the foods you eat, you have the greatest chance of obtaining the full range of nutrients. The Food Guide Pyramid (see Figure 2 and section below) offers information on the number of servings and amounts of various foods that are most healthful to consume.

• *Balance the food you eat with physical activity and maintain or improve your weight.* Being overweight dramatically increases the risk for many diseases, such as high blood pressure, heart disease, stroke, diabetcs, cancer, arthritis, and breathing disorders. Since many adults have a tendency to gain weight with age, this guideline encourages weight maintanance or loss as a goal of good health.

• *Choose a diet with plenty of grain products, vegetables, and fruits.* These foods are the basis of a varied and healthy diet. They contain vitamins, minerals, complex carbohydrates, and other compounds that are healthful, and they are usually low in fat.

• *Choose a diet low in fat, saturated fat, and cholesterol.* Although some dietary fat is needed to ensure good health, most Americans consume way too much fat and cholesterol. Such high-fat diets raise the risk of obesity, heart disease, and cancer.

• *Choose a diet moderate in sugars.* As with fat, Americans tend to go overboard with sugar, which is high in calories.

• *Choose a diet moderate in sodium.* Sodium has been associated with high blood pressure. Sodium and sodium chloride (salt) are found in large amounts in processed and prepared foods.

• *If you drink alcoholic beverages, do so in moderation.* Alcohol is high in calories and typically devoid of nutrients and can cause a number of illnesses if consumed to excess. Moderation is defined as no more than one drink per day for women and two drinks a day for men.

THE FOOD GUIDE PYRAMID

For nutrition purposes, foods used to be conveniently divided into the basic four food groups: the milk group, the meat group, the fruit and vegetable group, and the bread and cereal group. These categories were first developed in the 1950s and included recommendations on the amounts of foods to be consumed from each group.

In the mid-1980s, however, the federal government abandoned the basic four food groups in favor of the Daily Food Guide. This guide was redesigned in 1992 as the Food Guide Pyramid and was created to help Americans adopt the recommendations contained in the Dietary Guidelines for Americans.

Both of these programs were developed based on the latest nutrition research and surveys of what Americans are eating, and go far beyond the tenets of the basic four food groups in establishing goals for healthy eating. Both programs focus on fat because most Americans consume too much fat in their diets. In addition, the Food Guide Pyramid is designed to assist you in making better food choices, while also guiding you to eat the right number of calories to maintain a healthy weight. (Remember, the pyramid is a *guide,* not a strict rule.) Vegetarian groups have developed their own Food Guide Pyramids.

FIGURE 2
The Food Guide Pyramid

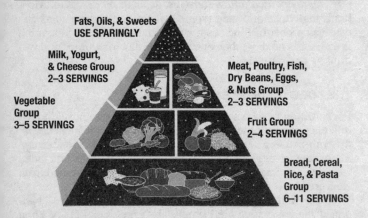

How the Pyramid Works

The Food Guide Pyramid is composed of four levels. Most of the foods you eat should come from the bottom two levels of the pyramid.

The bottom level, which is also the largest, is the bread, cereal, grain, and rice group. These foods should form the basis of every meal. Six to eleven servings per day are recommended for the complex carbohydrates they supply, which arc an important source of energy. These foods also contain fiber, vitamins, and minerals.

The next level contains the fruit group, from which you should try to consume two to four servings a day, and the vegetable group, from which you should try to eat three to five servings a day. Most people don't eat enough of these foods, which are major sources of vitamins, minerals, and fiber.

The second tier from the top contains the meat, poultry, fish, dry beans, eggs, and nut group. You should have only two or three servings of these foods a day. Also on this level is the milk, yogurt, and cheese group, from which you should have two or three servings a day. The foods in these groups are important sources of protein, calcium, iron, and zinc.

The top level contains the fats, oils, and sweets group, from which you should eat sparingly. Although you need a little fat in your diet to stay healthy, most of us consume too much of these types of foods. In addition, these foods tend to be high in calories. Their nutritional value is determined by the base ingredients from which the food is prepared.

Sample Calorie Levels

The Food Guide Pyramid offers recommendations for how many calories—and servings—you should eat each day depending on your age, sex, and activity level.

For sedentary women and some older adults, 1,600 calories a day is a good target for maintaining weight. That translates into six bread group servings a day, three vegetable group, two fruit group, two to three milk group, and five ounces from the meat group. For these people, a total of 53 g of fat and 6 teaspoons of added sugars are in the healthy range.

For most children (age 9 and older), teenage girls, active women, and sedentary men, 2,200 calories per day is the goal. That means nine servings from the bread group, four from the vegetable group, three from the fruit group, two to three from the milk group, and six ounces from the meat group. A total of 73 g of fat and 12 teaspoons of added sugars are okay.

For teenage boys, many active men, and some very active women, 2,800 calories a day is about right. That equals eleven servings a day from the bread group, five from the vegetable group, four from the fruit group, two to three from the milk group, and seven ounces of meat. Ninety-three g of fat a day and 18 teaspoons of added sugars are suggested.

Serving Sizes

American food portions have grown bigger and bigger over the years. Often, too, we eat larger portions of fatty meat and dairy products than we do of grains, fruits, and vegetables.

Many Americans are discouraged when they first read about the number of servings recommended in the Food Guide Pyramid. They believe they can't possibly eat six to eleven servings of grains a day, or three to five servings of vegetables. But the servings actually add up quicker and easier than you think—if you know the true size of a serving or portion.

Here's a guide:

- In the grain products group (bread, cereal, pasta, rice), one slice of bread, one ounce of cold cereal, or half a cup of cooked cereal, rice, or pasta equal a serving.
- In the vegetable group, one cup of raw leafy vegetables, half a cup of other cooked or chopped raw vegetables, or three-quarters of a cup of vegetable juice make up a serving.
- In the fruit group, one medium apple, banana, or orange, half a cup of chopped, cooked, or canned fruit, or three-quarters of a cup of fruit juice comprise a serving.
- In the milk group (milk, yogurt, cheese), one cup of milk or yogurt, one and a half ounces of natural cheese, or two ounces of processed cheese equal a serving.
- In the meat and beans group (meat, poultry, fish, dry beans, eggs, nuts), two to three ounces of cooked lean meat, poultry, or fish equal a serving. (Half a cup of cooked dry beans, one egg, two tablespoons of peanut butter, or one-third of a cup of nuts count as one ounce of lean meat.)

A typical daily menu designed to meet the minimal number of servings and 53 grams of fat listed in the Dietary Guidelines might look something like this:

BREAKFAST: ¾ cup of orange juice
              2 ounces of cereal with 1 cup of 2 per-
                 cent milk

LUNCH: 3 ounces of roast turkey in a sandwich
                 with 2 ounces of Swiss cheese and 1
                 tablespoon of mayonnaise, lettuce and
                 tomato
              8 ounces of diet soda

DINNER: 3 ounces broiled veal chop
              1 cup of salad with ½ tablespoon of
                 dressing
              ½ cup of seasoned rice
              ½ cup of broccoli
              1 roll with 1 teaspoon of margarine

                    1 large apple
                    1 cup of coffee with diet sweetener

How adequate is this carefully planned menu in meeting our daily vitamin needs? Let's see, using the FoodWorks computer program to analyze its vitamin and mineral composition: Compared with the RDA values for an adult, this menu is slightly lacking in copper and magnesium. It contains only half of the RDA for pantothenic acid and only 28 percent of the RDA for manganese.

Given that most people aren't eating as well balanced a diet or as many servings of fruits, vegetables, grains, and dairy products as described in the example, it's likely most Americans could benefit from taking supplements.

You can determine the vitamin adequacy of your own diet by using the same or a similar computer program, or by using the information found in the "Vitamin and Mineral Content of Foods" tables, beginning on page 397.

Special Needs of Women and Growing Children

The Dietary Guidelines for Americans indicate that growing children, adolescent girls, and women of childbearing age often need more calcium- and iron-rich foods than do adolescent boys and men.

Good sources of calcium include milk and milk-related products, cheeses such as mozzarella, cheddar, Swiss, and Parmesan, and yogurt. Canned fish with soft bones, such as sardines, anchovies, and salmon, as well as dark green leafy vegetables (kale, mustard greens, turnip greens) are also good sources of calcium. Tofu, if it's processed with calcium sulfate, and corn tortillas, if they're made from lime-processed corn, can be sources, too.

Good sources of iron include meats (beef, pork, lamb, liver, and other organ meats), poultry (chicken, duck, turkey, liver), fish (shellfish, sardines, anchovies), leafy green vegetables (broccoli, kale, turnip greens, collards), legumes (lima beans, green peas), dry beans and peas (pinto beans, black-eyed peas, canned baked beans), yeast-leavened whole-wheat breads and rolls, and iron-enriched white bread, pasta, rice, and cereals.

How to Order Copies of U.S. Nutrition Pamphlets

You can obtain copies of the fourth edition of the Dietary Guidelines for Americans (Home and Garden Bulletin No. 232) and the Food Guide Pyramid (Home and Garden Bulletin No. 252) by calling the USDA at 202-208-2417. The pamphlets are free.

TIPS ON BUYING, STORING, AND COOKING FOOD

Buying food knowledgeably, storing it carefully, and using cooking methods that preserve vitamins and minerals can greatly enhance the nutritional value of the foods in your diet.

Buying

Buy cereals and breads made from whole grains rather than processed grains. Most of the vitamins and minerals are removed in the milling process. Some but not all of those nutrients are replaced if the grain is "enriched," and some nutrients, such as folic acid, are now being added to "fortify" grain and other products. If you can't find whole-grain products, try for an enriched product. Nonenriched, processed products are the least desirable.

Use only milk products that have been fortified with vitamins A and D. Since the natural vitamin A and D content of milk is lost during processing, it must be replaced before you buy the milk. Skim milk and nonfat dry milk products must also be fortified with A and D.

Frozen meats, fish, poultry, and vegetables are essentially equal to their fresh counterparts when it comes to vitamin and mineral content. The flash-freezing process used to prepare frozen foods does not result in vitamin losses, except for vitamin E. Frozen vegetables that you buy in a plastic cooking pouch are the best kind of frozen product. They maintain their full vitamin content through the cooking process because of the sealed pouch. Avoid packages that have ice crystals on the outside; that indicates they've been thawed and refrozen, which may mean they've lost nutrients and/or been contaminated with bacteria.

Avoid canned vegetables. Any water-soluble vitamins left in the vegetables after processing dissolve in the water used in the packing process and are lost for nutritional purposes. In addition, most people are better off without the salt and sugar that may be added to canned goods to preserve them and make them taste better.

Never buy cans that have dents, bulges, or are rusting. They may be contaminated with bacteria.

Fresh and frozen fruits are preferable to canned fruits because of potential losses of their water-soluble vitamin content during storage. Fresh fruits may take several days or weeks to reach you, during which time they can begin to lose vitamin content. Still, we believe that fresh fruits should be your first choice—the fresher the better! Frozen fruits are a good second choice since they maintain their vitamin content in the same way as frozen vegetables do. Canned fruits are a poor third choice.

Color may be an indicator of vitamin content. For example, vitamin A is orange in color, and those foods with a high vitamin A content, such as carrots, reflect that color. When buying fresh fruits and vegetables, look for those with a deep, rich color.

Don't keep fresh fruits and vegetables around the house until they are overripe. The continuing enzymatic process of fruit ripening can lead to the loss of valuable vitamin content. If you buy fresh produce, buy only enough to last a few days (and no more than a week).

Homegrown fruits and vegetables are not nutritionally superior to the kind you can buy in your supermarket. However, they usually taste better because they are allowed to ripen naturally before you pick and eat them. And they may not contain pesticides, if you choose to and can grow them without using such products.

Storing

Make sure your freezer maintains a temperature of 0° F or less. If the temperature rises above that level, the frozen products may begin to thaw and lose some of their vitamin content. In addition, some frozen products have been found to lose vitamin content after prolonged storage of a year or more, so you should not store them for more than two or three months before use.

Vegetables should be stored unwashed in a sealed plastic bag in the vegetable crisper drawer. The refrigerator should be set at 35 to 40° F. Today's frost-free refrigerators are the worst thing for fresh vegetables because they automatically withdraw moisture from the air in the refrigerator, and water-soluble vitamins will be lost with the moisture extracted from the vegetables. Placing produce in sealed plastic bags in the crisper drawer will help to maintain the vitamin content for a few days.

Canned foods should not be stored in a very hot environment. The breakdown of vitamins is a chemical process. Like all chemical processes, this breakdown is more rapid when temperatures are higher. Therefore, maintaining your pantry in a cool place will minimize vitamin losses in canned foods.

Store milk and bread away from the sun or strong light, which can destroy their riboflavin content (and milk's vitamin A content, too). Clear plastic milk bottles should not be used for this reason.

Orange juice will begin to lose vitamin C after it has been stored in your refrigerator for several days, regardless of the container in which it is stored. Don't keep more than you will be able to use in a week's time. Powdered drinks with supplementary vitamin C will hold their vitamin content for a long time and may be an acceptable alternative to fresh or frozen juice products for some people even though they have no other nutrients.

If you pick tomatoes before they are ripe, allow them to ripen in a cool (not cold), dark place. They can be easily ripened by storing them in a paper bag at room temperature, never in the refrigerator. Ripening under any other conditions will result in the loss of some of their nutrients.

Preparing and Cooking

Use the minimum cooking time necessary. High temperatures over short periods of time are preferable to low temperatures over longer periods of time. Foods maintain their nutrients better with brief cooking.

The kind of pot used to cook your vegetables or meat does not significantly affect the vitamin content of the final product and may add some of its metal component to your food. Copper, iron, brass, or alloy metals may destroy some vitamin C in the foods being cooked, but the small losses attributed to the pot are unimportant.

Vegetables, including potatoes, retain more vitamins if they are cooked whole than if they are cooked in pieces. The smaller the pieces, the more vitamins lost.

Don't soak fresh vegetables or rice for prolonged periods of time before you cook them. You may soak the water-soluble vitamins right out of them. If you must soak your vegetables, reuse the water in heating produce or in soups, gravies, or sauces.

Prepare salads and cut vegetables just before you intend to eat them. This will reduce the loss of vitamin C.

Scrub all fruits and vegetables with a vegetable brush and diluted dishwashing liquid to remove as much pesticide residue as possible. Remove and throw out the outer leaves of lettuce and other greens. Buy produce grown locally—it's less likely to have as much pesticide on it as other produce—or buy organic produce.

Do not thaw frozen vegetables before cooking.

Vegetables will lose the most vitamins if boiled; steaming is not as harmful with respect to vitamin loss. Cooking your vegetables in a pressure cooker or microwave are the best ways to avoid vitamin losses because you need only a small amount of water in the process.

If you do boil fresh vegetables, use a minimal amount of water and bring the water to a boil before you add the vegetables. Whenever possible, reuse the same water for sauces, gravies, or stock, because this water retains many of the vitamins from the vegetables cooked in it.

Meats that are stewed or braised lose more vitamins than those that are fried or broiled. Stewing or braising allows water-soluble vitamins and some fat-soluble vitamins to be removed in the gravy. Rare meat has more thiamin, a heat-sensitive vitamin, than meat cooked for longer periods of time.

Precooking foods and storing them in the refrigerator for reheating can result in the loss of a lot of their vitamin C. This is a significant problem for some people because vitamin C is not found in a wide variety of common foods.

If you follow the practices we recommend for cooking foods to minimize vitamin losses, you will also minimize mineral losses. Avoid boiling foods for long periods of time, and use the cooking water as part of your meal. Steaming will cook foods equally well and minimize nutrient losses.

4

WHO NEEDS SUPPLEMENTAL VITAMINS AND MINERALS?

It may sound reasonable for average, healthy adults to assume that most of their vitamin needs are met by their regular diet, but this is often not so. The only way to estimate your own vitamin and mineral status is to critically examine the nutrients contained in the foods you eat every day. Also, see the checklist at the end of this chapter to determine if you are likely to need a nutritional supplement.

You must also take into account the fact that your normal need for vitamins and minerals is increased in some circumstances. Growing children need more vitamins and minerals; illness and changes in diet or activity level are also reasons to review and adjust your nutritional needs. In looking at situations that can increase your need for vitamins and minerals, we will first talk about people of different ages and then about categories of people that cut across age groups. Finally, we will consider some instances when illness and medication use can affect your vitamin and mineral needs. Table 7, at the end of the chapter, summarizes the various circumstances that indicate a need for supplements.

We believe that the available evidence supports the use of a multivitamin/mineral product and antioxidant supplement by all Americans. Apparently many physicians also believe this, though some are more reluctant than others to advise their patients to take a supplement until all of the data are in. A nationwide survey of 181 cardiologists found that while 44 percent took antioxidant supplements, only 37 percent of them recommend such supplements to their patients!

We advise you to read and absorb the information in each vitamin and mineral profile before you ask your physician or pharmacist for guidance. Ultimately, though, you must make your own decision about whether supplementation is right for you.

SUPPLEMENT NEEDS: INFANCY TO OLD AGE

Infants and Young Children

Infants and children under the age of eleven have special vitamin needs. Although children use more vitamins per pound of body weight than adults because they are growing and burning calories faster, their overall need for vitamins and minerals is generally less than adults' because they are physically so much smaller. Some notable exceptions to this rule are vitamin D, calcium, and iron.

Vitamin D plays an important role in the processing of calcium and phosphorous in the body, two major components of bone. Growing infants and children must have enough vitamin D and calcium for the development of strong bones and teeth. A greater appreciation of the need to build bone in childhood has emerged in recent years. This is why children ages nine to eighteen are advised to take in more calcium than some adults (1,300 mg versus 1,000 mg for adults nineteen to fifty years old). The DRI for vitamin D is 5 mcg (200 IU) for people from childhood to age fifty.

Iron is a component of hemoglobin, a protein that carries oxygen throughout the body as a part of red blood cells. An infant grows so rapidly that it uses much more oxygen per pound of body weight than an adult. So infants need at least as much iron as an adult, despite their smaller size. Many pediatricians prescribe vitamin supplements with iron to be sure that children get enough during these critical years.

The RDA/DRIs for infants are based on the known content of mother's milk. Since infants thrive when breast-fed, setting the RDA/DRIs at this level was a natural step. Some physicians feel that breast-fed infants should receive fluoride supplements to prevent dental cavities since they don't drink much fluoridated water. Indeed, the DRI committee is concerned with fluoride consumption and set fluoride Adequate Intake levels and Tolerable Upper Intake Limits for the first time in 1997. Supplemental vitamins D and K, as well as iron, also may be advised in some cases.

Infants fed a commercially prepared formula typically do not need supplemental vitamins because their formulas contain enough extra nutrients to be considered vitamin supplements. These formulas are designed to provide everything the infant will need to grow and be healthy. Just be sure the product label says that it contains vitamin D and iron. Using whole milk and an iron-fortified cereal does not work as well as an infant formula with iron.

There is some disagreement among nutritionists about how well the vitamins and minerals, especially zinc, in commercial formulas are absorbed by an infant when compared to those found in mother's milk. Although the commercial formulas have more nutrients in them, those nutrients are absorbed less efficiently than those obtained from mother's milk. Despite this difference in absorption, infants fed by either method will thrive.

Young children can present a more difficult problem than infants because of the food choices they make. Children usually refuse to eat the variety of foods that would provide the basic nutrients required for growth and development. A vitamin supplement is advisable for children who do not eat a balanced diet. When choosing a vitamin supplement for your child, don't forget to select one that includes iron, if iron-rich foods are not a part of his or her diet.

Try to vary the foods offered to your child, choosing from those that can be particularly good sources of vitamins and minerals. Many vegetables, fruits, grains, and milk products are enjoyed by young children and serve as the basis for a sound diet.

Teenagers

Teenagers have special vitamin needs because of their tremendous growth and the normal changes in their bodies that come with sexual maturation and the influence of sex hormones. Boys usually grow by adding muscle and bone, and they are sometimes more active than girls. Girls also add muscle and bone, but a larger percentage of their body weight goes to fat. In addition, girls develop uniquely female nutrient needs with the onset of menstruation.

Every teenager requires more phosphorous and calcium than the average adult because of the growth spurt that occurs between the ages of eleven and eighteen years. This need is directly related to the process of building strong bodies and teeth.

Teenage boys need slightly more of several of the B-complex vitamins than girls. This makes sense when we realize that the B vitamins play a key role in our energy-generating system.

Teenage boys and girls need more iron than they did at a younger age, but for different reasons. Teenage girls need more iron because of the the loss of iron with their menstrual period each month. Teenage boys need extra iron because they must supply more oxygen to rapidly growing tissues. Girls' need for extra iron (15 mg) continues through adulthood until they reach menopause, at about age fifty. A teenage boy's daily need for iron decreases from 12 mg to 10 mg at age nineteen, signaling that he has stopped growing and, often, reduced his level of activity.

Like young children, teenagers' eating habits often interfere with their ability to obtain the vitamins and minerals they need. Many adolescents snack to excess, especially on junk foods and fast foods. Teenage girls tend to eat less, sometimes a lot less, than teenage boys. Reducing food intake can be a way to maintain one's figure, but it does nothing to establish a solid nutritional base. When considering the need for a vitamin/mineral supplement for your teenager, remember that eating less food means that vitamin and mineral intake will also be reduced.

Offer your teen a variety of foods that are rich in vitamins and minerals. Fruits, grains, milk and milk products, and vegetables are especially good. A multivitamin/mineral supplement with iron is a good way to ensure that minimum requirements are met, but you should not depend upon it as the sole source of nutrients for your teenager. Nothing can replace good food as a source of good health.

Mature Adults

Adults need fewer vitamins and minerals than teens because they are no longer growing. Good nutrition remains a challenge, however, as adults strive to maintain their weight while eating highly nutritious foods that are low in calories.

Senior Citizens

Unfortunately, the RDA recommendations for vitamin and mineral intake are subdivided into age groups that end with fifty. Adults beyond the age of fifty are currently lumped into one category. The new DRIs have added categories for adults ages fifty-one to seventy, and ages seventy and up.

As you get older, the percentage of fat in your body increases. This fat replaces muscle, which has a greater need for energy (calories). Because of this change, your basal metabolism—the rate at which the body uses energy—is lowered. To complicate matters, many people tend to engage in less physical activity as they get older, lowering energy requirements even further.

When you reduce metabolism and physical activity, your need for food energy drops, though your requirement for vitamins and minerals generally stays the same. Eat the same amount of food while using fewer calories each day and your body will store the excess energy as fat. You must eat less food to avoid gaining weight as you age. Of course, when you eat less, you also get smaller amounts of vitamins and minerals. The upshot of all of these changes is that the need for a general-purpose vitamin and mineral supplement increases with advancing age.

Other factors also point to a need for supplemental vitamins and minerals among senior citizens. Older adults make less of the natural gastrointestinal enzymes and acids needed to digest food, and some older adults cannot chew their food properly. This leads to poor or inefficient digestion and the incomplete extraction of available nutrients from our food, most notably vitamin B_{12}.

In addition, nutritional problems among senior citizens can originate from social, economic, and psychological factors. For instance, losses of close family ties or spousal illness or death can cause depression, which may lead to a loss of interest in food and thus improper nutrition. There are also many older Americans who don't have the money to buy nutritious foodstuffs. And many are taking medications that interfere with the absorption of nutrients from foods.

There have been many studies on the vitamin status of older adults who do not supplement their diets with extra vitamins and minerals. One interesting study revealed that 95 percent of senior citizens are deficient in at least one nutrient. Ninety percent had low levels of thiamin (vitamin B_1) and vitamin C. When these people were given a supplement including B-complex and vitamin C, their vitamin status improved and they showed a major improvement in physical and mental condition.

Recent evidence points to the need for calcium supplementation in older adults, especially postmenopausal women, to maintain good bone health and prevent the bone-thinning disorder osteoporosis. The new DRIs recommend that adult men and women over age fifty-one consume 1,200 mg of calcium a day—an increase of 500 mg over the RDA set in 1989.

There is also some good evidence emerging to suggest that antioxidant vitamins—most notably C and E—can help ward off some of the effects of aging, such as heart disease, cancer, and cataracts. In addition, it appears that folic acid can reduce levels of the clot-producing amino acid homocysteine in the body, which is now considered to be a risk factor for heart disease and stroke. See Chapter 7 for further details on antioxidants and the individual vitamin and mineral profiles in Part 2.

The most reasonable and least costly way for older people to be sure of getting enough vitamins and minerals is to take a well-balanced multivitamin/mineral supplement. Many seniors prefer this solution because it saves them the time and effort of planning and preparing a balanced, lower-calorie diet. It is economical, and helps prevent overeating. Of course, it is still important for older adults to eat a variety of foods so that they obtain nutrients other than vitamins and minerals.

One note of caution: It is quite easy for vitamin A to build up to toxic levels that can damage the liver in the body of an older individual, so be sure not to consume more than 5,000 IU in supplements. It is also wise to consume vitamin A in the form of beta carotene, which has not been shown to be harmful.

SUPPLEMENT NEEDS: WOMEN OVER A LIFETIME

Young and Middle-Aged Women

Despite the fact that girls stop growing at around age eighteen, adult women still require a nutritionally balanced diet. Calcium is particularly important until age twenty-five because you want to ensure that your bones reach their maximum density before they begin to naturally lose mass in the early thirties and there-after. Iron deficiency remains a problem among menstruating women because of monthly losses during menstruation.

Many women diet excessively. In addition, calorie needs decline as women progress from young adulthood through middle age, which requires that they eat less food to maintain their weight. Both factors can lead to inadequate nutrition.

Pregnant Women and Nursing Mothers

Although there is general agreement that pregnant and nursing women need more of every vitamin and mineral, there is no consensus as to specific requirements, despite the fact that this area of vitamin research has been given much attention in recent years.

Vitamin and mineral amounts recommended by the National Academy of Sciences and included in the RDA/DRI tables are based on the increased energy needs of pregnant women. The academy estimates that a pregnant woman requires about 300 additional calories per day, or 80,000 extra calories during the full term of her pregnancy. Naturally, extra vitamins and minerals are needed to support the metabolism of these 80,000 calories and the growth of the unborn child.

After delivery, a nursing mother normally produces about 26 ounces of milk each day for a single infant. About one-third of the energy needed to make this milk comes from the extra fat stored during pregnancy, but the remaining energy needs to come from the mother's diet, as much as an extra 500 to 600 calories or more per day. In fact, daily energy needs during breast-feeding can actually exceed energy needs during pregnancy.

Studies have shown that pregnant women who do not take vitamin supplements may have reduced blood levels of vitamins A, B_{12}, and C, niacin, and pyridoxine. Consequently, recommendations for increased daily intake of these vitamins during pregnancy and breast-feeding vary between 25 percent and 65 percent above normal adult RDA/DRI levels, depending on the vitamin. If you examine the listings for the vitamins and minerals for which an RDA/DRI has been assigned, you will find that pregnancy and lactation are special cases in which the need for supplementation has been well documented in virtually all cases.

Here is a brief summary of women's special nutrient needs during pregnancy:

• *B vitamins.* Since the B vitamins are involved in different phases of the system used to generate energy from glucose (sugar), it makes sense that pregnant women, who use more energy, need significantly more B vitamins to assist in the provision of that energy. In fact, many RDAs are based directly on the number of calories we metabolize each day.

• *Folic acid.* Pregnancy makes great demands on body stores of folic acid (folate). If folic acid stores are low at the beginning of pregnancy, there is a good chance that a blood disorder called megaloblastic anemia will develop at some time during the pregnancy. There is also a chance that low stores of folic acid early in pregnancy will lead to neurologial birth defects such as spina bifida. It's even been suggested that inadequate folic acid stores may result in premature births. Folic acid levels are so important during early pregnancy that the United States Public Health Service recommended in 1992 that all women of reproductive age consume 400 mcg of folate each day. Women need to begin building up their stores of this B vitamin a month before conception, but because we have a very high rate of unplanned pregnancy in the United States and many women don't know they're pregnant until several weeks into the pregnancy, it's smart for all women to make sure they get enough folate daily.

In 1997 the March of Dimes reported that although 66 percent of two thousand women surveyed said they knew they should be supplementing their intake of folic acid, few were actually doing so. That's one reason why grain products are now fortified with folic acid. However, only 140 mcg of folate is added per every 100 g of cereal or grain product; depending on a woman's consumption patterns, this may not be sufficient to meet the 400-mcg-per-day requirement.

• *Vitamin D.* Vitamin D helps to form strong bones and teeth by mediating the body's use of calcium. Pregnant and breast-feeding women need extra vitamin D to ensure their child's proper skeletal development.

• *Calcium.* Like vitamin D, calcium is essential in building bone and teeth in fetuses and infants. Although calcium is typically included in vitamin/mineral supplements for pregnant and lactating women at a dose of 125 mg to 300 mg, the amount contained is nowhere near enough to meet your daily requirement of 1,000 mg per day. This is especially true of pregnant teenagers, who need 1,300 mg of calcium, according to the new DRI.

• **_Iron._** Iron is a special problem for pregnant and lactating women of all ages because it is difficult to get enough iron from your diet to meet the special needs during this time. Hence, your supplement formula should have 30 mg of iron in it.

These are only a few examples of the need for extra vitamins and minerals during pregnancy and breast-feeding. Women who don't take a vitamin supplement especially designed for this period of physical stress are more likely to develop severe vitamin and mineral deficiencies. These deficiencies can affect the course of the pregnancy, the unborn child, or the mother's general health after the child has been born, since many of the nutrients the baby needs are drawn from the mother's body. Thus, a woman who does not take in sufficient vitamins and minerals may give birth to a healthy baby but be left in an extremely deficient nutritional state herself. There is also evidence to suggest that a vitamin-deficient mother may be at higher risk of delivering a child with birth defects.

On the other side of the coin, too much vitamin A may be cause for concern during pregnancy because it has been associated with birth defects. In 1995 a study published in the _New England Journal of Medicine_ found that when pregnant women consume 10,000 IU or more of vitamin A—200 percent of the Daily Value (DV) of 5,000 IU—the risk of birth defects at least doubles. A fetus is most vulnerable to vitamin A damage during the first trimester, when a woman may not realize she is pregnant.

Based on this study, the United States Food and Drug Administration issued a warning to women of childbearing age about consumption of foods rich in vitamin A and supplements. The agency stated:

> Only a form of the vitamin known as pre-formed vitamin A is of concern. Pre-formed vitamin A is found in liver and other animal products and may be included in fortified cereals and dietary supplements. Look for ingredients such as retinyl palmitate and retinyl acetate on the label and limit your intake to about 100 percent of the DV for pre-formed vitamin A from these sources.
>
> Beta carotene, which is converted into vitamin A by the body, is a safer choice as a source of vitamin A. It is primarily found in plants and it is less toxic than pre-formed vitamin A.

Tally your intake of vitamin A from all sources, including foods and vitamin supplements, and make sure you're not receiving more than the DV for this nutrient.

For further details on prenatal supplements, see pages 108–109.

Pregnant Teenagers

Pregnant teens present a special challenge. In addition to the nutrients they need to support their still-growing bodies, they require additional nutrition to support their pregnancies.

The DRIs establish recommended nutrient intake levels of calcium, magnesium, phosphorus, vitamin D, and fluoride for pregnant teenagers. The other vitamin and mineral needs of a pregnant adolescent are typically calculated by adding the RDAs for fifteen- to eighteen-year-old girls to those of a pregnant woman. This practice, of course, requires that teenagers both eat more food and supplement their diet to ensure they reach the RDAs.

Unfortunately, a teenager may be less likely than an adult to eat foods rich in the nutrients she needs to ensure the healthy growth of her baby. Nutritional counseling that stresses the importance of diet and supplemental vitamins and minerals is often helpful in getting the message across to pregnant teenagers.

Women Who Take the Pill

Eight out of ten American women use oral contraceptives at some point during their reproductive lives. Pill use reduces the level of some nutrients in the body, especially if it is taken for a long time. Women who are on the pill should consider a vitamin/mineral supplement that includes vitamin B_6 and other B vitamins, folic acid, vitamin C, vitamin E, vitamin K, and zinc.

Body levels of iron and copper may be *increased* during pill use, thanks to a smaller volume of menstrual blood flow each month.

Postmenopausal Women

After the reproductive phase of life ends, typically around age fifty, women need less iron than they did in their younger years (10 mg instead of 15 mg) and slightly less of some B vitamins, according to the RDA tables. However, they still need the same amounts of most of the other vitamins and minerals as they did during middle age. Calcium requirements actually increase! The DRI for women over age fifty-one is 1,200 mg, compared to 1,000 mg for younger adults. This requirement may be met through diet and by consuming calcium supplements, such as tablets or Tums.

In addition, because adequate levels of vitamin D are essential to the absorption of calcium and some older women may not be exposed to enough sunlight to obtain vitamin D naturally, the DRI for women ages fifty-one to seventy is 10 mcg (400 IU)—double that of younger women. The DRI for women seventy and over is 15 mcg (600 IU), triple that of younger women. Many surveys have documented the fact that older women and men are deficient in vitamin D and that this is a major contributing factor in the development of osteoporosis.

SUPPLEMENT NEEDS: OTHER SPECIAL GROUPS

Athletes

You need more vitamins when you use more energy because vitamins are among the raw materials needed for the provision of energy to every cell in the body.

It's not possible to improve athletic performance by taking in more vitamins than the body can possibly use, but an athlete should be taking somewhat more of the water-soluble vitamins than an inactive person. Most important are vitamin C, thiamin (vitamin B_1), riboflavin (vitamin B_2), and nicotinic acid (niacin). There are several reasons for this. One is the fact that athletes tend to be more muscular than nonathletes, and so their regular energy demands are higher. Also, metabolism is directly linked to body temperature. Strenuous exercise causes a measurable increase in body temperature and with it an increase in the rate of metabolism. When this happens, the need for the raw materials of metabolism, including vitamins, also increases.

Finally, perspiration results in small losses of all normal body constituents that are ordinarily dissolved in the sweat, including water-soluble vitamins. For the serious athlete, even normal levels of vitamin intake coupled with very high levels of physical activity can result in some vitamin-deficiency diseases. Perspiration can also result in loss of excessive amounts of the electrolyte minerals sodium and potassium. In fact, the problem of electrolyte loss is so great among professional athletes and weekend warriors that special electrolyte replacement solutions containing sodium, potassium, and excess glucose have been developed to permit athletes greater surges of energy and extended periods of athletic activity. The first of these products was Gatorade, but similar formulas are made by several companies. They are not recommended for routine or regular use.

Other minerals that are important for physically active people are iron, chromium, zinc, calcium, and magnesium.

Observations in the early 1990s made by the "father of aerobics," Dr. Kenneth Cooper of the Cooper Aerobics Center in Dallas, suggested that, while moderate exercise is highly beneficial for many reasons, people who exercise to excess—those who appear to be the healthiest of all—still develop cancer and heart disease. Dr. Cooper theorized that elite athletes who run more than fifteen miles a week, for instance, are causing their bodies to release damaged oxygen molecules called free radicals that harm healthy cells. These findings have been verified by studies at other institutions. Dr. Cooper also realized that some of this free-radical damage could be prevented by increasing the dietary intake of the antioxidants vitamins C, E, and beta carotene and by taking antioxidant supplements.

Dr. Cooper recommends the following antioxidant supplement regimen for heavy exercisers: 1,000 mg of vitamin C and 400 IU of vitamin E. He also recommends beta carotene supplementation, which we do not.

Dieters

The association between vitamin and mineral intake from food and calories is an unavoidable relationship. If you eat less and exercise more, which is the only way to shed pounds for good, the possibility of vitamin deficiency becomes more real than ever. After all, regular exercise only increases your need for some vitamins and minerals, as discussed above, and reducing the number of calories in your daily diet carries an automatic reduction in vitamin and mineral intake.

As Table 6 demonstrates, most of the currently popular diet plans we analyzed using the Food Works nutrient analysis software are deficient in a number of nutrients. The New Beverly Hills Diet, which instructs you to eat only three or four food types a day (pineapple, corn on the cob, and salad for the day we analyzed), is the worst of the bunch. Compared with the RDAs, it is low in vitamins A, E, B_2, B_5, B_6, and B_{12}, niacin, calcium, iron, phosphorus, zinc, and magnesium. Dr. Atkins' New Diet Revolution doesn't meet the RDAs for vitamins B_1, B_2, B_5, and B_6, niacin, and magnesium. The Carbohydrate Addict's Diet is lacking in vitamins B_1, B_2, B_5, B_6, and E, folic acid, calcium, zinc, and magnesium. The Zone plan is low in vitamins B_1, B_2, and B_5, calcium, and zinc.

In addition, the Atkins, Carbohydrate Addict, and Zone diets are high in fat. The Weight Watchers International diet, designed to mimic the government's Food Guide Pyramid, is best, but even this diet is low in vitamins E and B_5, as well as zinc.

TABLE 6
Nutrient Content of Popular Weight-Loss Diets
(1-Day Menu)

As Compared with the RDAs and Analyzed Using the Food Works Nutrient Analysis Software

Diet	A	C	E	B_1	B_2	B_5	B_6	B_{12}	Niacin	Folic Acid	Calcium	Iron	Phosphorous	Zinc	Magnesium
Dr. Atkins' New Diet Revolution	A	A	A	X	X	X	X	A	X	A	A	A	A	A	X
Carbohydrate Addict's Diet	A	A	X	X	X	X	X	A	A	X	X	A	A	X	X
New Beverly Hills Diet	X	A	X	A	X	X	X	X	X	A	X	X	X	X	X
Weight Watchers	A	A	X	A	A	X	A	A	A	A	A	A	A	X	A
The Zone	A	A	A	X	X	X	A	A	A	A	X	A	A	X	A

A = Adequate amounts (90 percent or more of the RDA) of this nutrient can be obtained by following this diet.

X = The amount of this nutrient supplied in this diet does not meet its RDA. Supplements are needed to maintain daily requirements.

Given the deficiencies of these popular diets, it is advisable to take a vitamin/mineral supplement while on a weight-reduction plan to ensure that you are receiving the full complement of vitamins and minerals your body needs. That's one of the reasons why several of the diet plans, including Weight Watchers International, encourage daily consumption of a multivitamin.

Vegetarians

Most vegetarians who include animal products in their diets do not need vitamins or mineral supplements, primarily because they are so conscientious about their nutrition. Vegans, who don't eat any animal products, may, however, need additional calcium, iron, zinc, riboflavin, and vitamins D and B_{12}, since these nutrients are largely obtained from animal products. Use of fortified foods can provide some of the missing nutrients, but supplementation is often needed. Makers of vitamins for vegetarians include Pathway, Twinlab, Country Life, and Apothecary.

Alcoholics

Alcoholics need more of the B vitamins, particularly thiamin, because alcohol decreases the absorption and utilization of thiamin, riboflavin, pyridoxine, and folate in the body. Alcoholism can also alter vitamin A balance in the body and is often associated with vitamin D deficiency. Another important reason for vitamin and mineral deficiencies among alcoholics is the fact that alcohol often replaces solid food at mealtimes. This leads to obvious deficiencies of all essential nutrients. While supplemental vitamins and minerals won't cure an alcoholic or allow him or her to go on without worrying about the dire consequences of alcohol abuse, they may be able to replace some of the nutrients missing from a daily diet.

Smokers

Smokers use more vitamin C than nonsmokers because their metabolism is speeded up. This has been verified by studies showing that the usual concentration of vitamin C in the blood of smokers was lower than that of nonsmokers. This difference was maintained even after vitamin C injections were given to both groups. Some experts have estimated that each cigarette burns 2.5 mg of vitamin C and that heavy smokers can lose as much as 50 mg per day of that vitamin. Hence, smokers should consume 120 mg of vitamin C a day, twice the DV for vitamin C.

Smokers may be deficient in beta carotene (a form of vitamin A), folic acid, and vitamin B_{12}. Particularly relevant to women who smoke is the fact that smokers have lower levels of calcium in the blood; combined with a tendency toward earlier menopause in women who smoke, this may mean that a female smoker has an increased risk of osteoporosis.

Besides a multivitamin/mineral formulation that includes calcium, smokers may also benefit from antioxidant supplement therapy—taking the vitamins C and E—to protect them against the free-radical damage to their cells caused by their cigarette habit. *Beta-carotene supplementation by smokers is not recommended;* see page 147 for more information on this topic.

SUPPLEMENT NEEDS: MEDICAL PROBLEMS

Difficulties Absorbing Vitamins and Minerals

Some people cannot absorb vitamins and minerals from their food or from supplemental sources as efficiently as others. The most common causes of this problem are intestinal inflammations such as colitis, bile duct blockage (which affects only the absorption of fat-soluble vitamins), cystic fibrosis, diarrhea, and aging.

If you have an absorption problem, you may gain from vitamin supplements simply because increasing the amount of vitamins presented to the gastrointestinal tract means that more will be absorbed into the blood. The possible benefit offered by vitamin supplements will not be as great, however, if you have permanent absorption problems as opposed to a temporary problem, such as diarrhea. People with severe absorption problems may have to take their vitamins by injection.

Injury, Severe Burns, Trauma, Surgery, Infection

Each of these situations involves a set of circumstances in which the body is stressed and attempting to heal itself. The healing process requires intense activity on the part of all body systems, especially those involved with the provision of energy and growth of body tissues. Since vitamins and minerals are integrally involved in these processes, it is logical to assume that vitamin and mineral supplementation will help. In fact, physicians treating hospitalized patients recovering from surgery, severe burns, prolonged infections, and other extended illnesses have long known that nutritional supplementation is one of the basic keys to successful recovery. Today, even oral and plastic surgeons are recommending vitamin regimens prior to and after outpatient surgery to enhance healing.

Many patients have been fed intravenously with mixtures of glucose, amino acids, vitamins, trace minerals, and fats. This technique, known as total parenteral nutrition (TPN) or hyperalimentation, is a good temporary source of nutrition in people who can tolerate only small amounts of food and the sole source of nutrition for many people recovering from major surgery, burns, and so on.

Disease

Your mother probably told you two things: Always wear clean underwear and eat balanced meals. Generations of mothers have known that good nutrition not only prevents illness but also helps you get well sooner if you do fall ill.

Research has shown that mothers really do know best. Any physically stressful situation increases the rate at which your body uses vitamins. Since disease is another form of stress to which your body is exposed, it makes sense to use a vitamin supplement whenever a disease or other physically stressful situation presents itself.

It is also known that deficiencies in vitamins A or C tend to make you more susceptible to such ailments as the common cold. With a smaller supply of these vitamins, your body is less able to carry out those functions that protect it against invading viruses. Taking at least the RDA for both of these vitamins may help to speed your recovery if you are stricken with a bacterial or viral illness.

Drug Therapy and Vitamins

There are many drugs that can affect the action of vitamins, and vitamins that can affect the action of drugs. Here are some of the ways a drug can affect a vitamin.

A drug can interfere with the chemical action of a vitamin (one example is the effect of chloramphenicol, an antibiotic, on folic acid, one of the B-complex vitamins), or interfere with vitamins being absorbed into the bloodstream from the stomach or intestine (examples of this are the effect of neomycin, an antibiotic, on vitamin B_{12}, and that of mineral-oil laxatives on the absorption of vitamins A, D, E, and K).

A drug can increase the amount of vitamin absorbed, as colchicine, a drug used to treat gout, does with vitamin B_{12}, or can have the opposite effect, leading to vitamin deficiency, as with hydralazine, a drug used for high blood pressure, and pyridoxine (vitamin B_6). Oral contraceptives can also lower blood levels of vitamin B_6 in women, potentially leading to a deficiency.

A drug can also increase the rate at which a vitamin is eliminated from the body. An example of this is the effect of phenytoin, a drug used to treat epilepsy, on vitamin D.

Likewise, vitamins can affect drugs in the body in several different ways. For example, a vitamin can counteract or inhibit the effect of a drug. The best example is the effect of vitamin K on oral anticoagulant (blood-thinning) drugs. Vitamin K is used as an antidote to the effects of oral anticoagulants.

Vitamins can also influence the absorption of drugs through their own effects on body processes. Examples of this are the effect of vitamin C on oral iron supplements and the effect of pyridoxine (vitamin B_6) on I-dopa, a drug used to treat Parkinson's disease. Vitamin C increases the absorption of iron, and B_6 increases the rate at which I-dopa is broken down.

Large doses of vitamins can raise drug levels in the blood. Researchers have noted that doses of vitamin C exceeding 1,000 mg a day can raise estrogen levels among users of birth-control pills, in effect turning low-dose pills into high-dose pills. The latter, of course, are associated with more side effects than current low-dose oral contraceptives.

Vitamins can also affect a number of diagnostic tests. Large doses of vitamin C can affect certain blood tests for diabetes. Vitamin D can interfere with cholesterol and other blood tests. And potassium and iron can cause bleeding in the gastrointestinal tract that can skew the results of a fecal occult blood test (performed to check for colorectal cancer).

A complete table of known interactions and influences of vitamins on drugs and laboratory tests can be found in Part 6, "Vitamin, Mineral, and Herbal Drug Interactions." In addition, each vitamin and mineral profile includes a discussion of such problems, if applicable.

CHECK YOUR NUTRIENT INTAKE

Go through this checklist, designed for adults, to evaluate how well your daily diet stacks up to your nutrient needs.

1. *Do you consume two to four fruit servings in a typical day?*
   a. yes
   b. no

2. *Do you consume three to five vegetable servings each day?*
   a. yes
   b. no

3. *Do you eat two to three milk, yogurt, or cheese servings in an average day?*
   a. yes
   b. no

4. *Do you eat six to eleven servings of grain, bread, cereal, rice, and pasta a day?*
   a. yes
   b. no

5. *Do you eat two to three servings of meat, poultry, fish, dry beans, eggs, or nuts daily?*
   a. yes
   b. no

6. *Do you have at least two meals a day?*
   a. yes
   b. no

7. *Do you have an illness that has made you change the amount or types of food you eat?*
   a. yes
   b. no

8. *Do you consume more than one to two alcoholic drinks a day?*
   a. yes
   b. no

9. *Do you smoke cigarettes?*
   a. yes
   b. no

10. *Do you have tooth or mouth problems that make it difficult for you to eat?*
    a. yes
    b. no

11. *Do you take three or more different prescription or nonprescription drugs per day?*
    a. yes
    b. no

Scoring: Give yourself one point for each yes answer to questions 1 to 6, and one point for each no answer to questions 7 to 11.

• If you scored 8–11 points, your diet is probably ample and varied enough to meet your nutritional needs without turning to a supplement. We still, however, recommend taking a multivitamin/mineral product and the antioxidants C and E.
• If you scored 4–7 points, you could definitely benefit from a multivitamin/mineral supplement and vitamins C and E. Either you're not eating a broad enough variety of foods in the needed amounts, or your health habits or physical condition are affecting your body's ability to use the nutrients you are consuming.
• If you scored 0–3 points, you're in dire need of a better diet, a multivitamin/mineral supplement, and antioxidants in order to maintain or improve your health.

TABLE 7
Who Needs Supplements?

People whose vitamin/mineral intake is inadequate due to:

Dieting
Heavy alcohol use
Economic disadvantage
Old age
Illness

People who have extra vitamin/mineral needs:

Infants
Young children
Teenage boys and girls
Pregnant women
Breast-feeding women
Pregnant teenagers
Women taking the Pill
Smokers
Strict vegetarians
People undergoing major or outpatient surgery
People subject to severe injury and trauma
People suffering from disease or prolonged infection

People who have difficulty absorbing vitamins due to:

Bile duct blockage
Chronic diarrhea
Chronic disorders of the stomach and intestine
Effects of aging

People who are taking drugs that interfere with vitamins (see Part 6, "Vitamin, Mineral, and Herbal Drug Interactions")

5

VITAMINS AND MINERALS AS DRUGS

Interest in using vitamins and minerals as a medicine has exploded since the publication of the first edition of *The Vitamin Book*. American consumers have become enthusiastic about using large doses of these nutrients to ward off the effects of aging and to prevent chronic diseases. Some of this use is supported by medical evidence, but much is based on hope and hype, rather than on true scientific data.

One thing is clear. Vitamins, minerals, and related compounds such as coenzyme Q_{10} and carnitine will probably play a significant role in the prevention and treatment of many illnesses in the future. Despite the current lack of hard data, many medical experts believe that the evidence—especially on the antioxidant vitamins C and E and on folic acid—is so promising that it is better to supplement today than wait until tomorrow for definitive studies. As we noted previously, many experts even take supplements themselves, though they may not tell their patients to do so. This contradiction may have developed because, as scientists, they feel absolute proof is necessary before a therapy can be recommended to a patient, not because they believe supplementation is harmful.

THE SELF-CARE TREND

Even though professional health care is relatively easily available to most Americans, many of us still prefer self-help remedies and treatments. Close to 60 percent of all health problems in this country are self-treated with a nonprescription drug. This is partly a result of the ever-increasing cost of health care and partly due to the American determination to "do it ourselves."

Vitamins and minerals play an incredibly popular role in this social and psychological phenomenon.

It is generally recognized by health authorities that doses between three and five times the average adult RDA may be required from time to time. Such doses may be needed to correct a vitamin deficiency symptom, when someone has a chronic illness that limits nutritional intake or places a great demand on vitamin use, or when someone is not eating properly. Once you begin to take vitamins or minerals to treat a condition not related to vitamin deficiency, you have stepped into different territory. Now you are taking a vitamin or mineral for its effect as a drug.

When vitamins and minerals are used as medications, they are frequently taken in megadoses (see section on megadosing in Chapter 2). A megadose is generally defined as a dose of a nutrient that is ten or more times greater than the average adult RDA. If no RDA has been assigned, then a megadose is considered to be ten times the reference daily intake (RDI) or Daily Value (DV) listing required on food and vitamin labels. The latter are deemed to be the established safe and adequate daily intakes. In addition, the DRIs establish Tolerable Upper Intake Levels for some nutrients that should serve as a guide for vitamin enthusiasts and critics alike.

You must consider both the safety and the efficacy of taking vitamins as drugs. Since vitamins are chemicals that have an effect on the body, taking them in excessive doses may cause the system to become unbalanced. If that happens, vitamins may cause harmful effects that can far overshadow any possible benefits.

Proponents of vitamin therapy for nondeficiency diseases invariably base their claims on surveys and studies of some sort, but many of these guidelines are, in our opinion, not valid. When we evaluated studies for inclusion in this book, several important criteria had to be met before the study and its conclusions could be considered valid.

- Each study had to demonstrate clearly that the benefit could be traced to the vitamin under consideration.
- Sampling methods and other experimental procedures had to meet established scientific criteria.
- The methods of analysis had to be appropriate for the particular study method and the information collected.

Examples of how the facts can be misinterpreted and misrepresented are included in each vitamin and mineral profile in Parts 2 and 3 under the heading "Unsubstantiated Claims." These sections include therapeutic uses that have not yet met the rigorous requirements of scientific testing and confirmation. Table 8, at the end of this chapter, also provides a summary of current scientific knowledge about the therapeutic uses of vitamins and minerals. In some cases—including the use of vitamin E to enhance sexual performance, vitamin E as a treatment for muscular dystrophy, and vitamin C as a cancer cure—false claims have led millions of unwary Americans to use a vitamin supplement when it could not have helped or none was needed.

HOW FACTS CAN BECOME TWISTED

People who advance unproven theories of vitamin cure for the ills of mankind very often use faulty reasoning in drawing their conclusions. We will briefly review the most common kinds of errors and illustrate them with some of the most popular vitamin therapies. Often there is more than one error associated with each case of vitamin misuse, but we will focus on one error in each of the following discussions. More complete information may be found in each of the vitamin and mineral profiles.

Using Anecdotal Reports: Vitamin C and the Common Cold

This kind of faulty reasoning is based on taking the unverified and scientifically uncontrolled experience of one group of people and trying to apply it to everyone.

Vitamin C (ascorbic acid) has been widely promoted as a treatment for the common cold; see page 204 for more details. Reports in health and other popular magazines recommend vitamin C doses anywhere from 1,000 mg to 10,000 mg (10 g) a day. Unfortunately, the more vitamin C you take, the more likely you are to experience side effects. Even though such side effects are rare, they do occur, just as they would with any other drug.

Most of the current popularity of vitamin C can be traced to Dr. Linus Pauling, a Nobel Prize–winning chemist whose claims were based on his personal experiences and some early studies on the common cold. These early studies have been criticized by many scientists, who claim their scope and design were not broad enough to support the very general conclusion drawn—that vitamin C will prevent and treat the common cold.

Scientific attempts to verify the value of vitamin C treatment for the common cold have often not proven fruitful. When some positive results have been obtained, other investigators have not been able to reproduce them, and so the results are considered invalid.

Today it is widely accepted that regular high doses of vitamin C can't prevent a cold in most people. However, vitamin C may have some value in reducing cold symptoms if it's taken during the duration of a cold. Based on a recent reanalysis of twenty-one studies, Finnish investigators report that vitamin C at a dose of 1 g to 6 g a day may reduce the severity of cold symptoms by about 23 percent and shorten the duration of a cold by about a day. Although these results have also been questioned, many experts believe that it's probably not harmful, and may well be helpful, to increase your regular intake of vitamin C to between 500 and 1,000 mg a day, split into two doses twelve hours apart, when you feel a cold coming on.

Using Unverified Reports: Nicotinic Acid (Niacin) and Mental Illness

The practice of treating mental illness with vitamins has been called orthomolecular psychiatry. Orthomolecular practitioners often quote unverified reports and unreproductible results as the basis for their treatment. Generally, orthomolecular therapy, which has been around since the late 1950s, involves the use of large doses of nicotinic acid plus combinations of the B-complex vitamins and vitamin E. The American Psychiatric Association (APA) looked at the data on this therapy in 1973 and found that the claims of orthomolecular therapists were not valid and that the therapy was ineffective. However, orthomolecular therapy has survived in spite of the APA's negative assessment.

Many vitamin enthusiasts suggest that mental illnesses—including schizophrenia, which seems to have become the focus of many of these people—will respond to treatment with megadoses of some vitamins. Other claims for vitamin therapy having to do with mental health involve the treatment of depression, anxiety, and stress-related illnesses. Memory loss and confusion in older people is an exception to this rule. Such problems in fact may be caused by a vitamin B_{12} deficiency and may be highly treatable with supplementation.

It is interesting to note that psychiatrists and analysts who prescribe megavitamin therapy almost always combine other, more conventional forms of therapy (drugs, psychotherapy, and so on) with the vitamins. This obviously clouds the issue and makes it much more difficult to get a true picture of the effect of vitamin therapy. However, scientific evaluations of nicotinic acid as a treatment for schizophrenia conclude that improvements claimed by the purveyors of megavitamin therapies resulted not from the vitamins but from the conventional drugs and/or psychotherapy given together with the vitamins.

It may also be that some patients are being misdiagnosed as schizophrenics when they actually have bipolar disorder (manic-depression), a condition in which people exhibit periods of intense, frenetic, often bizarre activity alternating with periods of severe depression. The mineral lithium is the most effective and important agent used in the treatment of manic-depression. Manic-depressives being treated with products containing both nicotinic acid and lithium (even in the small amounts in which lithium can be found as a contaminant of the vitamin formula) may be experiencing benefit from the lithium alone.

Ignoring the Placebo Effect: Stress-Formula Vitamins

Placebos, or benign, inactive products (also known as sugar pills), are often given to patients to soothe and comfort them or to meet a patient's desire to take some medication even though a physician believes none is necessary. When this occurs, people may show an improvement simply because they are taking a pill. Sometimes people complaining of vague and nonspecific symptoms or those who are sad and depressed will show some improvement if given an inactive substance simply because they have been told they will get better. The placebo effect can account for 15 to 20 percent of the positive response to pain relievers and psychoactive drugs.

In the case of vitamins, the best example of a placebo effect is the so-called stress formula. All stress formula products contain at least three to five times the average adult RDA of the

B-complex vitamins and ascorbic acid, and some have added vitamin E and minerals. They have been widely promoted as helping to relieve the symptoms of stress, and in some cases they may have done just that—not because of the vitamins and/or minerals, but because of the placebo effect.

The claim that vitamins relieve emotional stress, other than that associated with marginal vitamin deficiency, is simply not reasonable. High doses of vitamins do not have a tranquilizing effect on the central nervous system. Nevertheless, many manufacturers of multivitamin products have developed a "stress formula," which might be represented by the following typical formula:

Vitamin	Dose	Percent of Adult RDA
Ascorbic acid	500 mg	833
Thiamin	10 mg	809
Riboflavin	10 mg	669
Nicotinic acid (niacin)	100 mg	566
Pyridoxine (B_6)	5 mg	213
Vitamin B_{12}	15 mcg	650
Pantothenic acid (B_5)	20 mg	200*
Vitamin E	30 IU	200

*There is no RDA for pantothenic acid; the Daily Value for adults is 10 mg.

The rationale for this formula is that someone under stress is experiencing a series of physical changes. When we are stressed, we may not be eating properly, getting enough sleep, exercise, or relaxation, or otherwise leading our normal life. This special combination of vitamins is supposed to compensate for these problems, despite the fact that logic tells us we cannot continually push ourselves beyond reasonable physical limits without suffering some adverse consequences.

One interesting argument often used by megavitamin proponents is the fact that surgical patients and those undergoing stressful treatments in a hospital are often given nutritional supplements that contain vitamins. It is acknowledged that these patients do better when they have been nutritionally supported, but it is unreasonable to draw the conclusion that the same vitamins that help a surgical patient to heal more quickly will help relieve your daily stresses. In the first case, the vitamins are contributing to the reconstruction and healing of tissues, and in the second, they are being taken to help reconstitute a stressed and worn psyche.

Since there have been no conclusive reports to substantiate the stress formula theory, we suggest that stress management be accomplished only under the guidance of qualified medical personnel and not with megadoses of megavitamins taken as a self-help measure.

Misapplying Animal Data to People: Vitamin E and Chromium

Some proponents claim that vitamin E increases human sexual function. This claim is based on the observation that rats deficient in vitamin E had reproductive problems. When the rats were given supplemental vitamin E, they were able to reproduce normally.

Vitamin E will probably not help your sex life unless you're a rat. Human studies have shown that megadoses of vitamin E in the range of 400 IU to 800 IU per day can, in some instances, cause side effects that include stomach upset, diarrhea, dizziness, bleeding in people taking oral anticoagulant drugs, and reduced gonad (reproductive) function in men. That's right—those megadoses of vitamin E can do exactly the *opposite* of what you are hoping to achieve.

Another example of improperly applying animal studies to people is the promotion of chromium, an essential mineral, as a way to slow or stop the aging process. Animals in which a chromium deficiency was artificially produced had difficulty metabolizing glucose, fats, and protein. They were smaller and died younger than their counterparts given chromium in the diet. These data have led vitamin and mineral enthusiasts to claim that chromium supplements can slow the aging process. Chromium, in the form of a complex with protein, does play a role in metabolizing glucose, but there is nothing to suggest that supplemental chromium pills can keep you young. In fact, chromium may do the opposite; another animal study suggested that chromium picolinate, a form of the mineral designed to enhance absorption, may actually damage chromosomes and potentially lead to cancerous changes.

HOW TO EVALUATE A MEDICAL STUDY

Not every published medical study is worth considering, although it seems that studies with the most interesting or controversial results end up in the newspaper or on the network news. In contrast, almost every study does represent another piece in an expanding puzzle. The best advice we can give about medical and nutrition studies is simply to avoid changing your behavior based on the findings of one study. Results need to be confirmed in further tests to ensure that they are not the result of chance or bias, but that a true connection exists between the items being studied and that the facts all point in a similar direction.

Here are some tips for discriminating the wheat from the chaff when it comes to medical studies:

• *Where was the research conducted? Is a respected institution involved?* That is usually a sign of a better study. Studies from little-known medical schools or private groups may not be as reliable. Studies from third-world countries may not apply to Americans.

• *Was the study done by researchers employed by a pharmaceutical company or vitamin manufacturer?* If so, you'd be wise to cast a suspicious eye on the results. Medical research costs are high and there is a strong incentive to only publish and promote studies with positive results, especially in a field that is as poorly regulated as nutritional supplements.

• *Was the study conducted in test tubes, animals, or humans?* Test-tube and animal data are always preliminary, and there's a chance that the same findings won't hold true in humans. The results of lab studies must be confirmed in people.

• *How was the study conducted?* The gold standard for clinical studies is the randomized, placebo-controlled, double-blind clinical trial. This is a trial in which the active agent (the vitamin) is compared against an inactive placebo in groups of people who are as closely matched in terms of age, sex, health status, and other factors as possible. Further, it is essential that no one who is directly involved with the study know which person is taking the vitamin and which is taking the inactive placebo. Under these conditions, many extraneous factors that could affect the study outcome will have been removed, and so the results are likely to give a truer picture of the vitamin's real effects. Some studies try to compare a vitamin with other active treatment, but this methodology is fraught with difficulties and usually open to severe criticism.

• *Was it a cohort or case-control study, where physicians simply observe two groups of people over time and how they respond to a specific therapy?* Cohort studies are prospective, meaning they enroll patients at the beginning of an "exposure" to a therapy and follow them forward in time to assess how frequently a certain outcome occurs. Case-control studies are retrospective, starting with a certain outcome and then looking backward at how a group may have ended up with this outcome. The major problem with these approaches is that the assessment of a response is based on the judgment of an individual physician or researcher, rather than on a database generated from information gathered on a large number of study subjects. This approach is less reliable than the gold-standard approach.

• *Was the study based on individual (anecdotal) case reports?* These studies, which describe the characteristics of individual patients who experience a specific outcome, are the least reliable form of clinical report. They typically involve a small number of patients and do not control for individual bias or other things that might inadvertently alter study results. It is virtually impossible to draw conclusions based on these types of reports.

• *How many people were studied?* It's best if a study sample is large, though the appropriate size of a well-done clinical trial can vary from hundreds to thousands, depending on many factors. In studies of only a few people, the chances are great that the results will be somehow skewed and not applicable to other people.

• *How long did the study last?* Typically, better studies take longer to do because they give researchers more time to study both the positive and negative effects of the test substance.

• *Where does the study fall in the spectrum of evidence?* Is the study the first of its kind? Or is it trying to confirm or refute the findings of a previous study? Preliminary studies are the first pieces in a puzzle; they're not the be-all and end-all of research. These studies must be repeated and results confirmed, or the findings shouldn't be considered valid. Oftentimes, study results flipflop, confusing doctors and consumers alike, before a clear picture begins to emerge. A good example of this is the controversy over the effect of salt intake on high blood pressure and risk of death.

• *Where was the study published?* If a study was published in a respected journal that requires all submissions to be reviewed by other health care professionals and revised if necessary prior to publication, the chances are better that the research is sound.

SOME FINDINGS FROM RECENT, VALID VITAMIN AND MINERAL STUDIES

The good news is that there is an expanding bank of well-designed, well-executed clinical trials evaluating the effects of various nutrients on preventing and treating disease. Here are highlights of some of the most recent, exciting studies. (You can find out more about each of these topics in the individual vitamin/mineral profiles.)

Antioxidants

The medicinal wonders of vitamins C, E, and beta carotene (a form of vitamin A) appear to be wide and varied. Several studies point to the ability of these nutrients—which fight damage to cells—to enhance immunity, reduce the risks of heart disease, cancer, and cataracts, and stall other effects of aging. But while the data compiled to date are largely promising, they don't present a very clear picture. Studies have flipflopped, particularly on the benefits of beta carotene, which was shown to actually worsen health in a couple of studies. For example, a large Finnish study called the Alpha-Tocopherol, Beta-Carotene (ATBC) Lung Cancer Prevention Trial showed that male smokers who took 20 mg a day of beta carotene for five to eight years had 18 percent more lung cancer and an 8 percent greater risk of death than men who didn't take the supplements. And a large U.S. study of beta carotene and vitamin A—the Beta Carotene and Retinol Efficacy Trial (CARET) study—looking at whether these two nutrients could prevent lung cancer in people at high risk for the disease was actually stopped early because preliminary results indicated the supplements weren't doing the subjects any good and might actually be causing harm. On the other hand, the Physicians' Health Study of 22,071 male physicians reported that beta carotene supplementation caused no harm but conferred no benefit in protecting men from cancer or heart disease.

What recommendations can be made on the basis of these beta carotene studies? It's probably a good idea to forgo mega-dose beta carotene supplements until the controversy is decided. However, the amounts found in multivitamin products aren't a cause for worry. Until the research comes in, be sure to eat foods rich in beta carotene such as carrots, apricots, peaches, collard greens, spinach, tomatoes, and cantaloupe. These products also contain other carotenoids, such as lycopene, that are likely to be protective of health. And avoid beta carotene supplementation if you are a smoker. All of the subjects in the Finnish study were smokers; a third of the subjects in the CARET study were former smokers; and 11 percent of the subjects in the Physicians' Health Study were current smokers, while 51 percent were former smokers.

Studies of vitamin E have also flipflopped. Some studies have shown that this vitamin provides protection against cancer, while others have not. In the Finnish ATBC study, which looked at prevention of lung and other cancers, smokers who received 50 mg of vitamin E, alone or in combination with 20 mg of beta carotene, did not seem to be helped by the vitamin E and might even have been harmed a bit. But a 1998 publication of more data from the ATBC database indicated that male smokers who took 50 mg (75 IU) of vitamin E a day for five to eight years had 23 percent less cancer and 41 percent fewer deaths from prostate cancer than men who did not. Since the ATBC study has been assailed by critics because it dealt solely with smokers and thus isn't applicable to the population at large, vitamin E's cancer-preventive effects are still in question. On the heart disease front, however, vitamin E is now accepted as a potent weapon. There's enough evidence to suggest that it's safe and wise to take about 400 IU of vitamin E a day—good news, considering that it's impossible to get enough vitamin E from foods unless you eat way too many calories. Vitamin E is primarily found in nuts and oils, which are full of fat. There is also some preliminary evidence to suggest that vitamin E can improve immunity in the elderly and may slow the progression of Alzheimer's disease.

Numerous investigations into the antioxidant effects of vitamin C (ascorbic acid) have shown that it offers some protection against heart disease, high cholesterol levels, and cancer, and boosts the immune system. None of the studies have wowed researchers or doctors, but since vitamin C at doses up to 1,000 mg appears safe, many doctors and their patients are taking it.

The bottom line is that a wealth of evidence points to supplementation of vitamins E (100 IU to 400 IU) and C (250 mg to 1,000 mg) as a good idea for all Americans. It's also been suggested by some studies that the performance of these vitamins are enhanced when they're taken together. Beta carotene supplementation, however, should be avoided until further clinical data becomes available.

Magnesium and Migraine

Early basic studies conducted at the New York Headache Center in Manhattan indicate that about half of migraine headache sufferers are deficient in the biologically active form of the mineral magnesium (called ionized magnesium). A special, though expensive, blood test can determine if you have a low level of this mineral; if so, an intravenous infusion of magnesium at a headache doctor's office or an emergency room may cure your migraine within minutes. In one trial, half of forty patients with migraine were found to have low ionized magnesium levels; when treated with intravenous magnesium, migraine pain was relieved in 86 percent of this subgroup of patients and lasted for at least twenty-four hours.

Oral magnesium to prevent migraine headaches is also being explored. However, current preparations may not help you, even with high doses, because they are not well absorbed into the blood. Still, since magnesium is a relatively benign mineral, a one- to two-month trial at 400 mg to 600 mg a day may be worthwhile. At worst, if you're otherwise healthy, you may experience diarrhea on this regimen. Higher doses, however, may cause an irregular heartbeat.

Zinc for Colds

Several studies have looked at the value of zinc gluconate lozenges as a way to shorten the duration of colds and lessen their severity. In the most widely reported of these studies, published in the *Annals of Internal Medicine,* researchers at the Cleveland Clinic found that zinc reduced cold suffering by an average of three and a half days. Among fifty people with early signs of a cold who sucked on four to eight zinc gluconate lozenges daily (52 mg to 104 mg), colds lasted four days—compared with seven and a half days for fifty cold sufferers who didn't get zinc lozenges. This trial was far from perfect. Its results are supported by a few other studies and haven't been supported by a handful of others.

Our advice: Try zinc lozenges if you want to, but be aware that there's a downside to them. You must suck on them to get the full benefit, and they may irritate your mouth or upset your stomach if you don't eat before taking them. And you shouldn't use them for more than a few days, since megadoses of zinc can be harmful.

Chromium for Diabetes

Although most of the news about the trace mineral chromium of late has involved claims that it will help you to lose fat and build muscle—studies show it offers negligible benefits in this regard and only if you exercise like a fiend—chromium's real benefits are in the area of lowering blood sugar. Studies indicate that chromium increases the efficiency of insulin, which helps deliver glucose (blood sugar) to the muscles to be converted into energy. Therefore, it's been suggested that megadoses of chromium (1,000 mcg versus the 50 mcg to 200 mcg recommended by the RDA panel) may lower elevated blood sugar levels in diabetics and perhaps even prevent the disease in those susceptible to it. However, a laboratory study at Dartmouth College suggested that when combined with picolinate—a compound that improves absorption of the mineral—chromium damages chromosomes. Until further studies offer definitive proof of chromium's ability to safely fight high blood sugar, there appears to be little reason for most healthy people to supplement with it.

Selenium for Cancer

Selenium is a mineral with a great deal of promise for helping to fight cancer. Indeed, early studies even indicate that a low selenium level might actually predispose one to cancer. But studies have shown conflicting results on how much protection it offers. One four-year Harvard University study of a thousand women found that those with high selenium intakes (150 mcg a day) had no less cancer than women with low selenium intakes (60 mcg a day). What's more, the small number of women (forty-one subjects) who took selenium supplements actually had twice the risk of cancer—though it wasn't clear if selenium was the culprit.

A four-year, randomized, placebo-controlled intervention trial at the University of Arizona of 200 mcg of selenium a day in 1,300 adults found that it didn't protect against skin cancer recurrence. In fact, selenium supplementers actually had a slightly greater chance of skin cancer. The researchers stopped this study three years early, despite the lack of protective effect against skin cancer, because they were shocked to find that selenium supplements appeared to halve the risk of developing prostate, colon, and lung cancer—and to reduce death rates from these cancers besides.

Before you go taking selenium supplements, remember that this is just one study—and one that was designed to research a totally different subject. In addition, it was conducted in the southwestern United States, where many Americans' diets are lacking in selenium. The results might have been different if the study was done in people with a selenium-rich diet. And the study population was composed of people who had already had one bout of skin cancer.

Further studies are needed, and in particular the findings of the Harvard or Arizona studies need to be replicated, before we can consider recommending selenium supplements for these purposes.

Folic Acid for Strokes, Cervical Cancer, and Birth Defects

Folate, a B vitamin, has been proven to prevent certain neural-tube birth defects such as spina bifida when women take it at a dose of 400 mcg in the first trimester of pregnancy. The government has recommended that *all* reproductive-age women consume 400 mcg (instead of the 180 mcg listed in the RDA) of folate from foods or supplements—just in case they become pregnant unexpectedly. This way, there will be enough folate in their bodies early in pregnancy to prevent these defects.

There are also some limited data that suggest folate may protect against cervical and colon cancer.

But the most exciting news about folic acid has been the mounting evidence that a folate deficiency may be implicated in heart attacks and strokes. If there's not enough folate, as well as vitamins B_6 and B_{12}, in the body, an amino acid called homocysteine can accumulate and, because it participates in the process of forming atherosclerotic plaque, clog blood vessels leading to the heart or brain. The buildup of homocysteine may be caused either by your genetic makeup or by your diet. A high level of homocysteine doubles your risk of heart disease and stroke, which is as much or more than high cholesterol or smoking does. In a European study of seventy-two people published in the *Journal of the American Medical Association* in 1997, supplementation with folate and vitamins B_{12} and B_6 reduced the risk of artery clogging by 62 percent compared to a control group who didn't receive the supplements. This study is just one of several that have shown a positive link between vitamin supplements and reducing homocysteine levels; still, doctors say more research is needed to definitively prove the connection.

Calcium and Vitamin D to Prevent Osteoporosis

Numerous studies have established the ability of calcium and vitamin D to help stall the rate of bone loss that occurs with aging, particularly in postmenopausal women, but also in older men.

Since many young men and women don't consume enough dairy products or leafy vegetables to reach the DRI of 1,000 mg—a level considered optimal for achieving peak bone mass—supplementation is often recommended. Likewise, supplementation is wise for older adults, who may not get enough calcium in their diet or absorb calcium well enough to achieve the DRI of 1,200 mg. Vitamin D supplementation should also be considered for older adults, especially those who don't go outside very much and aren't exposed to much sunlight.

Calcium to Relieve Premenstrual Syndrome (PMS)

A small study of seventy-three women conducted at Columbia Presbyterian Medical Center in New York City suggests that calcium supplements can relieve PMS symptoms and menstrual cramps. Further study is needed to confirm the link, but it is expected that Tums—an antacid that is mostly calcium carbonate—will soon be marketed for PMS.

Niacin for High Cholesterol

It's long been known—and well proven—that niacin in the form known as nicotinic acid and at high doses of 3 g to 6 g is a potent cholesterol-lowering agent. It's inexpensive and very effective. But it also carries a risk of some uncomfortable side effects such as flushing of the face and neck and itching, and some serious ones such as liver toxicity. Hence, nicotinic acid should be used to lower cholesterol only under a doctor's advice and guidance.

Potassium for High Blood Pressure

Most of the studies conducted on this subject have been small or nonrandomized and noncontrolled, with conflicting results, so potassium supplementation has been considered controversial. However, a recent Johns Hopkins University review of thirty-three previous randomized, controlled trials with 2,609 subjects showed that the mineral can reduce systolic blood pressure by 3.11 points, on average, and diastolic blood pressure by 1.97 points. The results were particularly compelling in people who ate a lot of salt. Besides reducing blood pressure, the authors of the review stated that there is evidence to support the idea that even small doses of potassium either from the diet or oral supplements may be able to delay the onset of high blood pressure. Our advice: Ask your doctor about taking potassium supplements if you have high blood pressure, and increase your dietary consumption of this mineral. But be careful. Some high blood pressure medicines should not be mixed with potassium supplements. More about this in Chapter 13.

VITAMIN/MINERAL OVERDOSES

Many people take megadoses of vitamins and minerals without truly understanding the potential problems associated with them. The possible side effects of megadose therapy with vitamins and minerals are discussed in each of the vitamin and mineral profiles. Some of these nutrients, such as vitamin A, vitamin D, thiamin, pyridoxine, calcium, chloride, magnesium, potassium, sodium, iron, copper, zinc, fluoride, manganese, and molybdenum, can be toxic when taken in megadoses. Extreme caution must be exercised when considering megadose therapy, especially when minerals are involved. You should not take megadoses of vitamins as medicines unless prescribed by your doctor to treat a specific problem or unless a therapeutic use has been scientifically substantiated. The fact that the press or a public figure has publicized the use of one vitamin or another does not make it effective therapy or protect you from possible harmful side effects.

PSEUDOVITAMIN PRODUCTS

Many Americans are now discovering vitaminlike substances such as DHEA, melatonin, coenzyme Q_{10}, and glutathione, and various herbal remedies. Despite the fact that these substances and others have been characterized as having antiaging and other properties for decades, their purported effects are still more speculation than fact.

The fervor to find the "fountain of youth" in a pill led to the National Institute of Aging (NIA) issuing a warning in 1997 advising consumers not to take these products—no matter how much they're hyped. Although the NIA acknowledges that futures studies may reveal important health benefits for some or all of these compounds, there is currently no evidence to show they can prevent or reverse the aging process. Also, scientists are worried that they may have long- or short-term side effects not yet realized.

For more information about vitamin-like compounds and herbs, see Parts 4 and 5 of this book.

TABLE 8
Therapeutic Effectiveness of Vitamins and Minerals

VITAMIN/MINERAL	SUGGESTED MAJOR USES	EFFECTIVE	SLIGHTLY EFFECTIVE	NOT BENEFICIAL	INFORMATION LACKING
Water-Soluble Vitamins					
Vitamin B₁ (thiamin)	Beriberi prevention and treatment		X		
	Treatment of inborn errors of metabolism		X		
	Nerve tonic	X			
	Insect repellent			X	
Vitamin B₂ (riboflavin)	Conjunctivitis (red eye)	X			
	Skin diseases	X			
	Migraine				X
Vitamin B₃ (nicotinic acid)	High cholesterol	X	X		
	Heart disease	X			
	Mental illness/schizophrenia				
	Pellagra (prevention and treatment)		X		
Vitamin B₅ (pantothenic acid)	Relief of itching/soothing of wounds		X		
	Healing of wounds	X			
	Graying of hair			X	
	Stress	X			
Vitamin B₆ (pyridoxine)	Depression due to use of oral contraceptives				X
	Treatment of inborn errors of metabolism		X		
	Carpal tunnel syndrome			X	
	Reduce breast milk				X
	Morning sickness				X
	Premenstrual syndrome		X		
Vitamin B₁₂ (cyanocobalamin)	Pernicious anemia	X			

VITAMIN/MINERAL	SUGGESTED MAJOR USES	EFFECTIVE	SLIGHTLY EFFECTIVE	NOT BENEFICIAL	INFORMATION LACKING
Folic Acid	Tiredness			X	
	Confusion/memory loss in the elderly		X		
	Megaloblastic anemia		X		
	Cervical cell changes and anemia resulting from a low folic acid level due to use of oral contraceptives				X
	Birth defects such as spina bifida		X		
	Stroke and heart disease				X
Vitamin C (ascorbic acid)	Scurvy		X		
	Wound healing		X		
	Herpes cold sores		X		
	Cold symptoms			X	
	Preventing the common cold				X
	Preventing infection	X			
	Genital herpes	X			
	Periodontal disease	X			
	High cholesterol	X			
	Cancer				X
	Mental illness				X
	Heart disease			X	
	Alcoholism				X
	Drug abuse				X
	Rectal polyps				X
	Bedsores				X
	Cataracts				X
	Alzheimer's disease				X
Beta carotene	Cancer				X

VITAMIN/MINERAL	SUGGESTED MAJOR USES	EFFECTIVE	SLIGHTLY EFFECTIVE	NOT BENEFICIAL	INFORMATION LACKING
Fat-Soluble Vitamins					
Vitamin A (and retinoic acid)	Cataracts				X
	Heart disease				X
	Cancer				X
	Acne		X		
	Psoriasis		X		
	Night blindness			X	
Vitamin D	Rickets	X			
	Osteomalacia (adult rickets)	X			
	Malfunctioning parathyroid gland	X			
	Fanconi's syndrome	X			
	Psoriasis			X	
Vitamin E	Cystic breast disease				X
	Intermittent severe leg muscle pains				X
	Nighttime leg cramps				X
	Healing of wounds		X		
	Protection of the body's cells from the effects of oxidation	X			
	Sexual function		X		
	Heart disease	X			
	Athletic performance			X	
	Scars			X	
	Cardiac problems due to chemotherapy				X
	Hemolytic anemia due to G6PD deficiency				X
	Glutathione synthetase deficiency				X
	Environmental hazards such as lead poisoning			X	

VITAMIN/MINERAL	SUGGESTED MAJOR USES	EFFECTIVE	SLIGHTLY EFFECTIVE	NOT BENEFICIAL	INFORMATION LACKING
Vitamin K	Cancer				X
	Cataracts				X
	Immunity				X
	Alzheimer's disease				X
	Bleeding prevention in newborn infants	X			
	Antidote to oral anticoagulants	X			
Other vitamins					
Choline	Alzheimer's disease		X		
	Liver damage due to alcoholism			X	
	High cholesterol		X		
Inositol	High cholesterol		X		
	Arteriosclerosis			X	
	Stroke			X	
	Heart disease			X	
	Cirrhosis			X	
	Dizziness			X	
PABA	Sunscreen	X			
Laetrile (vitamin B$_{17}$)	Cancer			X	
Essential fatty acids (vitamin F)	Intravenous feeding	X			
Bioflavonoids (vitamin P)	Bleeding			X	
	Cold symptoms			X	
	Prevention of colds			X	
Essential Minerals					
Calcium	Rickets	X			
	Osteomalacia	X			
	Postmenopausal osteoporosis	X			

VITAMIN/MINERAL	SUGGESTED MAJOR USES	EFFECTIVE	SLIGHTLY EFFECTIVE	NOT BENEFICIAL	INFORMATION LACKING
Phosphorous	High blood pressure				X
	PMS				X
Magnesium	Laxative	X			
	Laxative	X			
	Antacid	X			
	Seizures due to toxemia of pregnancy	X			
	Migraine headache	X			
Iodine	Underactive thyroid and goiter	X			
Iron	Iron-deficiency anemia	X			
Potassium	Reduce blood pressure	X			
Zinc	Healing of burns	X			
	Healing of wounds and broken bones	X			
	Arthritis			X	
	Cancer			X	
	Common cold/symptoms		X		
Important Trace Minerals					
Copper	Heart disease			X	
	Arthritis			X	
	Prevention of aging			X	
Manganese	Dental cavities	X			
Fluoride	Postmenopausal osteoporosis		X		
Chromium	Type II diabetes		X		
	Weight loss			X	
Selenium	Cancer				X
	Prevention of aging				X

6

HOW TO BUY AND TAKE VITAMIN AND MINERAL PRODUCTS

As you face shelves of vitamin and mineral products, it will soon become obvious that the various formulas and forms vary widely, though more than one company may make the same formula. You will also note that there are many different claims made for each formula and that the jargon used by vitamin manufacturers is not standardized.

Your final decision to take a supplement and what product to take must include consideration of your personal habits, physical condition, eating habits, and medicines you take. Most people will do quite well with a regular multivitamin or a multivitamin with minerals—and additional supplements as needed to achieve the recommended 400 mcg of folic acid, 100 to 400 IU of vitamin E, and 250 to 1,000 mg of vitamin C. The real need for special therapeutic formulas, stress formulas, antioxidant formulas, or other formulas guaranteed to cure what ails you is questionable. Also, the decision to take vitamin products that supply more than 100 percent of daily requirements should be made only after taking it over with a knowledgeable health provider.

WHERE TO GET ADVICE ON YOUR VITAMIN NEEDS

The first health professional to consider is your family doctor. Many medical schools now teach the basics of nutrition. But most physicians in current practice, like other health professionals, have received virtually no training in the nutrition sciences during their education. Their background in this field has been gleaned from readings in the medical literature, personal experience, and exposure to nutritionists and other physicians who have extensively studied the subject. The best that the average doctor can offer in this area is extensive background and training in disease and its treatment, a knowledge of where to find nutritional information, and good common sense. When asked to recommend a vitamin or vitamin-mineral supplement, many physicians will simply recommend the brand of vitamins they or their patients take, or one that was the subject of a recent medical advertisement or sales pitch. Fortunately, their recommendation is usually as good as any other person's.

Some physicians, however, are more nutritionally oriented than others and may be able to recommend a vitamin regimen suited to your individual needs. For instance, obstetricians usually recommend a prenatal vitamin-mineral supplement for pregnant or breast-feeding women, because the required level of nutrient intake is almost impossible to meet by diet alone. Sports medicine specialists may recommend a variety of vitamins and minerals for their athlete patients. And cardiologists may suggest an antioxidant formula or vitamins E and C.

Other health professionals can offer solid advice about the role of nutrition and vitamins in specific body functions. For example, your dentist is probably the only person who closely examines your mouth. In doing so, he or she may come upon a sign of vitamin deficiency (B_1, B_2, or B_{12}) or a drug side effect by noting the appearance of your mucous membranes, tongue, and gums. Don't exclude your dentist from nutritional discussions; he or she may have some interesting information to offer.

Your pharmacist is the most accessible and most affordable source of health care information and advice. When it comes to vitamin products, most pharmacists are more than willing to offer consultation, but, like other health professionals, the level of nutritional knowledge varies from one pharmacist to the next. Pharmacists are exposed to only basic nutritional information during their professional education, and those who have become expert in this field have done so through postgraduate study. While many pharmacists have made the effort to do this, others have not. This means that you must choose your pharmacist as carefully as you do a doctor. A pharmacist who takes the extra time to be sure his or her professional expertise is current is worth the search, even if that pharmacy charges a few pennies more for prescriptions or vitamins.

Dieticians and nurses are also good information sources

when it comes to nutritional matters, although only the dietician has extensively studied nutrition. However, these usually salaried employees of a hospital or clinic offer their services only to patients of those facilities. In recent years, though, many registered dieticians have gone into private practice as nutritional counselors. They and others specializing in nutrition therapy can be found in the yellow pages under "Nutritionists." Look for a person with some professional credentials, such as the abbreviation *RD* (Registered Dietician) after his or her name.

Last, but certainly not least, are the thousands of people who own, operate, and work in health food stores or vitamin centers. Quite a few of these people provide commonsense information about balanced diets, proper nutrition, and vitamin use, but too many of them feel that vitamins are the cure-all for our daily problems, from the common cold to cancer. If the medical establishment (including the pharmaceutical industry) had the answers to these illnesses, they would have been making and selling them long ago at a substantial profit. Unfortunately, the remedies for many of the ailments that plague us are not known to anyone, including the "vitamin jockeys." Be extremely cautious when someone tells you about vitamins that can save or replace your hair or perform some other equally miraculous feat, the miracles of natural (versus synthetic) vitamins, or the aphrodisiac powers of this pollen or that vitamin. These statements are typically untrue and should be considered a form of modern medical quackery.

We are not saying you should ignore everything you hear in a health food or vitamin store and pay attention to anything you hear in your doctor's office or a pharmacy. We believe that all health-related information, regardless of the source, should be viewed as information to be verified and then acted on. Beware of instant cures and miracles.

One final point: Health food and vitamin stores are in existence because there is a tremendous (more than $3.5 billion per year) market for the products they sell. We don't want to suggest that the sole motive of these people is to sell you as much as they can without regard to your needs, but keep in mind that if they don't sell you something, they can't stay in business.

UNDERSTANDING VITAMIN AND MINERAL JARGON

When shopping for a vitamin formula, remember that the people who make and market these products sell them in the same way as they would sell detergents, food products, toothpaste, or any other consumer good. Market surveys of vitamin and other health product purchasers have shown a strong preference for products labeled as *natural, high-potency, complete formula, super,* or with other terms that convey a sense of strength or a link with "natural goodness."

Since these words do not have a specific definition, they can be used in whatever context the manufacturer wishes. Some products give the impression of being high-potency but are really the same as regular multivitamins or multivitamins with minerals. Other products are given names that imply they are stress or therapeutic formulas but do not fit the profile for these products.

The only way we can suggest to deal with these marketing practices is to ignore them and follow these simple steps:

- Decide what kind of vitamin supplement you want to take (multivitamin with or without minerals, antioxidant formula, prenatal formula, and so on).
- Compare labels, on which the content of each vitamin must be expressed along with the percentage of the Daily Value it represents.
- Compare prices among products.
- Avoid products with gimmicky names, claims, or ingredients.
- Buy the product that meets your needs at the lowest price.

HOW VITAMINS ARE MEASURED

One of the things many people find confusing about buying vitamins is the units used to measure them. Most vitamins and minerals are measured in terms of how much they weigh, and since vitamins and minerals are usually needed only in very small quantities, the units of weight of each are very small.

The largest unit of weight you will come across in this book is a gram. One gram is equivalent to about one-fifth of a teaspoon. The abbreviation for *gram* is *g*.

Most vitamins and minerals are measured in milligrams. One

milligram is equal to one-thousandth of a gram. The abbreviation for *milligram* is *mg*. However, some vitamins are needed in such small quantities that they are measured in units equal to one-thousandth of a milligram, or one-millionth part of a gram. This unit is called a *microgram,* and its abbreviation is *mcg* or *μg*.

Several vitamins—notably A, D, and E—are measured both in terms of international units, or IU, based on measures of biological activity, and in terms of weight (mg). Because one or the other measure may be listed on a particular product or reference, this can be confusing unless you know the equivalents. They are:

Vitamin A (retinol)* 3.3 IU = 1 mcg

Vitamin D (cholecalciferol)** 400 IU = 10 mcg

Vitamin E 15 IU = 10 mg

NATURAL OR SYNTHETIC VITAMINS?

A major decision faced by the vitamin consumer is whether to buy a "natural" or "synthetic" product.

Time and time again, one hears claims that vitamins from "natural" sources such as plants or other materials found in nature are actually of higher quality, more effective, and better for you than those manufactured in the laboratory. This is simply untrue.

Since vitamins are identifiable chemicals, the source of the chemical is not nearly as important as the purity and quality of the chemical in determining whether it will be able to do its job. Although the words *natural* and *organic* are in vogue, the only important difference between natural and synthetic vitamins is cost. Natural vitamins must be extracted from plants and in-

---

*All substances with vitamin A activity are included here. Their vitamin activity is expressed in terms of retinol equivalents, which is one form of vitamin A.
**All substances with vitamin D–like activity are included here. Their vitamin activity is expressed in terms of cholecalciferol equivalents, which is one form of vitamin D.

volve a complicated, often costly, process. These costs are passed on directly to you in the form of a higher purchase price.

The only vitamin that you might consider purchasing in its natural form is vitamin E. Why? Because natural vitamin E (d = alpha tocopherol) may get into cells and body fluids more efficiently than does synthetic vitamin E (dl-alpha tocopherol).

BRAND-NAME OR GENERIC VITAMINS?

Today, brand-name and generic vitamins with the same ingredients are equivalent in potency and quality. Generics simply tax your pocketbook less. Many drugstore and supermarket chains market supplements under their own names; these are usually comparable to national brands and typically less expensive.

TIME-RELEASE VITAMINS

Time-release vitamins are, in general, just another marketing gimmick. There's no evidence that time-release multivitamin/mineral or antioxidant supplements are better than the standard formulas. In fact, the coatings around the pills may actually make it harder for the body to absorb fat-soluble vitamins.

COLLOIDAL MINERALS

These products are sold under a variety of different brand names, and most notably through an audiotape called *Dead Doctors Don't Lie*. A colloidal mineral preparation is a clay with a high content of minerals that is suspended in a liquid solution. The content of the clay varies—some products may even contain dangerous concentrations of aluminum or other minerals. The products are also expensive, and there's no evidence to back up their claims. (One of the claims on the tape is that our soil is depleted of minerals thanks to overfarming. We don't believe that to be true.)

Our advice: Avoid them.

CHELATED MINERALS

A claim made by some vendors of multivitamin/mineral products is that chelated minerals—minerals that are attached to an amino acid—are more rapidly and completely absorbed into the system than nonchelated minerals. Some have gone so far as to say that products with minerals that are not chelated are the same as those with no mineral content at all. While this may sound reasonable, there is no scientific evidence to support such a claim. And when a chelated mineral is digested, it is separated from the amino acids, so chelation does not aid in absorption. Indeed, chelated minerals might even be less well absorbed than other minerals.

The only proven value of chelated mineral products is their ability to separate the purchaser from more dollars than the purchaser of traditional vitamin-mineral formulas. Again, we suggest you avoid them.

SINGLE VITAMINS VERSUS MULTIVITAMIN PRODUCTS

Is it better to take an all-inclusive product or to determine your individual needs and take each component as a separate pill? Ideally, one might suspect that it would be best to determine *exact* vitamin and mineral needs and then buy each ingredient as a separate product.

While there is nothing wrong with this approach, it is not the easiest way to be sure of meeting minimal nutritional requirements. And it can be dangerous, too—say, if you take too much vitamin A. Therefore, we recommend that individual supplements be used only when they are specifically indicated (such as for high doses of C and E). Possible reasons to take individual vitamin supplements may be found in the individual vitamin and mineral profiles. If you do decide to buy each vitamin as a separate product, you need not worry about most vitamins or minerals interfering with each other. Important vitamin, mineral, and herbal interactions are listed beginning on page 385.

EXPIRATION DATES AND STORAGE

Vitamins lose potency over time, so be sure to check the expiration date when you buy a new bottle to ensure you'll have enough time to finish it before it loses power. If there is no expiration date, ask your pharmacist if there's a code on the bottle that can tell him or her the date. Or, as a last resort, mark your date of purchase on the bottle and use it for up to a year before discarding any remaining pills.

Keep your vitamins and other supplements in a cool, dry place. (The medicine chest in the bathroom, by the way, is not a good choice.) *And make sure supplements are out of the reach of children and pets.* Since some vitamin products look and taste like candy to children, they may be tempted to eat them like candy. Iron is the most dangerous compound in adult vitamins for children and is one of the leading causes of poisoning deaths among children under the age of six in the United States.

STAMP OF APPROVAL

One way to tell a quality vitamin or mineral product is to look for the U.S. Pharmacopeia (USP) stamp on the label. The USP sets voluntary quality standards for vitamin and mineral supplements. To use this stamp, manufacturers must produce a product that meets USP's strict standards.

In a related area, the FDA is taking steps to ensure that their Good Manufacturing Practices (GMP) are followed by vitamin/mineral manufacturers. A final GMP program may soon be put into place, requiring manufacturers to adhere to certain standards for making supplements, but it is not yet known if this will be mandatory.

CHOOSING A MULTIVITAMIN PRODUCT

There are several hundred different brands of multivitamin/mineral combinations from which to choose. The major types are described here (there is some overlap between categories) and the vitamin and mineral content of some of the most popular brands is listed in Table 10, at the end of this chapter.

General Multivitamins

Multivitamin formulas contain several vitamins, no minerals, and meet most people's vitamin needs. Usually included in these formulas are vitamins A, C, D, E, thiamin, riboflavin, pyridoxine, and nicotinic acid (niacin) in amounts that approximate and in some cases (often, for example, for vitamin C) exceed the RDA/DRIs for each of these nutrients. Some multivitamins contain other ingredients, such as B_{12}, calcium pantothenate, pantothenic acid, and folic acid; quantities are usually in the RDA ranges. If you choose a formula with folic acid, you will be sure to meet your RDA/DRIs for all vitamins for which there are RDA/DRIs since manufacturers must meet these minimum requirements.

General multivitamin combinations are usually among the least expensive of all vitamin products. Theragran offers a complete vitamin formula. Some other brands are Centrum, One-a-Day, and Unicap. There are also many generic multivitamin brands available at substantial savings over some of the brands mentioned. A word of caution, however: Generic multivitamins may not be suitable as prenatal supplements or as vitamins for breast-feeding women (see page 108).

Multivitamins with Minerals

These formulas contain both vitamin and mineral ingredients. The quantity of each ingredient is generally close to the RDA/DRI, where one has been established, although once again it is virtually impossible to classify the specific ingredients of products in this group. Multivitamin/mineral products are promoted as general-purpose nutritional supplements. The sales pitch here is simply: "As long as you're taking a multivitamin, why not take some minerals, too? After all, it's just as easy to take a multivitamin/mineral product as it is to swallow a vitamin." The need for daily supplementation of these elements is questionable, but sales of products in this class attest to their popularity.

A typical multivitamin with minerals product contains vitamins A, C, D, E, thiamin, riboflavin, pyridoxine, folic acid, sodium or calcium panthothenate, cyanocobalamin, iron, calcium, copper, magnesium, manganese, zinc, and iodine. Some members of this group have added trace elements such as selenium, chromium, molybdenum, and biotin to their formulations. Selenium is part of our antioxidant defense system. If you believe you would benefit from including minerals in your supplement, make sure that the product includes selenium. Most, but not all, vitamin/mineral combination products contain 10 to 40 mcg selenium per tablet or capsule, which is enough for most people.

A popular multivitamin and mineral combination often recommended by doctors and pharmacists is Theragran-M. Other brands include Centrum, Myadec, One-A-Day Maximum, and Unicap-M. Generic equivalents are available.

Multivitamins with Iron

Dietary surveys have shown that a substantial number of Americans are deficient in iron. This has led to the development and use of a wide variety of formulas with between 10 mg and 27 mg of iron per tablet or capsule. Many people believe if you need extra vitamins, you probably also need extra iron. If you accept this theory, be sure to choose a product that provides you with your age- and gender-specific RDA for iron. (The RDA for females between the ages of eleven and fifty years is 15 mg; for males between the ages of eleven and fifty, it is 10 mg. The RDA for adult men and women over the age of fifty is 10 mg.) If you think your vitamin intake is fine but believe you need iron, take an iron supplement alone.

Be aware, though, that standard multivitamins plus iron are not suitable for pregnant women—they don't contain the RDA for iron, which is set at 30 mg during pregnancy. In addition, be sure not to *overdo* it with iron. An excess supply has been linked to a potential increased risk of heart attack and colon cancer, and in people who have an unusual genetic disease called hemochromatosis, iron supplements may lead to the dangerous buildup of iron in the body.

Popular brand names of multivitamins with iron (which often contain other minerals as well) include Theragran-M, Allbee C-800 Plus Iron, Centrum, Sigtab-M Tablets, Stresstabs + Iron, and Unicap Plus Iron.

Therapeutic Multivitamins

Therapeutic formulas contain the same vitamins as those in the groups we call multivitamins and stress formulas (discussed below under "B-Complex Formulas") but in larger quantities. They can usually be identified by the letter *T* or the word *therapeutic* in their name. The levels of vitamins found in these formulas can approach the megadose range (ten times the RDAs).

Products in this group are often recommended for older people or for those who are extremely deficient in one or two vitamins. The feeling is that, since all vitamins are obtained from food, if you are deficient in one, you are probably deficient in several others. Therefore, a therapeutic multivitamin is recommended. Most of the contents of any therapeutic formulation will be either saved in the body or eliminated via the urine, so you should consider carefully the regular use of one of these products.

The premier therapeutic multivitamin product is Theragran. As with other multivitamins, there are low-cost versions of this formula sold through many vitamin outlets and pharmacies, and they may even be labeled as being "equal to Theragran." Caution should be used when selecting generic products to ensure they are equivalent in their content to name brands.

Therapeutic Multivitamins with Minerals

Products in this class usually contain the same basic ingredients as multivitamins with minerals. Again, the only difference is that products labeled therapeutic usually contain larger (one and a half or two times) concentrations of each ingredient. Since the extra quantities provided in the so-called therapeutic formulas are probably not necessary, the superiority of these formulas over other vitamin mixtures should be questioned.

Two of the more popular therapeutic vitamins with minerals are Theragran-M and Unicap T.

B-Complex Formulas

These products are usually promoted to people who want to be sure they can build red blood cells, keep their blood vessels and nervous systems functioning, and maintain normal body metabolism at a high level of efficiency.

B-complex formulas contain only the B vitamin group in quantities that approach the RDAs, although there is a tremendous range of vitamin concentrations among the various B-complex formulas. Some brands are Allbee, Geritol Liquid, Incremin with Iron Syrup, and Lipotrol. Some companies add a variety of other ingredients, including biotin, PABA, lecithin, choline, and inositol. Despite these added ingredients, these products remain in the B-complex category.

B Complex with C (Stress Formulas)

B complex with C formulas are the original "stress" formulas. They are essentially the same as the B-complex vitamins, but have added vitamin C.

Some manufacturers have added other nutrients to their formulas. The amounts of vitamins contained in most "stress formulas" exceed the RDAs by several times, but the choice of ingredients and dosage strengths does not seem to follow any logical pattern.

The best known stress formulas are Theragran Stress Formula, Allbee with C, Bee-T-Vites, One-A-Day Stressgard, Sigtab Tablets, StressMates, and Stresstabs Advanced Formula.

Many manufacturers have patterned their stress formulas after Allbee with C because of its commercial success. This raises an interesting question. Obviously, people who make and sell vitamin products do so because they are interested in making money. But the promotional efforts behind many of these products cannot be justified by their possible benefits to the consumer. Have they added extra vitamin C and other ingredients to their formulas to make their products nutritionally more complete or to keep up with the latest vitamin or mineral rage? Whenever a new ingredient is added to a vitamin product, often the name is changed to reflect that addition. This allows the manufacturers to advertise their "new, improved" formula. A stress formula to which additional nutrients, such as desiccated liver, brewer's yeast, zinc, magnesium, and folic acid, have been added is Allbee C-800 Plus Iron.

Stress formulas are promoted for people who find themselves under tremendous emotional stress, despite the fact that no medical evidence supports claims made for these formulas. We do not use more vitamin C than normal when we are in an *emotionally* stressful situation, and the normal amount needed is far less than that found in stress formula vitamins. The idea is based on the proven need for additional nutrition after *physical* stress, such as surgery or injury. See the profile on vitamin C in Part 2 for further information on your actual needs for this vitamin.

Antioxidant Vitamin Formulas

In recent years, special antioxidant brands have been created to capitalize on the research that suggests megadoses of vitamins C and E and beta carotene are protective against heart disease, cancer, and possibly other diseases, too. Many of the formulations also contain selenium, manganese, chromium, and other minerals.

Popular brand names include Nature Made Antioxidant Formula, One-A-Day Antioxidant Plus, Protegra Antioxidant Vitamin & Mineral Supplement, and Alive Antioxidant Formula.

Antioxidant formulations created to encourage eye health and ward off cataracts and other eye problems are also on shelves. Brand names include Ocuvite, Opti-Vue, Ocu-Care, and Ocu-Guard. While there is actually some evidence that antioxidants can protect against these conditions, it appears there's little reason to take an antioxidant supplement solely designed to boost eye health. A general antioxidant formulation should be adequate for this and other health problems.

Vitamins for Women and Men

A number of male- and female-specific formulas have been developed to meet the differing needs of the two genders. Some products are also age-specific. For instance, there are formulas for menopausal women, as well as for men over fifty.

Women's formulas may contain extra calcium, iron, zinc, and folic acid. Men's formulas may contain extra B vitamins, antioxidants, trace minerals, and no iron.

If you prefer, you can use one of these products instead of an adult's multivitamin and mineral supplement. However, be aware that some of these products contain herbs and other compounds, such as evening primrose oil, ginseng, chamomile, bee pollen, ginger, yohimbe, and saw palmetto. These are supposed to add "extra value" to the products—saw palmetto, for instance, is touted to be good for a man's prostate—although their benefits in these low doses are questionable and unsupported by scientific studies. What the addition of these compounds and their special packaging really do is add to the price of the product.

Popular brand names include Femiron Multivitamins and Iron, One-A-Day Women's, One-A-Day Men's, Mega Men, and Rejuvex.

Pediatric Vitamins

The main things that differentiate pediatric vitamins from general multivitamins of the one-a-day variety or multivitamins with minerals are the form in which they can be purchased and some of their lower-than-adult doses. The most successful pediatric products are those made and sold in the shape of animals or popular cartoon characters and flavored to taste like candy. Many children will not take vitamins unless they are flavored, can be chewed, and resemble some familiar character. So if you want your child to take a daily multivitamin, these products may be your only choice.

The chewable multivitamins that have added minerals to their formulas can provide added benefits to the child who does not eat properly, but they cannot be considered a replacement for good nutrition. One of the latest mineral additions to children's chewable vitamins is calcium, but the amount of calcium (around 100 mg) in these products is insufficient to meet the child's DRI (800–1,300 mg) for that important mineral. Your child will still have to obtain calcium from dietary sources. Another mineral, fluoride, is included in some prescription-only formulas, and your doctor may suggest one of these formulations to prevent cavities if the water supply in your area is not fluoridated.

Popular children's vitamins include Bugs Bunny Chewable Vitamins, Centrum Jr. Children's Chewable Vitamins, Flintstones Chewable Vitamins, Poly-Vi-Sol Chewable Tablets and Drops, and Sunkist Children's Chewable Multivitamins.

Infants are often given a liquid product, such as Tri-Vi-Sol, containing vitamins A, C, and D. These products are meant to supplement the vitamins supplied in mother's milk or infant formulas. Some pediatricians will switch a child to a more comprehensive vitamin product once the infant has stopped nursing or taking prepared formulas; others will simply tell you to stop giving your child a supplement on the assumption that the baby is getting all required nutrients from its food. Do not accept the doctor's recommendation on blind faith. If you know that your child is a good eater, he or she probably does not need a vitamin supplement. If, however, your child is a fussy or poor eater, he or she may need supplemental vitamins. Remember, no one knows your child better than you!

Prenatal Vitamins

The needs of the pregnant or breast-feeding woman have been studied in greater detail than those of almost any other group. Therefore, the types and amounts of micronutrients found in these formulas are more standardized than the ingredients in any other product class. Your doctor will probably recommend a specific prescription-only prenatal formulation, but several products will meet your needs. When evaluating prenatal vitamins, bear in mind that they should meet all the RDA/DRIs specified for pregnant or lactating (breast-feeding) women. That means they should contain larger quantities of just about every vitamin and mineral than formulations designed for adults.

All prenatal vitamins contain extra folic acid. The RDAs indicate that pregnant women should be receiving at least 400 mcg (0.4 mg) per day of folic acid and breast-feeding women should receive 260 mcg to 280 mcg (0.26 mg to 0.28 mg). Most nonprescription prenatal vitamins contain 800 mcg, while most prescription-only prenatal vitamins contain 1 mg of folic acid, as added insurance.

Other differences among prenatal formulas to be considered are these:

- Some prenatal vitamins don't provide enough vitamin A. Pregnant women need 800 mcg (4,000 IU) a day, and those who are nursing need 1,200 to 1,300 mcg (6,000 to 6,500 IU). On the other hand, be sure you're not consuming more than 10,000 IU of vitamin A from dietary and supplement sources, as high doses have been linked to birth defects.
- Mineral content varies tremendously. The amount of calcium in prenatal vitamins varies from 125 mg to 250 mg per pill, but none meets the DRI (1,000 mg–1,300 mg) for calcium because of the physical difficulty of packing all that calcium into a single tablet. You must get extra calcium from milk, milk products, or other food sources.
- Pregnant women should take 30 mg of iron every day, and most of the products provide more than that amount.
- Some prenatal products have added a stool softener (to prevent you from becoming constipated) or amino acids (supposedly because they are the building blocks of DNA) to the basic formula.

The names of some commonly prescribed prenatal vitamins include Materna, Nestabs, Niferex, Precare, Prenate, and Zenate. Natalins, Prenatal-S, Prenavite, and Stuart Prenatal are nonprescription prenatal vitamins.

Mature Adults' and Seniors' Formulas

The graying of America has given birth to a whole new class of vitamin products—Centrum Silver, Geritol Extend, Geriplex-FS, One-A-Day 50 Plus, Unicap Sr.—marketed especially for mature adults, those over the age of fifty. But when you compare these formulas with other vitamins and mineral products, you will find that the nutritional benefits they offer to mature adults vary greatly. Often the formula is similar to that for adults, with more of some vitamins and minerals and less of others. Many do, however, contain less or no iron compared with other adult formulas, since iron needs may decrease with age (especially after women go through menopause and stop menstruating).

There are, however, two nonnutritional features of some geriatric formulas that may be considered pluses. One is a stool softener, which some manufacturers have incorporated into their products. An example is Geriplex-FS, to which docusate sodium, a fecal softener (hence the suffix "FS") has been added to prevent constipation while this product is being taken. Iron, an ingredient sometimes found in these and other formulas, can be constipating and particularly troublesome to anyone with bowel problems. Another unique feature is that some geriatric vitamin formulas are sold as liquids, allowing them to be taken more easily (and at considerably greater cost per dose) by those who cannot or do not wish to swallow capsules.

If you are a senior citizen, consider using any vitamin/mineral formulation that meets your RDA/DRI requirements. Do not restrict yourself to a geriatric formula.

Other Formulas

Some manufacturers sell mixtures of vitamins and minerals especially for men who are losing their hair, men with potency problems, athletes, women who wish to enhance the appearance of their hair or skin and nails, and anyone looking for more energy. Many products today even contain amino acids, herbs such as ginseng, and any number of other nutritional compounds. These formulas are said to be specially prepared to meet the nutritional requirements of people in each of these categories, although the doses seem rather arbitrary (as they often do in the other categories as well). One might ask, "Should a balding man with sexual problems take three different vitamin supplements?" The answer to this question is a resounding no!

There is no evidence to indicate that any of these special vitamin/mineral products can produce the kind of results claimed on the package labels and in the advertising for these formulas. These formulas are excellent examples of the unsubstantiated claims that are reviewed in each vitamin and mineral profile.

TABLET, CAPSULE, LIQUID, SPRAY . . .

When selecting a dosage form, you will want to pick the one that is most convenient and pleasant for you to take, while providing all of the vitamins and minerals you want. This is a very personal decision and one that can be made only by taste testing and considering the recommendations of others who have taken specific products.

All manufacturers are aware of the role that convenience, tablet size, and taste play in the selection of their products. You can be sure that each of them strives to provide you with the best-tasting, most convenient product possible. The only axiom for you to remember here is that the larger the number of vitamins and minerals and the more of each that is contained in a tablet, the larger the tablet. That's why so many of the new, all-inclusive products, the ones with everything under the sun, are large enough to be considered true "horse pills."

Here is a brief rundown of the most common dosage forms.

Tablets and Capsules

Most vitamins are sold as tablets or capsules simply because this is the most convenient way for manufacturers to pack all those nutrients into a single dosage unit. Other dosage forms usually contain less nutrient per dosage unit.

Chewable Tablets

These are special formulas for young children and others who cannot swallow traditional tablets or capsules. Multivitamins, multivitamins with minerals, and multivitamins with iron come in this dosage form. The major differences among these products lie in their taste and shape, both of which may be important to the person actually chewing and swallowing the product.

Many children and adults enjoy taking vitamin C as a chewable table, wafer, or gum, but this type of formulation is actually harmful to your teeth, since the acid in vitamin C can destroy teeth enamel. Opt for regular vitamin C tablets that you swallow instead.

Liquids

Liquid vitamin products were originally developed as another convenience for people who are unable to swallow tablets or capsules. Generally they contain relatively small amounts of nutrients in a dosage unit—usually a teaspoon or tablespoon. This is because vitamins can be difficult to dissolve and are unpalatable to some people, even at modest dosage ranges. Most liquid vitamins also contain a healthy dose of alcohol, needed to dissolve some of the vitamins.

Powders

If you're a purist, then vitamin powders are for you. However, your total daily vitamin and mineral needs would just fill a teaspoon, so it would be impractical for you to measure daily doses of supplemental vitamins and minerals. In fact, the only vitamin sold widely in power form is C, and this grew out of the practice of taking megadoses in the range of 5 to 10 g per day for the common cold.

Wafers and Other Food Products

A few vitamins are available as wafers, shakes or drinks, or other food products. These are simply more convenient ways for people to take a vitamin supplement. There is even a breakfast cereal, Total, that has enough vitamin content to meet

100 percent of the adult Daily Values for ten vitamins and minerals. The manufacturers of that product have used that fact as a major part of their advertising campaign.

Sprays

Vitamin sprays have recently appeared on the market. The first spray of its kind, Vitamist, is available without a prescription and is designed to be squirted into the mouth four times a day. The manufacturer claims that a spray formulation is absorbed via the mucous membranes in the mouth and that a spray is healthier than a pill, which may have waxes or binders in it.

However, there are no studies that have compared the two forms of administration—sprays to pills—and so there's no evidence that sprays work better than the traditional vitamins. But sprays, since they're so "innovative," do tend to be more expensive than pills.

WHEN AND HOW TO TAKE VITAMIN AND MINERAL SUPPLEMENTS

Vitamins and minerals may be taken at any time, generally without regard to food or meals. The body will extract everything it needs, regardless of dosage form or time of day. It is, however, a good idea to get into the habit of taking your vitamins at the same time every day; this establishes a routine and helps you to remember to take them. Many people take their vitamins with breakfast; others prefer lunchtime, coffee break, or bedtime.

In general, however, it is best to take vitamin and mineral supplements with a large glass of water and food. Food can be helpful in affecting the rate of absorption of some minerals, such as iron. In these cases, the food delays the passage of the mineral through the intestines and allows more time for the mineral to be absorbed into your bloodstream through the intestinal tissues. Also, food may reduce the chances of your getting an upset stomach from vitamins or vitamin-mineral combinations. See Table 9 for some suggestions on optimal timing.

TABLE 9
Supplement Timing

Supplement type	How to take it	Why
Multivitamin with minerals	With a glass of water and food	Water and food help break down the vitamins and minerals so you absorb the maximum amount of nutrients.
Vitamin C	With food, preferably in separate doses of 500 mg or less	Although this water-soluble vitamin is well absorbed by the body even on an empty stomach, when it's taken with food you ensure the tablet will fully dissolve and you'll get the most benefit. The body theoretically can't handle doses larger than 500 mg at one time; if you take more, what it can't use will be excreted in your urine.
Vitamin E	With a meal that contains a little fat; don't take with an iron supplement	This fat-soluble vitamin is best absorbed in the presence of fat. Iron may destroy vitamin E.
Calcium	With dairy foods, preferably in separate doses of 500 mg or less; avoid taking iron and fiber supplements at the same time	Dairy foods improve calcium absorption; fiber and iron reduce absorption. And you probably won't fully absorb large doses.
Iron	With a citrus drink; don't take with coffee, tea, wine, or fiber supplements	Citrus (vitamin C) helps the body better absorb iron; tannins in coffee, tea, and wine reduce absorption, as do fiber supplements.
Zinc	With protein—eggs, beef, or lamb—but not with dairy foods, coffee, tea, wine, or fiber or calcium supplements	Food reduces the stomach upset zinc can cause. Protein increases zinc absorption; dairy products, tannins in coffee, tea, and wine, fiber, and high doses of calcium may reduce absorption.

VITAMIN AND MINERAL INTERACTIONS

Most vitamins and minerals at doses near the RDA/DRI values do not significantly affect the absorption of other vitamins and minerals. Sometimes, though, one nutrient will help another to be absorbed into the blood. For example, vitamin C assists in the absorption of iron. In contrast, vitamin E, in large doses, has been reported to counteract the effects of iron in treating infant anemia; hence, don't give your child large doses of vitamin E unless instructed to do so by your pediatrician. Also, increasing your calcium intake can affect zinc absorption, necessitating an increase in zinc consumption.

More information on the interactions of vitamins, minerals, and herbs are detailed in Part 6, "Vitamin, Mineral, and Herbal Drug Interactions."

HOW THE GOVERNMENT CONTROLS AND REGULATES VITAMINS

Government regulation of the manufacture and sale of vitamins and minerals lies within the jurisdiction of the United States Food and Drug Administration (FDA). Up until 1994, supplements were regulated as food products. This allowed the agency to take steps to ensure that dietary supplements were safe and wholesome, and that their labeling was truthful and not misleading.

A "supplement war" occurred in the early 1990s, when the FDA, as mandated by an act of Congress, took steps to ensure that supplement labels were accurate and didn't made health claims that weren't supported by hard scientific evidence. In response, dietary supplement manufacturers and vitamin supporters went into a tailspin. They suggested that the FDA was trying to pull their supplements off the shelves or to regulate them as drugs.

The end result of this tug of war was the Dietary Supplement and Health and Education Act (DSHEA) of 1994. Under this new regulation, vitamin and other dietary supplement products are no longer required to undergo premarketing safety evaluations, as is required for new food ingredients or for new uses of old food ingredients. *The FDA now trusts manufacturers to ensure their products are safe to market.* Manufacturers are, however, required to meet other safety provisions and to back up any claims they make.

In brief, the provisions of DSHEA are:

• All dietary supplements (vitamins, minerals, herbs and other botanicals, and amino acids) must have scientific evidence to back up all health or nutrition claims made on their labels. No more wild claims that supplements can cure cancer, AIDS, or prevent aging are allowed unless there is real proof that a product can, indeed, do what it says it can. Calcium to prevent osteoporosis and folic acid to prevent birth defects are two examples of the kinds of claims the FDA finds acceptable.

• All supplements must bear ingredient labels, and literature that is displayed where supplements are sold must be scientifically balanced and truthful.

• Good manufacturing practices are encouraged, including the imprinting of expiration dates on supplement bottles to ensure that a consumer is buying a still-potent product.

In addition, the DSHEA required that an Office of Dietary Supplements (ODS) be set up within the National Institutes of Health to research the health benefits of supplements. This office was established in fall 1995, with a $5 million budget. A Presidential Commission on Dietary Supplements was also established to perform a study and make recommendations on how best to regulate label claims and statements for dietary supplements—and how to approach the evaluation of these claims.

The creation of ODS was a landmark event for dietary supplements because it marked the official entry of government into the research process for these agents. The real advantage of ODS is that it offers those interested in pursuing dietary supplement-related research a place to seek government funding.

Although this bill was a step in the right direction in regard to supplement labeling, it is our contention that the dietary supplement industry remains largely unregulated and minimally supervised. Before the FDA can yank a product from the market, it must be aware that it is causing harm or being marketed in an improper way, and it must prove that it is unsafe. This places a great burden on the FDA, not only to monitor the vast supplement industry, but also to build a convincing case against dangerous products. This system is much more lax than the one used to regulate drugs and food additives, which must undergo extensive premarketing testing to prove they are safe before they can be marketed. Drugs must also be proven to be effective before they are released. Under the DSHEA, dietary supplements can be marketed without proof that they are safe or effective—*again, it is up to the manufacturers to make sure they are making a good product.*

There is, in effect, relatively little control over the methods vitamin and mineral manufacturers can use to try and convince you to buy and use their products. Nor is there much regulation of vitamin and mineral doses allowed in products. This is an unfortunate situation because it fosters outright quackery and may prevent a consumer from getting the true story about vitamins and minerals he or she may be buying as part of an overall health maintenance program.

TABLE 10
Contents of Popular Multivitamin Products

Product	Vitamin A (IU)	Vitamin D (IU)	Vitamin E (IU)	Vitamin C (mg)	Vitamin B1 (mg)	Vitamin B2 (mg)	Vitamin B6 (mg)	Niacin (mg)	Vitamin B12 (mcg)	Pantothenic Acid (mg)	Folic Acid (mcg)	Iron (mg)	Calcium (mg)	Other
Adult Multivitamins														
Allbee with C (Self-Care)				300	15	10.2	5	50		10				
Allbee C-800 (Self-Care)			45	800	15	17	25	100	12	25				
One-A-Day Essential Vitamins (Bayer)	5,000	400	30	60	1.5	1.7	2	20	6	10	400			
Stresstabs Advanced Formula (Self-Care)			30	500	10	10	5	100	12	20	400			Biotin 45 mcg
Surbex with C (Abbott)				250	6	6	2.5	30	5	10				
Theragran Advanced Formula (Mead Johnson)	5,000	400	30	90	3	3.4	3	20	9	10	400			Biotin 30 mcg
Unicap Softgel Capsules (Pharmacia & Upjohn)	5,000	400	30	60	1.5	1.7	2	20	6	6	400			

Adult Multivitamins with Minerals

Product	Vitamin A (IU)	Vitamin D (IU)	Vitamin E (IU)	Vitamin C (mg)	Vitamin B_1 (mg)	Vitamin B_2 (mg)	Vitamin B_6 (mg)	Niacin (mg)	Vitamin B_{12} (mcg)	Pantothenic Acid (mg)	Folic Acid (mcg)	Iron (mg)	Calcium (mg)	Other
Alive Vitamin Mineral Formula (GNC)	5,000	200	100	100	20	20	20	20	20	30	400		275	Beta carotene 10,000 IU (6 mg) Biotin 150 mcg Copper 1 mg Iodine 150 mcg Magnesium 100 mg Phosphorus 210 mg Zinc 25 mg Chromium 50 mcg Manganese 5 mg Potassium 30 mg + others
Centrum (Lederle)	5,000	400	30	60	1.5	1.7	2	20	6	10	400	18	162	Copper 2 mg Iodine 150 mcg Magnesium 100 mg

| Myadec (Warner Lambert) | 5,000 | 400 | 30 | 60 | 1.7 | 2 | 3 | 20 | 6 | 10 | 400 | 18 | 162 |

Phosphorus 109 mg
Zinc 15 mg
Chromium 65 mg
Manganese 3.5 mg
Potassium 80 mg
Selenium 20 mcg
Biotin 30 mcg
Vitamin K 25 mcg
+ others

Biotin 30 mcg
Vitamin K 25 mcg
Phosphorus 125 mg
Magnesium 100 mg
Zinc 15 mg
Potassium 40 mg
Iodine 150 mcg
Chromium 25 mcg
Selenium 25 mcg
Manganese 2.5 mg
+ others

Product	Vitamin A (IU)	Vitamin D (IU)	Vitamin E (IU)	Vitamin C (mg)	Vitamin B₁ (mg)	Vitamin B₂ (mg)	Vitamin B₆ (mg)	Niacin (mg)	Vitamin B₁₂ (mcg)	Pantothenic Acid (mg)	Folic Acid (mcg)	Iron (mg)	Calcium (mg)	Other
One-A-Day Maximum (Bayer)	5,000	400	30	60	1.5	1.7	2	20	6	10	400	18	130	Iodine 150 mcg Biotin 30 mcg Copper 2 mg Zinc 15 mg Phosphorus 100 mg Manganese 2.5 mg Potassium 37.5 mg Magnesium 100 mg Chromium 10 mcg Selenium 10 mcg Molybdenum 10 mcg Chloride 34 mg
Unicap M (Pharmacia & Upjohn)	5,000	400	30	60	1.5	1.7	2	20	6	10	400	18	60	Iodine 150 mcg Copper 2 mg Zinc 15 mg

													Additional
Ultra Mega (GNC)	5,000	400	100	200	75	75	75	75	75	400	18	100	Phosphorus 45 mg, Manganese 1 mg, Potassium 5 mg, Beta carotene 6 mg, Biotin 75 mcg, Iodine 150 mcg, Magnesium 7.2 mg, Zinc 15 mg, Copper 250 mcg, Selenium 10 mcg, Manganese 6.1 mg, Chromium 10 mcg, Molybdenum 10 mcg, Potassium 10 mg + others
Vitasana (Ginasana)	4,000	400	30	.120	2.4	3.4	4	30	2	400	18	200	Phosphorus 160 mg, Magnesium 20 mg, Zinc 2 mg, Copper 2 mg, Manganese 2 mg

Product	Vitamin A (IU)	Vitamin D (IU)	Vitamin E (IU)	Vitamin C (mg)	Vitamin B$_1$ (mg)	Vitamin B$_2$ (mg)	Vitamin B$_6$ (mg)	Niacin (mg)	Vitamin B$_{12}$ (mcg)	Pantothenic Acid (mg)	Folic Acid (mcg)	Iron (mg)	Calcium (mg)	Other
Multivitamins with Iron														
Albee C-800 Plus Iron (Self-Care)	45	800	15	17	25	100	12	25		400		27		Potassium 16 mg Ginseng extract 80 mg
Stresstabs Plus Iron (Lederle)	30	500	10	10	5	100	12	20		400		18		Biotin 45 mcg
Unicap Plus Iron (Pharmacia & Upjohn)	5,000	400	30	60	1.5	1.7	2	20	6	10	400	22.5	100	
Therapeutic Vitamins Plus Iron and Minerals														
Geritol Complete (Smith Kline)	6,000	400	30	60	1.5	1.7	2	20	6	10	400	18	162	Biotin 45 mcg Phosphorus 125 mg Iodine 150 mcg Magnesium 100 mg Zinc 15 mg Copper 2 mg

Product												
Abbott Surbex T		500	15	10	5	100	10	20	20			
Theragran-M (Mead Johnson)	5,000	400	30	90	3	3.4	3	8	10	400	18	40

Abbott Surbex T — also contains:
Selenium 15 mcg
Manganese 2.5 mg
Chromium 15 mcg
Molybdenum 15 mcg
Potassium 40 mg
Chloride 35 mg
+ others

Theragran-M — also contains:
Biotin 30 mcg
Phosphorus 31 mg
Iodine 150 mcg
Magnesium 100 mg
Zinc 15 mg
Copper 2 mg
Selenium 21 mcg
Manganese 3.5 mg
Chromium 26 mcg
Molybdenum 32 mcg
Potassium 7.5 mg
Chloride 7.5 mg

Product	Vitamin A (IU)	Vitamin D (IU)	Vitamin E (IU)	Vitamin C (mg)	Vitamin B_1 (mg)	Vitamin B_2 (mg)	Vitamin B_6 (mg)	Niacin (mg)	Vitamin B_{12} (mcg)	Pantothenic Acid (mg)	Folic Acid (mcg)	Iron (mg)	Calcium (mg)	Other
Unicap T (Pharmacia & Upjohn)	5,000	400	30	500	10	10	6	100	18	25	400	18		Vitamin K 28 mcg Iodine 150 mcg Copper 2 mg Zinc 15 mg Potassium 5 mg Selenium 10 mcg Manganese 1 mg
Ultra Mega II (GNC)	5,000	400	200	300	100	100	100	100	100	100	400	10	50	Beta carotene 3 mg Biotin 100 mcg Iodine 50 mcg Magnesium 7.2 mg Zinc 15 mg Copper 10 mcg Selenium 10 mcg Manganese 6.1 mg Chromium 10 mcg Molybdenum 150 mcg Potassium 10 mg + others

Men's Formulas

Men's Mega
(GNC)

5,000	200	100	300	30	30	30	30	30	30	30	400	275

Beta carotene
9 mg
Biotin 250 mcg
Phosphorus
210 mg
Magnesium
100 mg
Iodine 150 mcg
Copper 2 mg
Zinc 50 mg
Manganese 5 mg
Potassium 30 mg
Selenium 25 mcg
Chromium
50 mcg
Vitamin K mcg
Pycnogenol 1 mcg
Saw palmetto
50 mg
+ others

One-A-Day
Men's
(Bayer)

5,000	400	45	90	2.25	2.55	3	20	9	10	400

Iodine 150 mcg
Magnesium
100 mg
Zinc 15 mg
Selenium

Product	Vitamin A (IU)	Vitamin D (IU)	Vitamin E (IU)	Vitamin C (mg)	Vitamin B₁ (mg)	Vitamin B₂ (mg)	Vitamin B₆ (mg)	Niacin (mg)	Vitamin B₁₂ (mcg)	Pantothenic Acid (mcg)	Folic Acid (mcg)	Iron (mg)	Calcium (mg)	Other
														87.5 mcg Copper 2 mg Manganese 3.5 mg Chromium 150 mcg Molybdenum 75 mcg Chloride 34 mg Potassium 37.5 mg + others
Prime Time Men (Great American Nutrition)	10,000	400	60	200	15	15	25	20	25	20	400		200	Biotin 200 mcg Potassium 30 mg Magnesium 100 mg Chromium 120 mcg Molybdenum 25 mcg Chloride 18 mg Zinc 15 mg

Women's Formulas

Product														
One-A-Day Women's (Bayer)	5,000	400	30	60	1.5	1.7	2	20	6	10	400	27	450	Copper 1 mg, Manganese 2 mg, Selenium 100 mcg, Yohimbe 100 mg, Saw palmetto 200 mg, + others
														Zinc 15 mg
Rejuvex (Mindbody)		200	230	30	2	2	10	10		10	10			Magnesium 500 mg, Selenium 25 mcg, Manganese 2 mg
Women's Daily Pak (Leiner)	2,500	200	230	120	2	3	2	20	3	10	400	4	725	Beta carotene 5,000 IU, Vitamin K 10 mcg, Biotin 30 mcg, Phosphorus 50 mg, Magnesium 100 mg, Iodine 100 mcg, Copper 3 mg

Product	Vitamin A (IU)	Vitamin D (IU)	Vitamin E (IU)	Vitamin C (mg)	Vitamin B1 (mg)	Vitamin B2 (mg)	Vitamin B6 (mg)	Niacin (mg)	Vitamin B12 (mcg)	Pantothenic Acid (mg)	Folic Acid (mcg)	Iron (mg)	Calcium (mg)	Other
Women's Ultra Mega (GNC)	5,000	400	100	200	80	80	80	80	80	80	400	27	500	Zinc 20 mg Manganese 4 mg Potassium 40 mg Selenium 30 mcg Chromium 20 mcg Molybdenum 25 mcg Evening primrose oil 500 mg 7-day 18-mg iron strip + others Beta carotene 3 mg Biotin 80 mcg Phosphorus 225 mg Magnesium 200 mg Iodine 150 mcg Copper 2 mg

Antioxidant Formulas

				Others
Alive Antioxidant Formula (GNC)	10,000	300	800	Zinc 15 mg, Manganese 5 mg, Potassium 10 mg, Selenium 100 mcg, Chromium 100 mcg, Molybdenum 50 mcg, Dong quai 50 mg, Bee pollen 25 mg, Royal jelly 5 mg + others
One-A-Day Antioxidant Plus (Bayer)	5,000	200	250	Selenium 25 mcg, Manganese 2 mg, Zinc 7.5 mg, Copper 1 mg, Selenium 15 mcg, Manganese 1.5 mg
Protegra (Lederle)	5,000	200	250	Zinc 7.5 mg, Copper 1 mg, Selenium 15 mcg

Product	Vitamin A (IU)	Vitamin D (IU)	Vitamin E (IU)	Vitamin C (mg)	Vitamin B1 (mg)	Vitamin B2 (mg)	Vitamin B6 (mg)	Niacin (mg)	Vitamin B12 (mcg)	Pantothenic Acid (mg)	Folic Acid (mcg)	Iron (mg)	Calcium (mg)	Other
														Manganese 1.5 mg

Mature Adults' and Seniors' Vitamins

Product	Vitamin A (IU)	Vitamin D (IU)	Vitamin E (IU)	Vitamin C (mg)	Vitamin B1 (mg)	Vitamin B2 (mg)	Vitamin B6 (mg)	Niacin (mg)	Vitamin B12 (mcg)	Pantothenic Acid (mg)	Folic Acid (mcg)	Iron (mg)	Calcium (mg)	Other
Centrum Silver (Lederle)	5,000	400	45	60	1.5	1.7	3	20	25	10	400	4	200	Biotin 30 mcg Vitamin K 10 mcg Copper 2 mg Iodine 150 mcg Magnesium 100 mg Phosphorus 48 mg Zinc 15 mg Chromium 130 mcg Manganese 3.5 mg Potassium 80 mg Selenium 20 mcg + others
One-A-Day 50 Plus (Bayer)	5,000	400	60	120	4.5	3.4	6	20	30	15	400		120	Biotin 30 mcg Vitamin K 20 mcg

Unicap Sr.
(Pharmacia & Upjohn)

5,000 200 15 60 1.2 1.4 2.2 16 3 10 400 10 100

Iodine 150 mcg
Copper 2 mg
Zinc 22.5 mg
Magnesium 100 mg
Manganese 4 mg
Potassium 37.5 mg
Selenium 105 mcg
Chromium 180 mcg
Molybdenum 93.75 mcg
Chloride 34 mg
Iodine 150 mcg
Copper 2 mg
Zinc 15 mg
Phosphorus 77 mg
Magnesium 30 mg
Manganese 1 mg
Potassium 5 mg

Pediatric Vitamins

Product	Vitamin A (IU)	Vitamin D (IU)	Vitamin E (IU)	Vitamin C (mg)	Vitamin B1 (mg)	Vitamin B2 (mg)	Vitamin B6 (mg)	Niacin (mg)	Vitamin B12 (mcg)	Pantothenic Acid (mg)	Folic Acid (mcg)	Iron (mg)	Calcium (mg)	Other
Bugs Bunny Complete (Bayer)	5,000	400	30	60	1.5	1.7	2	20	6	10	400	18	100	Phosphorus 100 mg, Iodine 150 mcg, Magnesium 20 mg, Zinc 15 mg, Copper 2 mg, Biotin 40 mcg
Centrum Jr. Shamu & His Crew + Extra C (Lederle)	5,000	400	30	300	1.5	1.7	2	20	6	10	400	18	108	Magnesium 40 mg, Biotin 45 mcg, Vitamin K 10 mcg, Iodine 150 mcg, Copper 2 mg, Phosphorus 50 mg, Zinc 15 mg, Manganese 1 mg

														Additional
Flinstones Complete (Bayer)	5,000	400	30	60	1.5	1.7	2	20	6	10	400	18	100	Chromium 20 mcg, Molybdenum 20 mcg, Phosphorus 100 mg, Iodine 150 mcg, Magnesium 20 mg, Zinc 15 mg, Copper 2 mg, Biotin 40 mcg
Flinstones Original Children's Chewable Vitamins (Bayer)	2,500	400	15	60	1.05	1.2	1.05	13.5	4.5		300			
Sunkist Children's Chewable Complete (Ciba Self-Medication, Inc.)	5,000	400	30	60	1.5	1.7	2	20	6	10	400	18	100	Biotin 40 mcg, Magnesium 20 mg, Iodine 150 mcg, Zinc 10 mg, Manganese 1 mg, Phosphorus 78 mg, Copper 2 mg

Product	Vitamin A (IU)	Vitamin D (IU)	Vitamin E (IU)	Vitamin C (mg)	Vitamin B₁ (mg)	Vitamin B₂ (mg)	Vitamin B₆ (mg)	Niacin (mg)	Vitamin B₁₂ (mcg)	Pantothenic Acid (mg)	Folic Acid (mcg)	Iron (mg)	Calcium (mg)	Other
Unicap Jr. (Pharmacia & Upjohn)	5,000	400	15	60	1.5	1.7	2	20	6		400			Vitamin K 10 mcg

Pediatric Vitamins Plus Iron

Product	Vitamin A (IU)	Vitamin D (IU)	Vitamin E (IU)	Vitamin C (mg)	Vitamin B₁ (mg)	Vitamin B₂ (mg)	Vitamin B₆ (mg)	Niacin (mg)	Vitamin B₁₂ (mcg)	Pantothenic Acid (mg)	Folic Acid (mcg)	Iron (mg)	Calcium (mg)	Other
Centrum Jr. Plus Iron (Lederle)	2,500	200	15	30	0.75	0.85	1	10	3	5	200	9	54	Biotin 22.5 mcg Vitamin K 5 mcg Magnesium 20 mg Iodine 75 mcg Copper 1 mg Phosphorus 25 mg Zinc 7.5 mg Manganese 0.5 mg Chromium 10 mcg Molybdenum 10 mcg
Poly-Vi-Sol with Iron	2,500	400	15	60	1.05	1.2	1.05	13.5	4.5		300	12		Copper 800 mcg

Chewable Vitamins and Minerals (Mead Johnson)													Zinc 8 mg
Pediatric Vitamin Drops													
Poly-Vi-Sol Vitamin Drops (Mead Johnson)	1,500	400	5	35	0.5	0.6	0.4	8					
Pediatric Drops Plus Iron													
Poly-Vi-Sol with Iron (Mead Johnson)	1,500	400	5	35	0.5	0.6	0.4	8		10			
Tri-Vi-Sol with Iron (Mead Johnson)	1,500	400		35						10			
Prenatal Multivitamins													
Materna Tablets (Lederle)	5,000	400	30	100	3	3.4	10	20	12	10	1,000	60	250

Materna Tablets additional ingredients: Biotin 30 mcg, Iodine 150 mcg, Magnesium 25 mg, Copper 2 mg, Zinc 25 mg, Chromium 25 mcg, Molybdenum 25 mcg

Product	Vitamin A (IU)	Vitamin D (IU)	Vitamin E (IU)	Vitamin C (mg)	Vitamin B$_1$ (mg)	Vitamin B$_2$ (mg)	Vitamin B$_6$ (mg)	Niacin (mg)	Vitamin B$_{12}$ (mcg)	Pantothenic Acid (mg)	Folic Acid (mcg)	Iron (mg)	Calcium (mg)	Other
* Natalins Tablets (Mead Johnson)	4,000	400	15	70	1.5	1.6	2.6	17	2.5		500	30	200	Manganese 5 mg Magnesium 100 mg Copper 1.5 mg Zinc 15 mg
Nestabs FA (Fielding)	5,000	400	30	120	3	3	3	20	8		1,000	36	200	Iodine 150 mcg Zinc 15 mg
Niferex-PN (Central)	4,000	400		50	3	3	2	10	3		1,000		125	Zinc 18 mg
Prenate Ultra (Bock)	2,700	400	30	120	3	3.4	20	20	12		1,000	90	200	Iodine 150 mcg Copper 2 mg Zinc 25 mg Docusate sodium 50 mg
* Stuart Prenatal (Wyeth-Ayerst)	4,000	400	11	100	1.84	1.7	2.6	18	4		800	60	200	Zinc 25 mg
Zenate Tablets (Solvay)	3,000	400	10	70	1.5	1.6	2.2	17	2.2		1,000	65	200	Iodine 175 mg Magnesium 100 mg Zinc 15 mg

* These prenatal vitamins are available without a prescription. Natalins is also available in prescription strength.

7

ANTIOXIDANT VITAMINS

Everyone is talking about antioxidants! A major pharmaceutical company runs full-page ads in newsmagazines pointing out the dangers of oxidative stress while mentioning that three of their multivitamin products can protect you from excess oxidation. Sales of vitamins have been increasing by 20 to 30 percent per year, and much of the growth can be credited to antioxidant formulas. In the first edition of this book, we correctly pointed to the value of antioxidant vitamins, but now there is evidence to prove it. Animal studies and several large controlled human trials point to the wisdom of taking antioxidant supplements, especially vitamin E to help prevent heart disease and cancer.

It is useful to know what oxidative stress is and which compounds normally found in our bodies protect us from the damaging effects of oxygen. This demonstrates how antioxidants can be protective, and it can also help you decide what might be the most important antioxidants for you to take.

This chapter explains antioxidants in the context of a regimen for good health.

OXYGEN RADICALS

Only some microorganisms (and plants), known as anaerobes, can live without oxygen; most, including humans, need oxygen. Anaerobes make energy by breaking down preformed carbohydrates and proteins, but energy-wise this process is inefficient. Most microorganisms and all animals (including humans) use oxygen to "burn" or oxidize foods into carbon dioxide and water. A great deal of energy is produced as a result of this process. Metabolizing one molecule of glucose with oxygen produces about four *times* as much energy as could be produced if the same molecule were to be metabolized without oxygen. In our bodies, carbon from food is oxidized to carbon dioxide. Oxygen is chemically "reduced" during this process to superoxide. Then superoxide grabs electrons from a neighboring source and combines with hydrogen to form water. The reduction of oxygen is accomplished in special structures inside body cells called mitochondria. Carbon dioxide that results from this process is eliminated in our breath, urine, and sweat. Plants use the carbon dioxide we produce to make oxygen. This is a very nice ecosystem, and one we need to be careful not to disrupt.

But the system isn't perfect. Did you ever notice how rubber or plastic becomes brittle and cracks after some time has passed? This happens when these materials react with oxygen in the air to produce a modified plastic or rubber that is not as soft and flexible as the original. We live in an environment filled with oxygen, and this is exactly what happens to our bodies as we age. Our skin loses flexibility and starts to wrinkle; our organs don't work as well; our blood vessels get clogged with plaque, putting us at risk of a heart attack or stroke; and we are at a higher risk for cancer. Oxygen is not the only reason that our bodies deteriorate, but it is part of the picture.

Oxygen damages body tissues after long periods of exposure because tiny amounts of chemically reactive oxygen are produced in the everyday reduction of oxygen in the mitochondria. This reaction sometimes occurs in other parts of our bodies as well. Reactive oxygen molecules that cause the problems described above are called *free radicals*. They will reach out to whatever is close by and attach to it. Let's say, for example, that the free radical combines with a lipid (fat) molecule in a kidney cell membrane. The lipid molecule is now a reactive radical itself and can react with another oxygen molecule to form a lipid peroxide radical. Meanwhile, a neighboring radical reacts with oxygen in the same process. This can continue until the kidney cell is permanently damaged. In theory, a single radical could destroy us with this chain reaction!

Actually, there are many different kinds of oxygen radicals. The most important are superoxides, hydroxy radicals, and perhydroxy radicals. These are extremely reactive (especially the hydroxy radical) and will combine immediately with anything nearby. (Hydrogen peroxide is also highly reactive, and that's why it works as a wound antiseptic.) There is another reactive form of oxygen as well, called singlet oxygen.

Oxidative injury is implicated in a long list of diseases. Following are some of the more important examples.

DISEASES RELATED TO OXYGEN RADICALS

Hardening of the Arteries (Atherosclerosis)

We have "good cholesterol" and "bad cholesterol" in our bodies. Good cholesterol is attached to lipids called HDL (high-density lipoproteins). Bad cholesterol is attached to LDL (low-density lipoproteins). One reason that the LDL cholesterol is bad is that it can form plaques in our arteries. When a plaque cracks or is otherwise activated, a blood clot can form that blocks blood flow through the artery (atherothrombosis). If the clot is in an artery that supplies heart muscle, the blood supply to part of the heart is blocked. This leads to chest pain (angina) or a heart attack (myocardial infarction, or MI). If the clogged artery carries blood to the brain, a stroke or TIA (a temporary ministroke) can develop. If the clogged artery is in the leg, pain develops on exercise, and in very severe cases leg amputation may be needed.

In the past decade it has become apparent that the free-radical oxidation of LDL is important to the process of plaque formation. This is one of the most important findings for heart disease and stroke prevention to date and provides many ways for people to help decrease their risk of heart disease.

Unmodified LDL does not begin the process of plaque formation. It can be inappropriately oxidized in the artery wall, though. Once LDL reacts with an oxygen radical, it is seen as a foreign substance by body defense systems and is attacked by protective cells called macrophages. Unfortunately, the process can be destructive, and the oxidized LDL sets up an inflammation in the outer layer of the artery that leads to a "fatty streak" and, later, a plaque deposit. Both can start the process of blood clotting. Chemicals, including antioxidant vitamins, that neutralize free radicals can help block plaque formation and may reduce the risk of heart attack and stroke.

The Complications of Diabetes

High glucose levels in blood and tissue that result from diabetes lead to increased LDL oxidation. Diabetics have an increased incidence of coronary and vascular diseases, and antioxidants have the potential of decreasing some of the LDL oxidation associated with diabetes.

Cancer

Exposing DNA in our cell nuclei to free radicals may result in DNA strand breaks and mutations, leading to cancer. Chronic inflammation and injury generate free radicals as part of the process, which helps explain why these conditions increase the risk for the development of cancers. For example, the hepatitis viruses often cause a chronic liver infection that sharply increases the risk of liver cancer. The inflammation caused by inhaled asbestos results in a high risk of lung cancer. Antioxidants have the potential to decrease cancer risks by neutralizing the free radicals causing damage.

Inflammation

Body cells whose job it is to engulf and destroy bacteria and damaged tissue particles accomplish this by producing short bursts of hydrogen peroxide and superoxide. For reasons that are not well understood, the process can get out of hand and these chemicals set off reactions like the one outlined earlier, leading to tissue injury. The reaction products of free radicals are detected in synovial (joint) fluid. The chain reaction sequence described earlier is probably important in spreading the inflammation and damage. Arthritis is one example of this situation, and antioxidants have the potential to help prevent inflammation.

Reperfusion Injury

If blood flow to an organ or tissue is temporarily shut off and then restarted, the influx of oxygenated blood causes injury over and above that caused by the temporary oxygen loss. Apparently, a lack of oxygen reduces the ability of body tissues to neutralize radicals. When radicals are generated with the influx of oxygen, damage results. This is a problem in organ transplantation and heart surgery, where blood supply is temporarily interrupted during the procedure. Antioxidants have the potential to reduce this injury.

Aging

Radical reactions certainly play a role in declining body function as we age. The immune system weakens, blood vessels get stiff and clogged, and organ function begins to decline. DNA strand breaks result in mutations that may start cancers. Cigarette smoke, ionizing radiation, and certain chemicals all increase the amount of free radicals and accelerate the aging process. For example, the wrinkled facial skin of the longtime smoker is due to free radical damage to the fabric of the skin by way of reactions discussed here. Antioxidants have the potential to minimize some aspects of the aging process.

Eye Disease

Premature infants who receive life-saving oxygen sometimes suffer damage to the retina of their eyes because the protective systems that neutralize oxygen free radicals are not yet in place. Degeneration of the retina, common in the elderly, is thought to be due in part to the inability of eye tissue to neutralize free radicals. Antioxidants have the potential to help prevent certain eye diseases.

Other Diseases

We could cite many other examples of conditions where oxygen radicals are thought to play an important role. If oxygen radical reactions could be blocked or minimized by drug or vitamin treatment, we might not cure disease, but we would certainly have a valuable treatment and prevention strategy.

THE BODY'S DEFENSES AGAINST FREE RADICALS

If radical reactions went unchecked, we would all have a very short lifespan. Fortunately, we are well equipped to survive in an oxygen-rich atmosphere. The burning questions are: Can we further enhance these protective mechanisms with dietary supplements? If we accomplish this, will it result in better health? We believe the answer to both questions is a resounding yes.

First let us consider our natural protective mechanisms and then see how several vitamins (and minerals) fit in. The most direct way to block free-radical-induced damage is to neutralize the radical where it is generated. A critically important nutrient, vitamin E, is well poised to do this. The chemistry of vitamin E is nearly perfect for its task. It dissolves in fat, so it can move in and through the lipidlike cell membranes. It can pick up that lone unpaired electron from a carbon-centered or oxygen radical to form a less reactive vitamin E radical.

Vitamin E is considered a chain-breaking free-radical scavenger because it removes the radical and stabilizes it. The vitamin E radical is chemically much more stable than other radicals. As such, it doesn't do damage to neighboring molecules. Eventually, however, we need to regenerate the E and to neutralize the vitamin E radical. This is done with the help of another remarkable vitamin, vitamin C. Unlike vitamin E, vitamin C dissolves in water and can accept the unpaired electron from E sitting in the lipid membrane. Now the radical is the vitamin C in the fluid outside the cell membrane. The vitamin C radical is then reduced to ordinary vitamin C by enzymes with the aid of NADH, a coenzyme form of niacin (vitamin B_3). Now we are out of danger thanks to three vitamins.

More protective modalities exist as well. An enzyme called superoxide dismutase is also very important. This enzyme causes the inactivation of superoxide (a reactive oxygen radical) to form less reactive hydrogen peroxide and oxygen. There are two superoxide dismutase enzymes. One is in cell mitochondria and contains manganese. The other is found in fluid outside the cell and contains copper and zinc.

Hydrogen peroxide, generated by the breakdown of superoxide, requires either of two other enzymes, glutathione peroxidase or catalase, to convert the reactive hydrogen peroxide molecule to water and oxygen. You may have seen catalase in action if you have ever put hydrogen peroxide liquid on an open wound. The "fizz" is the oxygen released by the action of catalase in the wound on the added hydrogen peroxide.

Earlier we mentioned singlet oxygen as another reactive

molecule. The carotenoids, precursors (early forms) of vitamin A, are chemically designed to neutralize singlet oxygen. Beta carotene is the most well known carotenoid, but there are many others. Other chemicals in the body can also react with radicals to render them harmless. These include melatonin, coenzyme Q_{10}, bioflavonoids, lycopene, and uric acid, but their exact roles are less well established.

TABLE 11
Antioxidant Vitamins and Minerals

VITAMIN OR MINERAL	FUNCTION AS ANTIOXIDANT/ FREE-RADICAL REMOVER
Critically important	
Vitamin E	Fat-soluble; chain-breaking free-radical scavenger
Vitamin C	Water-soluble; free-radical scavenger and antioxidant
Dietary carotenoids	Neutralize singlet oxygen; antioxidant
Selenium	Essential for functioning of glutathione peroxidase, needed to stop polymerization
Less critically important	
Thiamin	Necessary for regeneration of glutathione
Riboflavin	Necessary for regeneration of glutathione
Niacin	Necessary for regeneration of glutathione
Copper, manganese, zinc	Necessary for functioning of superoxide dismutase
Of uncertain importance	
Melatonin	Strong fat-soluble antioxidant
Coenzyme Q_{10}	Strong fat-soluble and water-soluble antioxidant
Bioflavonoids	Common dietary antioxidants

And there are yet more protective mechanisms. Earlier we said that lipid peroxides are dangerous because they undergo complex reactions that can damage a cell or membrane. Several vitamins and one mineral are involved in stopping this dangerous reaction. An enzyme called glutathione peroxidase stimulates the conversion of organic peroxides to relatively harmless organic alcohols. This critical enzyme requires selenium to function. In the reaction, glutathione is oxidized to glutathione disulfide. In order to regenerate glutathione, a series of enzymatic reactions occurs involving thiamin, riboflavin, and niacin.

Oxidative stress is the term used to describe a risk for damage from oxygen radical reactions due to an imbalance between oxidants and antioxidants. Oxidative stress can lead to damage and disease. Table 11 presents a summary of the antioxidant vitamins and minerals and their role in protection from the damage of oxidative stress.

CAN ANTIOXIDANT SUPPLEMENTS PREVENT CANCER AND HEART DISEASE?

Cancer and heart disease kill more people than any other disease. Basic research indicates that oxidative stress plays a role in these diseases, and animal research has indicated potential for antioxidant vitamins to help in preventing them. Here we will focus on studies of the potential effects of antioxidant vitamins in heart disease and cancer. Radicals may be involved in the development of other diseases, but they will be discussed only briefly because evidence for their effect is more limited.

Epidemiological or population studies show generally that dietary antioxidant vitamins have value in preventing heart disease and cancer. In recent years several placebo-controlled human studies targeting this effect have been completed. The results of these specific studies are encouraging but not in uniform agreement; two large studies of the preventive benefit of beta carotene that produced negative results have caused considerable controversy on this issue.

Dietary Studies

Early epidemiological studies of dietary habits supported the idea that antioxidants from dietary sources (fruits and vegetables) were associated with a reduced risk of heart disease and some cancers, especially lung cancer. These studies rely on huge data collections from several study populations. The Framingham Study is an example. Here, a large segment of the population of Framingham, Massachusetts, has been followed for many years. Blood samples have been periodically taken, questionnaires completed, diets monitored, and the volunteers watched for changes in health status. This study and many similar studies from around the world consistently find that vegetable and fruit consumption is related to the risk for coronary heart disease and some cancers. That is, the more fruits and vegetables you eat, the lower your risk. At the high end of fruit and vegetable intake, risk decreased by more than 50 percent compared to those eating the fewest fruits and vegetables.

What is it in the fruits and vegetables that may be protective? When the diets are analyzed, intake of vitamin E, vitamin C, beta carotene, flavonoids, and the mineral selenium are related to disease risk, that is, the smaller the intake, the higher the risk. While these studies suggest a strong benefit for antioxidant vitamin intake, one of their limitations that it is impossible to control for all confounding variables. For example, it is possible that people eating a diet high in vitamin E have a lower risk for heart disease because they live a healthier lifestyle in general.

Population Studies of Vitamin Supplement Use

Several more recent large-scale human studies have looked not only at diet but also at vitamin supplements taken by the populations being studied. These results address the issue of antioxidant vitamin supplement value more directly, but there is still the question of whether people who take supplements also have other healthy lifestyle practices, which may account for some of the observed results. Nevertheless, the value of vitamin E supplements over and above the amount obtained from a standard multivitamin now seems apparent for help in the prevention of coronary disease.

For example, the Health Professionals Follow-up Study has followed 51,529 male health professionals since 1986. Participants filled out detailed questionnaires on their diet and supplement use. Based on the results of four years of observation, and after controlling for other risk factors, a lower risk of heart disease was noted with increasing vitamin E dietary intake in 39,910 men. Those at the high end of dietary intake had a 36 percent smaller chance of developing heart disease. Of special interest is the observation that people taking vitamin E capsules in daily doses between 100 and 250 IU per day had a 46 percent lower risk of heart disease compared to people who did not take a supplement. Supplements had to be taken for at least two years in order for them to have a protective effect. Dietary carotene (all forms of carotene, not simply beta carotene) intake did not have a protective effect, except in smokers and former smokers, nor did total vitamin C intake. Multivitamin use was only modestly protective and only in people who took multivitamins for more than ten years.

The Nurses Health Study of 89,245 nurses followed from 1980 to 1988 and showed that vitamin E had a similarly strong protective effect against heart disease. The greatest effect, a decrease in risk of almost 50 percent, was found in women who took more than 100 IU per day for at least two years, compared to those who took no vitamin E supplement. Vitamin C supplements and beta carotene intake were not protective. Again, taking a multivitamin was only modestly protective (about a 20 percent decreased risk compared to no use).

The final example is a study of 11,178 elderly people, ages 67 to 105 years, over a period of about ten years. In this population, at high risk for death from heart disease and cancer, vitamin E supplements had a striking effect. People who took vitamin E supplements separate from a multivitamin had a 37 percent lower risk of death due to heart disease. The risk for death due to cancer was 41 percent less in vitamin E users. Those who used both vitamin E and vitamin C supplements (separate from multivitamin use) were somewhat better protected, with a 52 percent smaller risk of disease.

There was a trend for people to benefit from the combination of vitamins C and E in reducing cancer death, but vitamin C use alone did not protect against death from heart disease, cancer, or other causes. This study is the best one to demonstrate an advantage of taking both vitamin E and vitamin C. Multivitamin use was not shown to be protective in this study.

Primary prevention studies

The previous studies provide reasonable evidence that antioxidant vitamins, especially vitamin E, are useful to help prevent heart disease. The evidence for protection against cancer is weaker. More definitive proof of protection is obtained from studies in which healthy people without any evidence of disease take a placebo or an antioxidant vitamin and are followed for a sufficient length of time or until disease develops. These studies are called primary prevention trials. As you might imagine, primary prevention trials are expensive and very difficult to conduct. As a result, these large vitamin studies are generally funded by government health agencies.

For example, the ATBC study followed 29,133 Finnish smokers for five to seven years. The volunteers received either 20 mg of beta carotene, 50 mg of vitamin E, both vitamins, or an inactive placebo. Neither vitamin alone nor the combination had a protective effect against lung cancer. In fact, more lung cancers were found in the beta carotene group. This study has been criticized because of the low dose of vitamin E, because of the fact that synthetic beta carotene was employed, and because the smokers tested may have already had cancer before they entered the study.

A second study (CARET) gave 18,314 smokers, former smokers, or people exposed to asbestos either a combination of 30 mg of beta carotene and 25,000 IU of vitamin A (retinol) or placebo. The study was stopped after four years because, as with the ATBC study, a significant increase in deaths due to lung cancer was seen in the beta carotene/vitamin A group.

A third study, the Physicians' Health Study, was remarkable in that 22,071 healthy physicians took either 50 mg of beta carotene or placebo every other day and were followed for twelve years. This study lasted longer and studied a healthier population than the other two. Beta carotene had neither a beneficial nor harmful effect in this study.

Another study, published by the same group of Finnish investigators who did the ATBC trial, looked at the effect of 50 mg (75 IU) of vitamin E on prostate cancer in male smokers studied in ATBC. The researchers found that men who took 50 mg of vitamin E for five to eight years had a 23 percent smaller risk of developing prostate cancer, and those who did get prostate cancer were 41 percent less likely to die.

These large studies were disappointing for beta carotene proponents. We cannot say much about vitamin E from these studies because either it was not tested, the dose used was too low, or the results, as in the prostate cancer study, need to be confirmed.

Secondary Prevention Trials

A secondary prevention trial looks at whether the treatment will prevent a second occurrence of the disease being studied in a group of people who have already experienced the disease or who are at proven risk of the disease. Vitamin E has been shown to provide a benefit in several of these secondary prevention studies.

For example, 2,002 patients with heart disease were given a placebo or 400 IU per day of vitamin E for seventeen months. The vitamin E group had about 80 percent fewer nonfatal heart attacks, but the number of fatal heart attacks was about the same for both the E-treated and placebo groups.

Another study followed 156 men who had previous coronary bypass surgery. Vitamin E, at doses over 100 IU per day, reduced the worsening of heart disease compared to placebo. No benefit was seen for vitamin C, for multivitamin use, or for increased intake of dietary vitamin E.

In another study, patients with a previous colorectal adenoma (potentially cancerous tumor) who had had their polyps removed received either 400 IU of vitamin E with 1 gram of vitamin C per day or an inactive placebo. There was no difference between the placebo and vitamin E groups in the number of patients who needed surgery to remove adenomas after one year of treatment.

EVIDENCE OF ANTIOXIDANT SUPPLEMENT BENEFIT IN OTHER DISEASES

In older placebo-controlled studies, vitamin E has also been shown to be of some help in people with intermittent claudication, a painful condition due to poor circulation in the limbs. The origin of this disease is the same as a heart attack or stroke, atherosclerotic narrowing of the arteries, so it is not surprising that vitamin E can be helpful by virtue of its ability to reduce plaque formation and to decrease platelet stickiness.

An exciting finding was that vitamin E treatment somewhat slowed the rate of progression of Alzheimer's disease. A total of 341 patients received a drug called selegiline, a very high dose of vitamin E (2,000 IU per day), both, or placebo. People taking vitamin E experienced a greater delay in disease progression than those taking selegiline alone or placebo. More recently, a study at New York's Memorial Sloan-Kettering Cancer Center found that one form of vitamin C, dehydroascorbic acid, can get through the blood-brain barrier, allowing large amounts of vitamin C directly into brain tissue. The researchers conclude that this technique may prove to be an important therapeutic advance in treating Alzheimer's disease and other conditions that result from damaged brain cells. Clearly, more studies of vitamins E and C in Alzheimer's disease are needed.

The final example has to do with the signs of aging. Free-radical reactions progressively damage the immune system as we get older. Investigators in Boston gave doses of 60, 200, or 800 IU of vitamin E per day or placebo to eighty-eight elderly subjects for four months. Tests of immune function and antibody response to vaccinations showed that vitamin E improved immune function. The effect was generally better in the group receiving 200 mg per day.

RECOMMENDATIONS FOR TAKING ANTIOXIDANT VITAMINS

Taking antioxidant vitamins is a modest and inexpensive action you can take to decrease the risks of cancer, heart disease, and other conditions associated with aging. The operative word here is *modest*. It is very important to bear in mind that the largest benefit of vitamin intake is smaller than the benefit that can be achieved by making important lifestyle adjustments such as stopping smoking, losing excess weight, and exercising. While there is disagreement over the value of antioxidant supplements, there is uniform agreement that a diet high in vegetables and fruit and fiber is protective. Your mother was right: Eat your vegetables.

Having improved your lifestyle, can you expect further benefit by taking high doses of antioxidant vitamins? We believe that the evidence says yes for vitamin E, yes for vitamin C in combination with vitamin E, and no for beta carotene; it's inconclusive for the other antioxidant supplements. Here are our recommendations for taking antioxidant vitamin supplements.

1. Take a multivitamin supplement with minerals every day. Make sure the supplement contains selenium and folic acid

and 100 percent of the RDA for each of the eleven vitamins. This product will provide all of the vitamins you need for optimum antioxidant status, except vitamins E and C, and will provide adequate amounts of selenium. A generic product containing 100 percent of the RDA value of all vitamins and selenium can be purchased for $4 to $8 per 100 tablets. This is inexpensive and safe insurance.

2. Take 200 to 400 IU of natural (d-alpha tocopherol) vitamin E every day. Higher doses are not needed and lower doses have proven to be less effective in human studies. Natural vitamin E is absorbed and utilized better that the synthetic form (dl-alpha tocopherol), though most clinical studies have used the synthetic. The label should say d-alpha tocopherol. If it does not or says dl-alpha tocopherol, it is synthetic vitamin E.

3. Take 250 to 500 mg of vitamin C every day. Generic, synthetic vitamin C is fine. As discussed, the vitamin C works together with vitamin E in removing damaging oxygen radicals. Vitamin C without vitamin E does not appear to be especially helpful.

4. Eat a few carrots every day and increase your intake of other vegetables. The carrots will provide a nice mixture of carotenoids, and the other vegetables will provide flavonoids shown to have protective antioxidant properties. Avoid taking a synthetic beta carotene supplement. Evidence from large human clinical trials says it does nothing for, or might be even harmful to, smokers or former smokers. Beta carotene, at least the synthetic variety, is not the magic ingredient in vegetables that provides protection.

5. Avoid specialty antioxidant products. They are expensive and often contain ingredients of unproven value.

6. Don't give up on this program. Studies show that vitamin E will benefit you only after you have taken it for many months.

Part 2

VITAMIN PROFILES

8

WATER-SOLUBLE VITAMINS

VITAMIN B$_1$ (THIAMIN)

Popularly known as the "energy vitamin," thiamin is actually one of several B-complex vitamins involved in metabolic processes necessary for the release of energy. Thiamin's discovery is closely tied to the debilitating disease beriberi, which has been known since antiquity but suddenly reached epidemic proportions in Asia in the nineteenth century. Not coincidentally, it was at that time that the practice of polishing rice was introduced. As the vitamin-rich covering of rice was removed, people who relied on this food as a staple were unwittingly deprived of thiamin. It was not until the 1930s that the substance that can prevent beriberi, now known as thiamin, was discovered in the residue of rice polishings. Once the chemical structure of thiamin was determined, a process for making it synthetically was developed, and today virtually all the thiamin we take is manufactured.

FUNCTION

Thiamin is primarily involved in carbohydrate (sugar) metabolism in the body. Carbohydrate metabolism is quite complex, and thiamin is a factor in three separate parts of the process, where it acts as a coenzyme (or catalyst). Coenzymes speed a chemical reaction or enable it to occur.

The first reaction for which thiamin acts as a coenzyme is called glycolysis. In glycolysis, sugars are converted to energy. In effect, glycolysis can be compared to putting logs on a fire. Without thiamin, we would not be able to release the energy from glucose stored in the body; we could not burn the log. The actual enzyme helped by thiamin is called pyruvate dehydrogenase. Pyruvate dehydrogenase links the chemical reactions that split large sugars into small ones to the reactions that burn the smaller sugars.

Second, thiamin is involved in the reactions that burn the smaller sugars produced by glycolysis. This, in turn, involves several different chemical reactions and is commonly known as the Krebs or citric acid cycle. In the Krebs cycle, thiamin acts as a coenzyme for an enzyme called alpha ketoglutarate dehydrogenase. If thiamin were not present, this enzyme could not function, and you would not be able to live because you would not be able to efficiently use carbohydrate (sugar) energy.

The third reaction that employs thiamin as a coenzyme involves an enzyme called transketolase. Transketolase cannot function without thiamin. It is involved in the production of ribose and NADP, two chemicals that are essential to the operation of every cell in the body because they are ingredients in the manufacture of the nucleic acids. Nucleic acids are the basis of your genes, which control all cell and body functions.

In addition, thiamin is involved in nerve impulse transmission throughout the body. We know that thiamin is involved in chemical reactions that provide energy to nerve cells, but its exact role in this process is not known.

DAILY REQUIREMENTS

Daily thiamin requirements depend on the number of calories eaten on an average day. You need 0.5 mg for every 1,000 calories of energy. If you normally eat about 3,000 calories, your daily requirement is about 1.5 mg; if you eat only 2,000 calories, your requirement is reduced to 1 mg.

People who normally expend large amounts of energy, such as athletes and construction workers and those who normally eat a high-carbohydrate diet, should consider supplementing their thiamin intake, according to the amount of energy involved.

DIETARY SOURCES

Fortunately, small amounts of thiamin are present in nearly all living things. Most Americans get their dietary thiamin from enriched flour, whole grains, and lean beef. Other good sources are listed in the accompanying table.

VITAMIN B_1 (THIAMIN) CONTENT OF SELECTED FOODS
(Average adult RDA is 1.2 mg)

FOOD	APPROXIMATE CONTENT (MG PER 3 OZ)
Beans	0.60
Beef	0.60
Brazil nuts	0.85
Brewer's yeast	1.60
Chickpeas	0.30
Corn	0.33
Eggs	0.16
Figs (dried)	0.90
Gooseberries (raw)	0.15
Liver	0.22
Oats	0.60
Peas	0.72
Peanuts	1.20
Pecans	0.79
Pork	0.60
Potatoes	0.10
Rice (enriched white)	0.30
Rice (brown)	0.45
Rice bran	2.30
Sesame seeds	0.90
Soybeans	1.10
Sunflower seeds	2.20
Wheat germ	20.00
White flour (enriched)	0.50
Whole wheat flour	0.50

Thiamin is stable when frozen and stored. When heated, thiamin is also stable in acidic fruits and in foods that are processed in acidic solutions such as vinegar. However, prolonged cooking of meats and nonacid vegetables can destroy significant amounts of thiamin. For example, roasting meat destroys 30 to 50 percent of its thiamin content, and canning or boiling vegetables destroys up to 40 percent of the thiamin present. Certainly we are not suggesting that everyone eat only raw vegetables, but rather that you pay attention to your total daily thiamin intake, assuming an approximate loss of 50 percent for cooking and processing. If you cannot eat fresh vegetables, you can minimize thiamin loss by using vegetables pickled in vinegar. Even better, use frozen vegetables.

If you eat large amounts of raw clams and fish, you should be aware of an enzyme in seafood called thiaminase, which destroys thiamin. This enzyme, however, is itself destroyed in cooking. This interaction is more important today because of the increased popularity of eating raw seafood as sushi or sashimi.

DEFICIENCIES

Given the role that thiamin plays in sugar metabolism, it should come as no surprise that thiamin deficiency can be dangerous and life-threatening. In the United States, refined white flour is enriched with thiamin (as well as riboflavin, niacin, and now folic acid) by law. Thus, even though most of the original B vitamin content of the flour is removed during processing, white flour represents an important source of dietary thiamin, and gross thiamin deficiencies are relatively uncommon where enriched white flour is used. Marginal thiamin deficiencies are much more common and usually associated with inattention to proper diet.

Deficiency Symptoms

Early signs of marginal thiamin deficiency include loss of appetite (which only worsens the problem of thiamin deficiency), weight loss, vomiting, nausea, weakness, fatigue, and mental problems such as depression, memory loss, difficulty concentrating and dealing with details, and personality changes.

Gross thiamin deficiency results in the disease beriberi,

which affects three distinct areas of the body: the heart (cardiac beriberi), brain and nerve function (central nervous system beriberi), and the stomach and intestines (gastrointestinal beriberi). The symptoms of each vary tremendously with the degree of deficiency, age of the patient, and speed with which the disease developed. If disease onset is more rapid, it is usually more serious. Physical signs of gross thiamin deficiency include muscle weakness, decreased reflex activity, fluid in the arms and legs, enlargement of the heart, nausea and vomiting, and nervous system problems similar to those associated with marginal deficiency.

Thiamin status can be tested in two ways. One is a relatively simple blood test your doctor can order, called transketolase function after the fact that the activity of the enzyme transketolase is directly related to levels of thiamin in the body. The other involves the level of pyruvic acid in the blood; people with a thiamin deficiency will have more pyruvic acid in their blood because of the changes in sugar metabolism that occur when sufficient thiamin is not present.

PEOPLE WHO MAY BENEFIT FROM SUPPLEMENTATION

Alcoholics

The alcoholic presents a special problem when it comes to thiamin. Not only is his or her diet usually deficient in thiamin, but alcohol interferes with the passage into the bloodstream of what little thiamin is eaten. Alcohol may even cause thiamin to be displaced from places in the body where it is needed. Ironically, alcoholics need more thiamin than the average person because of their very high carbohydrate intake (alcohol is a carbohydrate). They need the thiamin to break down and use all that extra carbohydrate.

A nerve disease called Wernicke-Korsakoff syndrome may occur in alcoholics as a result of their severe drinking and thiamin deficiency. There is also evidence that many alcoholics have a genetic tendency toward this condition. People with Wenicke-Korsakoff syndrome show symptoms of confusion, memory loss, and psychotic behavior, and some symptoms may remain even after the vitamin deficiency has been corrected. The cost of institutionalizing and treating Wernicke-Korsakoff patients has been estimated at more than $70 million per year in the United States alone, and it has therefore been suggested that small amounts of thiamin be added to alcoholic beverages to prevent the development of this syndrome. We believe this approach should be given serious consideration.

Diabetics

Diabetics with marginal thiamin deficiencies may develop a mild form of Wernicke-Korsakoff syndrome when taking their antidiabetes medicines. Diabetes treatment is aimed at reducing high blood sugar levels by providing extra insulin, stimulating the pancreas to make more insulin, or helping to improve body cell utilization of glucose. Once insulin gets into the blood, it stimulates glucose metabolism by the normal pathways, which involve thiamin. If the diabetic is already marginally thiamin-deficient, this process can accentuate vitamin deficiency symptoms and in a few cases has resulted in the development of Wemicke-Korsakoff syndrome. Diabetics can avoid this situation simply by taking a daily multivitamin or eating foods known to be rich in thiamin.

Other Special Groups

Others who should pay special attention to thiamin intake are senior citizens, those who have been consistently deficient in thiamin, and pregnant and lactating women, whose thiamin requirements are significantly greater because of their increased energy expenditure.

TOXICITY

Few adverse reactions to thiamin have been noted in the medical literature. It is generally thought of as safe and nontoxic when taken by mouth; thiamin injections have resulted in a few allergic reactions, but life-threatening situations are rarely encountered.

A small number of animal studies have shown that giving large amounts of thiamin over a prolonged period of time interferes with the animals' ability to eliminate some drugs and, perhaps, some cancer-causing chemicals. The importance of this observation to people who regularly consume excessive amounts of thiamin is not known, but we believe that long-term consumption of large amounts of *any* vitamin is ill-advised unless there are specific therapeutic reasons for doing so.

INTERACTIONS

Thiamin can interact with drugs used to relax muscles during surgery to produce excessive muscle relaxation, but no special precautions are needed.

THERAPEUTIC USES

Thiamin supplements may be given to counteract any symptom of thiamin deficiency reviewed earlier in this profile. Of course, such symptoms will not be relieved by thiamin unless they are, in fact, caused by vitamin deficiency.

In addition, thiamin can be used to treat certain rare metabolic defects present in small numbers of people in which the thiamin-dependent enzymes discussed under "Function" are abnormal and require inordinately large amounts of the vitamin.

These so-called inborn errors of metabolism are often first discovered in infants or children who exhibit learning disabilities. These disabilities develop because insufficient amounts of energy are provided to a developing nervous system. If the infant or child is treated with thiamin early and vigorously, the condition may improve dramatically. However, thiamin is not helpful in treating any other kinds of learning disabilities.

UNSUBSTANTIATED CLAIMS

Nerve Tonic

Thiamin had been used as a cure-all nerve tonic for many years, but modern researchers finally determined its ineffectiveness for this purpose. Nevertheless, thiamin's popularity as a nerve tonic continues solely because of individual testimonials and word-of-mouth endorsements. Also, vitamin manufacturers and marketers are still free to promote their products for this and other questionable uses because vitamins are still not as tightly regulated as drugs. The usual thought process is that if nervous system problems are a consequence of thiamin deficiency, thiamin must be a good treatment for all nerve problems, regardless of their origin. Obviously, this is fuzzy thinking. Thiamin can help only if the nerve problems are actually caused by thiamin deficiency.

Insect Repellent

Another invalid application of thiamin that has achieved some popularity among consumers over the years is its use as an insect repellent. The popularity of thiamin for this purpose stems from several isolated reports in the medical literature of successful use. The theory is that if you take large amounts of thiamin by mouth, insects will be repelled by the unpleasant taste and odor of thiamin in the perspiration and will not bite you. Despite the fact that studies of this claim have failed to prove its value, and the fact that the Food and Drug Administration determined that thiamin is ineffective as a repellent more than fifteen years ago, some people continue to recommend one 150 mg tablet of thiamin three or four times every day you will be exposed, beginning one day before you go into the woods. A dose in this range would probably not cause any harm, despite the fact that it approaches a hundred times the average adult RDA of thiamin. While laboratory tests do not support its use, we have talked with many who claim it does work under field conditions when the hiker is perspiring. We suggest that a brief test might be worthwhile, but be sure to bring a traditional insect repellent as a backup.

Other Uses

Thiamin has also been promoted for other uses for which its value has not been proven. We cannot recommend that you take this vitamin to treat motion sickness or pain. Thiamin will also not improve appetite, digestion, or mental alertness, nor will it promote growth unless you are thiamin-deficient. A small, well-controlled study showed benefit in schizophrenia from a combination of high-dose thiamin and acetazolamide, but this approach has not been explored by others. More work is needed. Consult your medical care specialist about the desirability of using high-dose vitamins for serious mental diseases.

AVAILABILITY

Thiamin tablets are available without a prescription in strengths of 5 mg, 10 mg, 25 mg, 250 mg, and 500 mg. Thiamin injections require a prescription from your doctor.

VITAMIN B₂ (RIBOFLAVIN)

Riboflavin has a bad taste and is yellow in color. In fact, the distinct taste of multivitamin products is caused by riboflavin. Like most B-complex vitamins, riboflavin is involved with energy production. But unlike the others, a lack of riboflavin shows itself primarily as skin sores and blemishes that affect the skin surface and the lining of the stomach.

FUNCTION

Riboflavin is converted in the body into two active forms, flavin mononucleotide (FMN) and flavin adenine dinucleotide (FAD). FMN and FAD are essential to cell function because they are coenzymes (catalysts) for chemical reactions that involve utilization of oxygen and liberation of energy. This energy is used to convert food into more energy, which cells then use to perform their designated body functions. Riboflavin is found in every body cell.

DAILY REQUIREMENTS

As is the case with thiamin, your daily riboflavin requirement is related to the number of calories you take in each day. More calories means more riboflavin will be needed to convert food to useful energy. You should be getting 0.6 mg of riboflavin for every 1,000 calories you eat. Thus, if you are on a 3,000-calorie diet, you will need 1.8 mg a day. If you eat 2,000 calories, you will need only 1.2 mg a day, and so on.

People who expend large amounts of energy every day, including athletes, construction workers, and others with heavy physical demands, should take care to supplement their daily riboflavin intake.

DIETARY SOURCES

Protein-riboflavin combinations are called flavoproteins and are important to all life forms. It is therefore logical that riboflavin is found in a wide variety of foods. Milk, cheese, chicken, lean beef, and pork are particularly rich sources. It has been estimated that about half of our riboflavin intake comes from dairy products. Other good sources are listed in the accompanying table. Riboflavin is stable when heated, and because it is bound to food proteins and other molecules, much of the vitamin content of foods cooked in water (about 80 percent) is retained in the finished product, even if the cooking water is discarded. Riboflavin is destroyed when mixed with chemically basic substances, like baking soda. It is also broken down by sunlight; therefore, you should keep riboflavin-rich substances away from direct sunlight. Normal room lights are not strong enough to cause much riboflavin destruction, although common sense would dictate that dark or opaque containers be used for cooking and storage in order to minimize vitamin losses.

VITAMIN B_2 (RIBOFLAVIN) CONTENT OF SELECTED FOODS
(Average adult RDA is 1.2 mg)

FOOD	APPROXIMATE CONTENT (MG PER 3 OZ)
Almonds	0.81
Apricots (dried)	0.15
Bee pollen	1.70
Beans	0.20
Boysenberries (frozen)	0.11
Brewer's yeast	3.40
Broccoli	0.18
Cheese	0.43
Chicken	0.34
Corn	0.17
Cottage cheese	0.23
Cream cheese	0.13
Dates (pitted)	0.09

FOOD	APPROXIMATE CONTENT (MG PER 3 OZ)
Eggs	0.17
Liver	3.60
Meats (lean beef and pork)	0.17
Milk	0.15
Mushrooms	0.30
Mustard greens	0.60
Parsley	0.23
Passion fruit	0.12
Pears (dried)	0.16
Peas	0.23
Prunes (dried)	0.20
Raspberries (red or black)	0.08
Spinach	0.17
Sprouts	0.17
Strawberries	0.07
Turkey	0.18
Veal	0.28
Wheat germ	0.60
White flour	0.05
White flour (enriched)	0.13
Whole wheat flour	0.13
Yogurt	0.16

Grains carry most of their riboflavin in the germ and bran coat. Bleaching and other refining processes used to produce white flour remove most of this vitamin from this important dietary staple. In enriched flour, riboflavin as well as thiamin, niacin, and now folic acid have been added to replace the amounts removed in processing. Enriched flour is better than nonenriched, but it makes sense to eat more unadulterated, vitamin-complete, whole-grain flour when possible.

DEFICIENCIES

Riboflavin deficiency may be difficult to recognize because it rarely occurs alone. It is normally accompanied by other vitamin deficiencies and is most commonly found among people whose diets are inadequate or consist mostly of carbohydrates.

A person who eats too little protein will force the body to break down its own proteins, including the riboflavin-containing flavoproteins. Thus, a diet very low in protein will lead to a riboflavin deficiency unless unusually large amounts of the vitamin are obtained from dietary or other sources, an unlikely prospect if protein intake is so low.

Considering the importance of riboflavin-dependent enzymes to energy production and body metabolic processes, it is remarkable that riboflavin deficiencies are not more serious and life-threatening. The reasons for this are not well understood but may be due to the widespread availability of riboflavin from foods; it would be very difficult to consume a riboflavin-free diet.

Deficiency Symptoms

Many of the symptoms that accompany riboflavin deficiency can be traced to a loss of the general ability to perform normal tissue repairs. The first deficiency symptoms are a general loss of facial color, sores at the corners of the mouth, and a sore throat. These may be followed by a magenta coloration of the tongue (called glossitis), red and raw lips, and skin sores (especially in cracks and around joints). A greasy, scaling rash may develop by the nose and can spread to involve both cheeks and the skin around the ears. Rashes in the genital area are common. People with severe riboflavin deficiency may become anemic or develop nerve disease, but these are relatively infrequent.

One interesting symptom of riboflavin deficiency is the invasion of blood vessels into the cornea of the eye. This produces an appearance that can be compared to red eye or conjunctivitis. The eye, in contrast to other organs, does not contain FMN or FAD. Rather, it contains free riboflavin. It is thought that free riboflavin in the eye may play a role in bringing oxygen to tissues that have no other obvious sources of oxygen. When there is not enough riboflavin in the eye, the body compensates by growing blood vessels into the normally clear cornea to supply needed oxygen.

Riboflavin levels in the body are best tested by measuring the amount of vitamin passed out in the urine over a twenty-four-hour period. People who lose less than 0.05 mg per twenty-four hours are probably deficient. People with riboflavin anemias will also begin to make new red blood cells and will experience an increase in blood hemoglobin level after taking the vitamin. This effect can be monitored by routine blood counts and hemoglobin levels. In addition, people who are riboflavin-deficient may have low levels of activity of an enzyme in red blood cells called glutathione reductase.

PEOPLE WHO MAY BENEFIT FROM SUPPLEMENTATION

Severe riboflavin deficiencies are rare in the United States, but marginal deficiencies involving many of the symptoms described above have been observed in alcoholics. Also, dietary surveys have revealed marginal deficiencies in some senior citizens, the poor, some urban teenagers who do not drink milk regularly, and smokers.

Pregnant and breast-feeding women need extra riboflavin to meet their increased energy requirements.

Scientists have noted that women taking oral contraceptives or thyroid hormone may be riboflavin-deficient. Also, animal studies indicate that those who take phenothiazine (antipsychotic) drugs such as chlorpromazine (Thorazine and others) or tricyclic antidepressants such as amitryptiline (Elavil and others) may have less riboflavin in their bodies than people not taking those medicines. The reasons for this are not known.

TOXICITY

Riboflavin is not considered toxic. Excess riboflavin is rapidly passed out of the body via the urine. Those who favor taking large doses of the B vitamins need only look at the bright yellow color of their urine, caused by riboflavin, to appreciate how much of their megadose they are flushing down the toilet.

THERAPEUTIC USES

Riboflavin supplements may be given to counteract any of the symptoms of riboflavin deficiency reviewed earlier in this profile. However, such symptoms will not be alleviated by riboflavin unless they are, in fact, caused by vitamin deficiency.

Riboflavin has no important therapeutic use other than relief or prevention of the deficiency state.

UNSUBSTANTIATED CLAIMS

Cure for Skin and Eye Diseases

Using riboflavin to cure "red eye" caused by vitamin deficiency has led to the use of riboflavin in doses of 5 to 10 mg per day to prevent or even cure various eye diseases. Riboflavin has also been used to treat skin disorders that mimic those seen in people with riboflavin deficiencies. These uses for riboflavin were popular earlier but have fallen into disfavor more recently. Unfortunately, riboflavin works in skin and eye diseases only when the reason for the disorder is the lack of riboflavin.

Other Uses

Vitamin B_2 will not prevent cancer or stress, or improve reproductive ability. It will not increase growth unless one is severely deficient in this vitamin.

AVAILABILITY

Riboflavin is available from various manufacturers as tablets in strengths of 25 mg, 50 mg, and 100 mg. It is an ingredient in most multivitamin products.

VITAMIN B₃ (NIACIN)

Niacin is the word most often used to describe chemical compounds having vitamin B_3 activity. Nicotinic acid (niacin) and nicotinic acid amide (nicotinamide) are both found in vitamin preparations. They are of equal nutritional potency. In the body, the forms of the vitamin that participate in biochemical reactions (called coenzymes) are nicotinamide adenine dinucleotide (NAD) and nicotinamide adenine dinucleotide phosphate (NADP). Nicotinic acid can be easily converted to nicotinamide and to NAD and NADP in the body. On the surface, niacin appears to be similar in function to thiamin (vitamin B_1), but the two vitamins are actually involved in energy metabolism in somewhat different ways.

Niacin deficiency is called pellagra. Epidemics of pellagra occurred in southern Europe in the mid-eighteenth century and in the midwestern and southern United States in the early 1900s. The corn-based diet then prevalent in those areas led to this debilitating and sometimes fatal deficiency disease. Corn is low in tryptophan, an amino acid that can be converted to niacin, and the niacin contained in corn is not easily assimilated by our bodies. Pellagra has virtually disappeared in the United States since white flour began to be enriched with niacin in 1939.

Nicotinic acid is *not* related to nicotine, as the name might imply.

FUNCTION

Niacin must be converted to NAD or NADP before it can affect your body. Both NAD and NADP are coenzymes (catalysts) for more than 150 different cellular reactions involved in generating energy for normal cell function. NADP is also important for many body reactions that manufacture necessary fatty acids and in the metabolism and elimination of drugs and chemicals from the body.

DAILY REQUIREMENTS

Daily niacin requirements depend on the number of calories you eat and the amount of energy you expend each day. At least 4.4 mg of niacin is required for every 1,000 calories of energy expended to prevent pellagra, but the RDA is set at 6.6 mg for every 1,000 calories. Your daily intake should *never* fall below 13 mg. People who expend large amounts of energy on a regular basis, including construction workers, athletes, laborers, and others with physical occupations, should consider taking extra niacin.

DIETARY SOURCES

The body gets niacin from food sources in two ways. One is by ingesting preformed niacin; some plants contain pure niacin and nicotinic acid amide, while meats have some preformed NAD and NADP. Also, your body makes niacin from a natural amino acid known as tryptophan, also found in many foods, but you must take in 60 mg of tryptophan to make the equivalent of 1 mg of nicotinic acid. In addition, the chemical reactions involved in converting tryptophan to nicotinic acid require pyridoxine (vitamin B_6). Thus, low B_6 intake can lead to reduced niacin activity, due to the reduced conversion of tryptophan to niacin.

Most people get about half their daily niacin requirement as the pure vitamin and make the rest from tryptophan. Fortunately, both niacin and tryptophan are found in a wide variety of foods, and this makes it relatively easy to satisfy your niacin requirement by dietary means. Some rich sources of this vitamin are liver, turkey, tuna, and peanuts. Niacin is also present in coffee and beer, but you would have to drink a quart of coffee or twenty-five to thirty bottles of beer a day to reach the RDA!

Additional good sources are listed in the accompanying table, where the niacin content is listed in terms of niacin equivalents. Thus, you don't have to think about whether your food has tryptophan or niacin; that has already been taken into consideration.

Niacin is very stable when heated or stored over long periods of time. However, this vitamin dissolves easily in water and will be lost if the cooking water is discarded.

NIACIN CONTENT OF SELECTED FOODS
(Average adult RDA is 16 mg. All concentrations are expressed in niacin equivalents.)

FOOD	APPROXIMATE CONTENT (MG PER 3 OZ)
Almonds	3.15
Barley	3.33
Beef	4.24
Brewer's yeast	32.30
Halibut	8.28
Liver	13.60
Mushrooms	3.80
Peaches (dried)	4.76
Peanuts	14.45
Pork	5.00
Potatoes	4.40

FOOD	APPROXIMATE CONTENT (MG PER 3 OZ)
Rice (brown)	4.30
Rice (white)	3.25
Salmon	11.70
Sardines	4.90
Shrimp	3.00
Sprouts	2.55
Swordfish	10.00
Sunflower seeds	5.00
Tuna	10.20
Turkey	9.35
Wheat	3.87
White flour	3.65
Whole wheat flour	3.65
Veal	7.00

DEFICIENCIES

Niacin deficiency has been seen in areas of the world where the basic dietary staple is corn or other unfortified cereals that are poor sources of both tryptophan and niacin. Other conditions that can contribute to niacin deficiency are gastrointestinal problems that interfere with the body's ability to absorb the vitamin, unusual dietary habits, infections, or an overactive thyroid. Since niacin needs are related to energy production, it is easy to understand how any condition that places extra stress on the body or demands energy expenditure will increase the need for niacin.

Niacin deficiency may develop in people with a rare disease called carcinoid syndrome, even though there is no problem with vitamin intake. In carcinoid syndrome, tumors develop that make large amounts of chemicals called 5-hydroxytryptophan and 5-hydroxytryptamine. The tumors use dietary tryptophan to make these chemicals, leaving little to be converted to niacin. Niacin deficiency can also develop in people with another rare condition called Hartnup's disease, a natural inability to absorb tryptophan from the gut.

Deficiency Symptoms

Symptoms of the classic niacin deficiency state, called pellagra, can be summarized by the "three D's": dermatitis, diarrhea, and dementia. Dermatitis (skin rash) is the most distinguishing feature of pellagra. The rash appears as scaling, flaking skin. Cracking and bleeding occur in more severe cases. It is usually located in areas where skin is stressed, such as the elbows, feet, hands, and areas of skin exposed to the sun, and these areas become noticeably darker than other areas of skin. Casal's necklace, one of the best-known signs of niacin deficiency, consists of darkening of the skin on the face, neck, and back; it appears as if the victim were wearing a dark necklace.

The diarrhea of pellagra can be quite severe and will only make the problem worse. It can cause loss of appetite, reducing still further the absorption of niacin from food. This diarrhea is probably caused by lesions in the stomach and intestinal tract due to the niacin deficiency. Other gastrointestinal tract symptoms are: upset and irritated stomach, a red and swollen tongue with sores on it, and enlarged salivary glands that produce excess saliva. Nausea and vomiting are common, and about half of the people who develop pellagra also lose their digestive juices until the disorder is corrected.

Dementia, the third D, is an unusual feature of vitamin deficiency and may be simply defined as a serious mental impairment with disorientation. If left untreated, the dementia can progress to the point where the victim enters a catatonic state and will die in a coma. Other symptoms of niacin deficiency involving the brain and central nervous system are irritability, memory loss, anxiety, hallucinations, and delirium.

Not everyone who is niacin-deficient will develop pellagra. The most common symptoms of marginal niacin deficiency, also known as subclinical pellagra, are diarrhea, headaches, nervousness, and a swollen and red tongue.

The easiest way to test for a niacin deficiency is to measure the level in your urine of methylnicotinamide, the final product of the body's metabolism of niacin. Low levels of this substance indicate a possible vitamin deficiency, but the test result is not always conclusive.

PEOPLE WHO MAY BENEFIT FROM SUPPLEMENTATION

Alcoholics, pregnant and breast-feeding women, people with infections or an overactive thyroid, smokers, and those under a great deal of daily physical stress may become niacin-deficient and should consider a routine supplement.

Women taking oral contraceptives require more than the usual 60 mg of tryptophan to make the equivalent of 1 mg of niacin because their conversion rate is reduced. They should increase intake of foods high in niacin or take a nutritional supplement.

TOXICITY

Doses of niacin of up to 100 mg per day usually cause no problems. However, patients taking more than 500 mg per day of nicotinic acid will experience significant adverse reactions to that therapy. Interestingly, it is nicotinic acid, not other forms of the vitamin, that causes the problems. However, as discussed later, only nicotinic acid has cholesterol-lowering abilities, so this is the form of the vitamin usually used in high doses. Virtually everyone taking high doses of nicotinic acid becomes flushed within two hours of taking the vitamin. The flush is usually confined to the face and hands and can be described as redness and a feeling of burning and stinging. Tolerance to this reaction develops in time, so that it often becomes less severe as time goes on. In addition, many people experience stomach upset, cramps, nausea, vomiting, and diarrhea. Liver damage can also be caused by nicotinic acid if it is taken consistently for an extended time; this is probably the most worrisome side effect associated with this vitamin. The damage is usually reversible but nevertheless worrisome. Other severe side effects of nicotinic acid overdose are difficulty metabolizing blood sugar (glucose), disturbed heart rhythms, a rash over large areas of the skin, and gouty arthritis. Some say the water-soluble vitamins are all nontoxic, but this is not true for nicotinic acid (and vitamin B₆) in high doses.

The adverse effects of nicotinamide are less severe, and it does not cause the flushing reaction. On the other hand, it does not lower cholesterol as effectively as nicotinic acid.

INTERACTIONS

Nicotinic acid interacts with clonidine, used to treat hypertension, and with certain blood and urine tests. See Part 6, "Vitamin, Mineral, and Herbal Drug Interactions."

THERAPEUTIC USES

Niacin supplements are given to counteract any of the deficiency symptoms reviewed earlier in this profile. However, such symptoms will not be alleviated by niacin use unless they are, in fact, caused by vitamin deficiency.

In addition to the prevention and cure of pellagra, it has been known for a long time that nicotinic acid, but not nicotinamide, when given in high doses, is capable of reducing both total cholesterol and an especially bad form of cholesterol called LDL cholesterol. It will also reduce levels of triglycerides, which are undesirable blood fats, and raise levels of HDL ("good") cholesterol, which is associated with a lower risk of heart attack and other circulatory problems. Nicotinic acid is now one of the recommended first-line agents for treating patients whose blood levels of cholesterol or triglycerides are too high. Importantly, nicotinic acid has been shown to reduce heart attacks and in the long run to reduce overall mortality in patients with previous heart disease. In combination with other lipid-lowering drugs, it has even reduced atherosclerotic lesions or plaques in blood vessels. And it is cheap, costing less than $5 per month for treatment.

What is the downside to nicotinic acid treatment for blood lipids? In brief, 1 to 5 g doses of nicotinic acid are required per day to achieve good lipid-lowering effects, and these high doses are associated with significant adverse effects. Keep in mind that the RDA value for niacin is 18 mg, so nicotinic acid treatment is using doses up to fifty times dietary levels.

Clearly this is a case of using this vitamin for its drug effects. Almost everyone taking more than 500 mg a day of nicotinic acid will experience flushing and some degree of stomach upset. Taking an aspirin one hour before the nicotinic acid dose will help reduce the flushing. Patients generally develop a tolerance to nicotinic acid, so the flushing gets less annoying with time. Other common side effects of nicotinic acid are headache, heartburn, diarrhea, and a warty skin rash. Liver toxicity, which has been observed in some patients on nicotinic acid, is of greater concern. This effect is reversible when treatment is stopped. Nicotinic acid can activate duodenal ulcers, upset glucose balance in diabetics, and make gout worse.

Manufacturers have attempted to reduce some of the gastric complaints by formulating nicotinic acid in slow-release forms. Unfortunately, while the special slow-release dose produced less flushing than conventional nicotinic acid, more liver toxicity was detected in one study.

Between 30 and 50 percent of people taking nicotinic acid have to give up the therapy because of adverse effects. One study has shown that individualizing the dose for each patient to the lowest effective level both reduced lipids and shrank the number of patients who had to drop nicotinic acid treatment.

Our recommendation is this: Nicotinic acid is an inexpensive and valuable drug for treating patients with high blood lipids, but it is not a vitamin that should be taken in high doses without the advice and care of a qualified health care professional. Don't self-medicate with high doses of nicotinic acid because of the chance of liver damage and other significant problems.

UNSUBSTANTIATED CLAIMS

Treating Mental Illness

High doses of nicotinic acid have been prescribed for mental illnesses, most notably schizophrenia, for which it was first used in the early 1950s. The theory behind this use came from the fact that niacin alleviated symptoms of mental illness caused by nicotinic acid deficiency. Some psychiatrists still prescribe doses up to 20 g a day, and hardly a month passes without the publication of another article extolling the virtues of nicotinic acid and other miracle nutrients in the treatment of mental illness.

Nicotinic acid was tested and found ineffective in the treatment of schizophrenia. The most comprehensive of these evaluations was conducted in 1971 by the Canadian Mental Health Association. Their studies were set up as a controlled multicenter evaluation, similar to that described for the evaluation of nicotinic acid for heart disease. The findings of these careful studies are best summarized by saying that the claims of nicotinic acid enthusiasts have not been confirmed. In a comparison of such factors as the length of hospitalization and the quantity of tranquilizers consumed, the niacin group even fared worse than the placebo group. There have been other, more recent controlled studies, but the results are not consistent and generally do not support the efficacy of nicotinic acid, or any other vitamin for that matter, as a treatment for mental illness.

In this context, we would also like to add a comment concerning the placebo effect. Nicotinic acid causes flushing of the face and a tingling sensation, which gives the impression that the drug is having profound effects on the body. A compassionate and enthusiastic therapist may use these symptoms to make patients think the drug is having an effect. It is attractive to many people to think that they can take psychiatric treatment into their own hands, avoiding traditional therapies. But we believe that using nicotinic acid without other medicines and/or psychotherapy can be dangerous.

Other Uses

We cannot recommend that you take this vitamin to treat bad breath, canker sores, deafness, dizziness, depression, hypertension, skin blemishes, or tiredness. Nicotinic acid also will not prevent migraine headaches or senility, nor will it improve digestion.

AVAILABILITY

Nicotinic acid (niacin) is available in tablets of 25 mg, 50 mg, 100 mg, and 500 mg. Timed-release capsules and tablets in similar strengths and an elixir with 50 mg in every teaspoonful are also available. These high doses are used to lower blood fat levels, as discussed above. Nicotinamide is available in capsules and tablets containing 50 mg, 100 mg, and 500 mg. Niacin injections are restricted to prescription-only use.

VITAMIN B₅ (PANTOTHENIC ACID)

The name of this vitamin (derived from the Greek word *pan*, meaning "all") means "from everywhere." Pantothenic acid does indeed live up to its name; it is found throughout our environment. As a result, this vitamin is unique in that severe human deficiencies have almost never occurred naturally. Symptoms of deficiency have been produced only under extreme or experimental conditions.

FUNCTION

Pantothenic acid is converted in the human body to a cofactor called coenzyme A. Coenzyme A is a high-energy compound used in the transfer of a variety of substances during normal body processes. These include the metabolism of carbohydrates, the breakdown and synthesis of fatty acids, the generation of glucose from glycogen (the form in which glucose is stored in the liver), and the body processes that make such substances as steroid hormones. Intermediates in the metabolic cycles that convert glucose (from the digestion of carbohydrates) to carbon dioxide and water and energy all have coenzyme A attached to them. Thus, if it were possible to remove all pantothenic acid from our bodies, we would die because we couldn't process food into energy and into the materials our bodies use to build tissues.

DAILY REQUIREMENTS

There are no established standards for pantothenic acid, and it is therefore not included in the RDA tables. However, the Food and Nutrition Board of the National Academy of Sciences has established 4 to 7 mg as a safe and adequate daily adult intake. These standards are only an estimate of daily requirements and cannot be taken as precise needs.

DIETARY SOURCES

Most Western diets contain more than enough pantothenic acid. Some of the richest sources are meats (especially organ meats), corn, lentils, eggs, nuts, and lobster. Additional good sources are listed on the accompanying table.

Cooking losses of up to 30 percent occur during prolonged heating of acidic foods. Also, much of the pantothenic acid content of whole wheat flour is lost during processing to white flour.

PANTOTHENIC ACID CONTENT OF SELECTED FOODS
(Average adult safe and adequate daily intake is 5.5 mg)

FOOD	APPROXIMATE CONTENT (MG PER 3 OZ)
Almonds	0.43
Apricot nectar	0.86
Avocadoes	0.94
Beans	0.34
Blue cheese	1.53
Brewer's yeast	9.35
Broccoli	1.20
Cashew nuts	1.11
Cheese	0.43
Chicken	0.77
Chickpeas	1.02
Corn	4.25
Eggs	1.96
Egg yolk	3.57
Lamb	0.50
Lentils	1.40
Lobster	1.28
Milk	0.34
Mushrooms	0.85
Peanuts	2.38
Peas	2.90
Pomegranate	0.54
Potatoes	0.50
Salmon	0.68
Sardines	0.77
Soybeans	4.42
Sunflower seeds	4.25
Tuna	0.43

FOOD	APPROXIMATE CONTENT (MG PER 3 OZ)
Turkey	0.77
Walnuts	0.77
Wheat germ	1.87

DEFICIENCIES

Volunteers fed a pantothenic acid–free diet under experimental conditions took ten weeks to develop deficiency symptoms. Others fed a similar diet and given a substance that counteracts the effects of pantothenic acid developed the symptoms in a shorter period of time.

Deficiency Symptoms

Deficiency symptoms consisted of nausea, numbness in the extremities, sleep disturbances, muscle spasms and cramps, poor muscle coordination, headache, fatigue, stomach pains, stomach gas and diarrhea, and occasional vomiting. Subsequent studies have shown that people deprived of pantothenic acid had fewer antibodies in their blood and were not as well protected against foreign substances such as bacteria.

During World War II, prisoners of war complained of "burning feet" syndrome, associated with tingling and numbness in the legs. These symptoms can occur in anyone who is malnourished and may represent a form of pantothenic acid deficiency, since they respond to vitamin treatment. However, a direct relationship has not been established.

The relationship between symptoms of pantothenic acid deficiency and its function is not always as apparent as that relationship is in other vitamins. However, pantothenic acid deficiency can lead to nerve and muscle disorders because of its role in fat and glucose metabolism; decreased immune response because of a decline in steroid metabolism; and gastrointestinal problems because of a decline in normal cell function in the gastrointestinal tract.

TOXICITY

Pantothenic acid is nontoxic. People have taken doses as high as 10 g (10,000 mg) a day with no known adverse effects.

THERAPEUTIC USES

Pantothenic acid supplements may be given to counteract the symptoms of pantothenic acid deficiency reviewed earlier in this profile. However, such symptoms will not be alleviated by pantothenic acid unless they are, in fact, caused by vitamin deficiency.

Pantothenic acid is also sold as dexpanthenol (D-pantothenyl alcohol), a lotion or cream to be applied to burns, cuts, or abrasions. This product relieves itching and is soothing to the wound. Experiments have shown that dexpanthenol can help speed up the healing process following minor surgery to the nasal sinuses. Topical use of pantothenic acid seems worthwhile for minor wounds and inflammation.

UNSUBSTANTIATED CLAIMS

Alleviation of Stress

Pantothenic acid has been promoted as an "antistress" vitamin. The origins of this alleged property lie in animal studies and the human experiments described under "Deficiencies" above. Advocates for this use of pantothenic acid feel that it will prevent stress and stress-related diseases because people in whom a vitamin deficiency was created were less able to respond to stressful situations. There is, however, no factual evidence that pantothenic acid will prevent or treat any other forms of stress.

Weight Reduction and Acne Treatment

Pantothenic acid has been promoted for use in weight loss programs. The rationale for this claim is that this vitamin facilitates a complete breakdown of fats, thus decreasing the amount stored. Proponents claim that hunger is reduced and stored fat is better metabolized during dieting. Large doses of pantothenic acid (over 1 g) are used. The same rationale is advocated for the application of pantothenic acid for acne treatment. Here, a more complete breakdown of fatty acids is proposed to decreasing the plugging of pores that starts the acne lesion. While these hypotheses are interesting, controlled studies are lacking to demonstrate benefits.

Other Uses

We cannot recommend that you take this vitamin to treat alcoholism, allergies, arthritis, constipation, fatigue, liver cirrhosis, shock, or stomach ulcers.

AVAILABILITY

Pantothenic acid is available without a prescription as calcium pantothenate. It comes in strengths from 25 mg to 500 mg. The alcohol derivative (dexpantothenol) is also marketed as a lotion or cream.

VITAMIN B₆ (PYRIDOXINE)

Vitamin B_6 actually consists of six substances: pyridoxine, pyridoxine phosphate, pyridoxal, pyridoxal phosphate, pyridoxamine, and pyridoxamine phosphate. All have the same potency. *Pyridoxine* is considered synonymous with *vitamin B_6*, but technically *vitamin B_6* is a better descriptive term because it encompasses all active forms of the vitamin. Although a great deal is known about the processes in which B_6 is involved in the body, there are still many unanswered questions about its importance and function in humans. With the discovery that B_6 is involved in eliminating homocysteine, more attention is being given to this vitamin because of possible implications in heart disease prevention. As discussed in the folic acid section, high blood levels of homocysteine are now considered a risk factor for atherosclerosis, blood vessel disease, and deep vein clot formation, all of which are key factors in the development of angina pains, heart attacks, strokes, transient ischemic attacks (TIAs, or ministrokes), and disease of leg arteries.

FUNCTION

Pyridoxal phosphate is the active form of vitamin B_6 in humans and is manufactured by our bodies from pyridoxine or from the other forms of the vitamin. People who are magnesium-deficient may be less able to make the active form of this vitamin, as magnesium plays an essential role in phosphate transfer reactions (see Chapter 10). Also, riboflavin is involved in the conversion of B_6 into the active form of the vitamin; riboflavin deficiency (itself rare) can lead to a B_6 deficiency.

Pyridoxal phosphate is required by at least a hundred different enzymes, including those involved in the formation and reactions of amino acids used as building blocks for protein. Pyridoxal phosphate is also needed for proper brain and central nervous system function, because many chemical transmitters, used by the brain for communication, depend on B_6 as a coenzyme (catalyst) in their formation from simple amino acids. B_6 deficiency can affect mental health and lead to convulsions.

Other important functions of this vitamin include catalyzing the manufacture of hemoglobin (responsible for carrying oxygen from the lungs to every cell in the body) and conversion of the chemical tryptophan to niacin. The latter is essential to normal body operation, because about half of our niacin comes from tryptophan converted by the body.

DAILY REQUIREMENTS

Daily pyridoxine requirements vary with the amount of protein in the diet. The more protein you eat, the greater your need for pyridoxine. The recommendation is 1.5 mg for every 100 g of dietary protein. The adult RDA value is 2 mg for males and 1.6 mg for females.

DIETARY SOURCES

B_6 is found as pyridoxine in vegetables; in animals and animal products, B_6 activity is supplied by pyridoxal or pyridoxamine. As indicated above, the various forms are identical in terms of vitamin B_6 activity. The vitamin is present in a variety of foods, and rich sources include meats, grains, fish, eggs, and carrots. Additional good sources are listed in the accompanying table.

There is no evidence to support the contention that B_6 deficiency is widespread in the United States. It can be found in many foods, and some usable B_6 is made by bacteria in the gastrointestinal tract.

VITAMIN B_6 CONTENT OF SELECTED FOODS
(Average adult RDA is 2 mg)

FOOD	APPROXIMATE CONTENT (MG PER 3 OZ)
Avocadoes	0.44
Bananas	0.31
Beef	0.26
Bran	0.90
Brewer's yeast	3.40
Carrots	0.17
Cashew nuts	0.36
Eggs	0.43
Fish	0.43
Hazelnuts	0.59
Lentils	0.41
Liver (calf's)	0.60
Peanuts	0.36
Pork	0.28
Potatoes	0.39
Rice (white)	0.76
Salmon	0.88
Soybeans	0.62
Shrimp	0.54
Sunflower seeds	0.98
Tuna	0.32
Turkey	0.36
Wheat bran	0.90
Whole wheat flour	0.51

Routine B_6 supplementation is probably not necessary as long as your diet is reasonable. Nevertheless, it is included in virtually every available multivitamin product. An exception may be made for the elderly, since marginal B_6 deficiencies have been noted in the elderly, especially elderly hospitalized patients. As discussed in Chapter 4, we recommend that all people over age sixty-five take a complete multivitamin/mineral supplement.

Pyridoxine is relatively stable in foods during processing, although as much as 25 percent of the vitamin activity may be lost during cooking. It is also quite stable when food is frozen or dehydrated, but it is destroyed by ultraviolet light, and so B_6-containing foods should be stored in dark or opaque containers. Other forms of the vitamin—pyridoxal, for example, found in meat—are even less stable when heated. The milling and refining of whole wheat destroys most of its pyridoxine content, which is not replaced in the enriched flour used by most consumers. Thus while the amount of B_6 in one's diet is highly variable, nevertheless it is usually adequate for prevention of deficiency symptoms.

DEFICIENCIES

Since pyridoxine is involved with brain function, the formation of hemoglobin in red blood cells, and the manufacture of body proteins, B_6 deficiency is reflected in the impairment of all these biological functions. While severe pyridoxine deficiency is rarely seen because of the widespread presence of B_6 in the diet, marginal deficiencies may be found in some special circumstances, including people taking several drugs that interact with pyridoxine. Therapy with the antituberculosis drug isoniazid is the best-documented case where signs of B_6 deficiency may be observed. Obvious deficiency states have also been produced under test situations by feeding volunteers 4-deoxypyridoxine, which counteracts vitamin B_6.

Deficiency Symptoms

Under test conditions, nervous system abnormalities such as irritability, confusion, nervousness, and numbness in the hands and feet were observed. Skin lesions similar to those seen with niacin (B_6 is needed for the body to synthesize niacin) and a magenta coloration of the tongue have also resulted after several weeks of a pyridoxine-deficient diet plus the vitamin antagonist 4-deoxypyridoxine. Convulsive seizures can develop if the vitamin is withheld for extended periods. Some time ago an incident occurred in which three hundred infants were mistakenly given pyridoxine-deficient baby formula. These children became nervous, and several of them experienced convulsions before the problem was discovered and corrected. Severe B_6 deficiency will cause anemia in humans, but this rarely occurs in people who are simply deficient in dietary B_6 intake. This anemia can be easily reversed by taking vitamin B_6. B_6-deficient patients also feel tired and listless.

It is possible to determine vitamin B_6 deficiency by giving a person a loading dose (a large dose all at once) of the chemical tryptophan by mouth. The patient will then pass a number of unusual metabolites of tryptophan out of his or her body via the urine. One of these, xanthurenic acid, is a convenient measure of B_6 deficiency. This test, however, is not routinely used. A blood test for the activity of a specific pyridoxal phosphate–dependent enzyme is a more convenient screening method.

PEOPLE WHO MAY BENEFIT FROM SUPPLEMENTATION

Pregnant women need extra pyridoxine for several reasons. The growing fetus requires a considerable amount of energy, extra vitamins, and other nutrients from the mother. Also, estrogenic hormones, present in larger-than-usual amounts during pregnancy, tend to change amino acid metabolism and increase the need for pyridoxine. Since abnormally low pyridoxine levels have been reported during pregnancy, expectant mothers should take a special prenatal vitamin formulation that provides about 2.5 mg of pyridoxine per tablet.

TOXICITY

B_6 is considered nontoxic in daily doses up to between 20 and 50 mg. However, there have been a small number of incidents of severe nerve disorders after taking vitamin B_6 megadoses. The doses taken were as high as 6 g (6,000 mg) per day, or three thousand times the average adult RDA. These people had difficulty walking, their hands became numb and difficult to control, they lost some sensory perception (touch, temperature, vibration, pinprick, and feeling of position), and they lost feeling in the area around their mouth. All improved after they stopped taking the vitamin, but the recovery took as long as seven months in some cases, and some symptoms remained even at that time. Since then, these symptoms have been noted in people taking as little as 50 mg a day of the vitamin, although adverse effects at doses below 500 mg per day are very rare.

Animal studies have shown doses equivalent to between 200 and 600 mg per day in humans will decrease blood levels of prolactin, a hormone involved in breast milk production. Some people have suggested that B_6 be avoided by nursing mothers, but there is no evidence that the amounts of pyridoxine contained in normal vitamin supplements can affect breast milk production.

INTERACTIONS

Pyridoxine can interact with barbiturates, levodopa (l-dopa, given for Parkinson's disease), phenytoin (for seizures), isoniazid and cycloserine (used to treat tuberculosis), hydralazine (for hypertension), penicillanime (a treatment for arthritis and Wilson's disease), oral contraceptives, and vitamin B_{12}. See Part 6, "Vitamin, Mineral, and Herbal Drug Interactions," for details.

THERAPEUTIC USES

Pyridoxine supplements may be given to counteract any of the symptoms of vitamin B_6 deficiency reviewed earlier in this profile. However, such symptoms will not be alleviated by pyridoxine unless they are, in fact, caused by vitamin deficiency.

In addition, pyridoxine has been found to have some therapeutic value for the following conditions.

Depression Associated with Oral Contraceptives

There is limited evidence suggesting that supplemental B_6 may be of some value in partially reversing the depression occasionally associated with the use of oral contraceptives. The reason for this is that the estrogenic component of the pill alters blood levels of pyridoxine and therefore increases the daily requirement. Pyridoxine is needed to form brain neurotransmitters, and it also binds weakly to steroid hormone receptors.

Large-scale controlled trials are lacking to confirm this observation. However, we recommend B_6 supplementation in doses of 25 to 100 mg per day for those women taking oral contraceptives who have experienced troublesome depression and not achieved relief from another therapy. Since this depression is specifically caused by B_6 deficiency, vitamin B_6 therapy should not be viewed as of general value in the treatment of any other form of depression.

Premenstrual Syndrome

Vitamin B_6 has also received publicity as a treatment for this common problem. The theory here is that the symptoms of premenstrual syndrome (PMS) are caused by a hormone imbalance associated with menstruation. Advocates of this therapy say that the situation is similar to oral contraceptive–related depression and the marginal deficiencies reported among pregnant women. Another possible mechanism of action may be the ability of high doses of B_6 to bind to steroid hormone receptors. In any event, there have been at least five small, randomized, placebo-controlled trials addressing the question of the usefulness of B_6 to relieve PMS. We can summarize the evidence by simply indicating that the results are not in agreement. Most studies show a small improvement with B_6 compared to placebo, and some women claim significant relief from PMS with B_6.

Our advice: B_6 may be worth a try if PMS is a problem. A dose of 100 to 200 mg per day (100 mg twice a day) should be used, but do not take over 200 mg per day due to toxicity risks. Take the B_6 only during the two weeks prior to menses, that is, during the time when PMS occurs. If after a test of one or two cycles it does not seem to be helpful, stop its use. B_6 seems to work only for some women, not all, and one cannot predict who will benefit and who will not.

Reduction of Breast Milk

Some European physicians have employed daily doses of 50 mg of pyridoxine to purposely suppress prolactin secretion and reduce milk production in women who have just given birth. High-dose pyridoxine has been hailed as a savior because it may replace the hormones that have been used for this purpose. There is not much information to support this use of B_6.

Treating Inborn Errors of Metabolism

There are at least six rare, inherited genetic defects that can be treated by giving high doses of vitamin B_6. Studies have shown that in most cases these defects are the result of a genetic error that leads to the manufacture of a defective enzyme. The defect is usually related to the enzyme's inability to bind tightly to its needed vitamin. If the enzyme cannot bind to the vitamin, it cannot function. Extraordinarily high vitamin doses may be able to "flood" the enzyme, so even though the vitamin is not tightly bound to the enzyme, it can still work.

These are not true vitamin-deficiency diseases. They are defects in a single enzyme that can be overcome by megadoses of the appropriate vitamin. The abnormally low enzyme activity can lead to a variety of symptoms, but usually the problem is revealed during early childhood in the form of mental retardation and failure to grow and thrive.

There are several examples of B_6-dependent inborn errors of metabolism. These rare but serious defects often respond seemingly miraculously to vitamin treatment. It must be emphasized that most cases of mental retardation or developmental problems *will not* respond to vitamin treatments. Only a specialist can pinpoint cases that will respond and the exact vitamin needed.

Carpal Tunnel Syndrome

The sheath of tissue that carries the tendons and the median nerve through the wrist to the hand is called the carpal tunnel, and for unknown reasons, the size of the opening can become reduced. When this happens, the nerves passing through become compressed, with resulting pain, loss of touch sensation, loss of strength, and tingling sensations in the hand. Carpal tunnel syndrome can accompany several disease states, but more commonly it appears as a result of repetitive motions of the hand and wrist. It is frequently seen in data entry personnel, carpenters, joiners, violinists, and writers, for example. Pain at night interferes with sleep, and loss of strength in the hand sometimes makes work impossible. The only sure treatment is surgery to open up the tunnel and to relieve pressure.

One well-known research group in Texas has published numerous reports on the successful use of vitamin B_6 to relieve carpal tunnel syndrome. They believe that carpal tunnel syndrome is related to vitamin B_6 deficiency. However, the published experiences of other investigators have not been so enthusiastic about the value of B_6 treatment. More recent clinical trials have indicated that B_6 therapy relieves pain to some extent but may not improve nerve conduction function. This implies that the B_6 is affecting pain thresholds and may not be doing much to improve the underlying reason for the pain. Thus inflammation and damage may be continuing, but you don't feel the pain as much.

B_6 therapy should be undertaken *only* with the guidance of a health care professional experienced in dealing with carpal tunnel syndrome. Doses of B_6 should be 100 to 300 mg per day and continue for at least three months. This is about two hundred times the RDA value. If signs of toxicity develop (numbness in the legs, for example), discontinue use immediately.

Relieving Morning Sickness

Pyridoxine has been combined with an antihistamine and promoted for the treatment of morning sickness. This combination was called Benedectin and was sold in the United States for almost two decades until it was withdrawn in 1982. The withdrawal was a voluntary action on the part of the manufacturer because the question was raised of this product's potential for causing birth defects. High doses of pyridoxine have caused birth defects in laboratory animals, and while this lab data cannot be directly translated to human beings, Bendectin was withdrawn because of the manufacturer's desire to avoid adverse publicity and the staggering cost of potential lawsuits. Thus, the issue was never resolved to anyone's satisfaction. There is evidence to support the role of pyridoxine in the treatment of morning sickness. But we recommend that pregnant or breast-feeding women take pyridoxine only for nutritional purposes, unless it is taken under medical guidance.

In addition, there is nothing to indicate this vitamin is valuable in treating nausea and vomiting caused by conditions other than pregnancy.

Cardiovascular Disease

In recent years, elevated blood levels of an amino acid called homocysteine have been associated with a higher risk of heart disease and blood vessel disease (atherosclerosis). Pyridoxine is one of three vitamins (the others are B_{12} and folic acid) that are involved in getting rid of homocysteine in the body. This is discussed in more detail in the section on folic acid, the most important vitamin in eliminating homocysteine. RDA levels of vitamin supplements will usually normalize homocysteine levels. Our message is simple: Take a multivitamin/mineral supplement that contains 100 percent of the RDA for B_6, B_{12}, and folic acid. Unless you have a rare inborn error of metabolism, this will keep homocysteine levels at an appropriate value.

UNSUBSTANTIATED CLAIMS

We cannot recommend that you take vitamin B_6 to treat arthritis, diabetes, mental retardation, numbness, or obesity. B_6 will also not prevent aging, fluid retention, or leg cramps, nor can it improve your vision or help you lose weight.

Vitamin B_6 has been used to treat a variety of mental disorders, including childhood learning disabilities, autism, schizophrenia, and Alzheimer's disease. The evidence for value of B_6 here is conflicting and inconclusive. Low levels of B_6 have not been found in mental disease patients.

AVAILABILITY

Vitamin B_6, as pyridoxine hydrochloride tablets, can be purchased without a prescription in strengths between 25 and 100 mg. Several timed-release preparations are also available, but the value of timed-release vitamins is questionable. Pyridoxine hydrochloride (100 mg) injection is available only on a doctor's prescription.

VITAMIN B₁₂ (CYANOCOBALAMIN)

Plants can make most B vitamins, but not B_{12}. The producers of B_{12} in nature are the bacteria in the environment. Ruminant animals (such as cattle) have huge bacteria populations in their gut that help digest the cellulose from the grass that they eat. The bacteria make vitamin B_{12} that gets absorbed and deposited in the tissues of the animal.

The B_{12}, made by the bacteria in the human gut, is not absorbed by the colon where most of the bacteria are located. However, if humans consume meat and dairy products, they will then obtain adequate amounts of B_{12} from their diet. B_{12} intake is therefore a concern for vegetarians. Additionally, some people have an impaired ability to absorb B_{12} so may become deficient even though their diet provides ample amounts. The inability to absorb vitamin B_{12} can result in a condition called pernicious anemia. Pernicious anemia is a life-threatening disease demanding immediate and vigorous treatment.

Cobalamin, which contains the trace mineral cobalt, is the natural form of B_{12}. But the commonly available form of B_{12}, cyanocobalamin, is not found in nature. It was accidentally discovered by a pharmaceutical researcher attempting to purify cobalamin. Cyanocobalamin is the most convenient way to supplement your B_{12} intake because of its stability. On the other hand, hydroxycobalamin, the chemical precursor to cyanocobalamin, is sometimes preferable to cyanocobalamin and offers some advantages to people with a proven B_{12} deficiency. It is absorbed more slowly than cyanocobalamin after injection into a muscle and is stored in larger quantities by the liver. Hydroxycobalamin produces a more sustained rise in B_{12} levels and is eliminated more slowly from the body.

FUNCTION

Vitamin B_{12} acts in concert with folic acid in body reactions that are critical to the process of normal cell division and are required for the synthesis of DNA and RNA, the architects of every cell and function in the body. Body tissue cannot divide and grow normally without vitamin B_{12}, and its role is particularly vital in the bone marrow, where blood cells are manufactured.

One coenzyme form of B_{12} is called methylcobalamin and with the help of folic acid, can donate its methyl group to convert homocysteine (high levels are a risk factor for heart disease) to methionine. The other, adenosylcobalamin, is involved in the breakdown of certain fatty acids and in the synthesis of an amino acid, leucine.

B_{12} also participates in the body's regeneration of folic acid. Without B_{12}, we would be unable to efficiently use the folic acid in our bodies and would require such massive amounts of that vitamin that we probably couldn't get enough from food sources. This regeneration reaction involves the metabolism of homocysteine and is discussed in more detail in the section on folic acid. Suffice to say that we need to get ample B_6, B_{12}, and folic acid so that damaging homocysteine does not build up in our bodies.

Another important function of B_{12} is its essential role in the metabolism of body fats. The body has a strange way of handling the many fats that contain odd numbers of carbon atoms. Normally, fats with an even number of carbon atoms are chopped into neat little two-carbon units, which are then fed directly into our main energy-producing mechanisms, the glycolysis and tricarboxylic acid cycles. Fats that have an odd number of carbon atoms in them are chopped up in the same way as even-numbered lipids until the process is almost completed. B_{12} facilitates the breakdown of the final three-carbon unit in the metabolic cycle.

Cobalamin appears to be important in another way as well. B_{12}, through its role in methionine and homocysteine metabolism, participates in the manufacture of a material called myelin, which sheathes and protects nerve fibers. People who are deficient in B_{12} produce faulty myelin and can, if the deficiency lasts long enough, develop damage to some peripheral nerves and portions of the spinal cord. This condition is called pernicious anemia.

DAILY REQUIREMENTS

The average adult RDA for B_{12} is 2 mcg, and most people obtain plenty in the diet if they eat some meat, eggs, dairy products, or fish.

This vitamin is an exception to the general rule that water-soluble vitamins are not stored in the body in large quantities for extended periods of time. The liver has an extremely efficient system to retain B_{12} and usually has about a thousand-day supply. Even if you were to completely stop taking B_{12}, it would take at least three years for deficiency symptoms to develop. A functioning intestinal absorption system for B_{12} is a must, of course, because some B_{12} passes into the gastrointestinal tract via the bile after it has been used and is then reabsorbed and used again.

DIETARY SOURCES

Most of us receive B_{12} as the cobalamin derivatives found in fish and shellfish, beef, and dairy products, though a little may be found in legumes—plants that have a special relationship with certain soil bacteria. Liver, clams, and sardines are by far the richest sources, but cheeses that are rich in bacteria, such as Camembert and Gorgonzola, are also good. Other good sources are listed in the accompanying table.

VITAMIN B_{12} CONTENT OF SELECTED FOODS
(Average adult RDA is 3 mcg)

FOOD	APPROXIMATE CONTENT (MCG PER 3 OZ)
Bass	1.10
Beef	2.70
Blue cheese	1.20
Camembert cheese	1.00
Chicken	0.43
Clam broth	8.50
Clams	17.00
Crab	0.72
Eggs	1.26
Flounder	5.10
Gorgonzola cheese	1.00
Halibut	1.10
Herring	4.30
Liver	77.40

FOOD	APPROXIMATE CONTENT (MCG PER 3 OZ)
Liverwurst	1.20
Lobster	1.10
Mackerel	8.50
Milk	0.34
Pork	0.51
Sardines	29.00
Sausage	0.94
Scallops	0.70
Shrimp	0.70
Snapper	7.50
Swiss cheese	1.70
Turkey	0.36

Foods containing vitamin B_{12} should be protected from light but are otherwise relatively stable; less than 30 percent of B_{12} content is lost during cooking.

DEFICIENCIES

The classic B_{12} deficiency disease, pernicious anemia, is rarely caused by inadequate amounts of dietary B_{12}. It is usually related to a problem in absorbing the vitamin from the small intestine. This complex process requires hydrochloric acid and a compound known simply as intrinsic factor. Intrinsic factor is a complex protein made by special cells in the stomach lining to facilitate the absorption of vitamin B_{12}. Enzymes made by the pancreas are also necessary to digest food and release the contained vitamin B_{12}. Pernicious anemia is more common in the elderly because their stomachs may not make enough hydrochloric acid or they may make a type of intrinsic factor that doesn't bind B_{12} very well, and thus nonbound B_{12} is not absorbed.

Deficiency Symptoms

The symptoms of pernicious anemia include a gradual and possibly permanent loss of reflexes, nerve sensation, and nerve function due to the lack of production of myelin sheaths. Renewal of myelin may or may not return after treatment with B_{12}. This damage is often felt as tingling and numbness in the arms and legs, unusual mood swings, memory losses, or visual difficulties, but it can show up in a variety of other forms, depending on the nerve or nerves damaged.

The diagnosis of pernicious anemia is based on an analysis of your blood and must be made by a doctor. Typically, an unusually large proportion of immature or abnormal red blood cells will be found because they cannot proceed through the stages of normal maturation.

The presence of abnormal propionic acid metabolites in the blood is an indication of inadequate B_{12} absorption. Tests for pernicious anemia also include tests of stomach function, to make sure that you have enough hydrochloric acid, and may include the Schilling test, which measures your ability to absorb the B_{12} available in your diet.

Other deficiency symptoms are those caused by megaloblastic anemia, which is usually associated with folic acid deficiency (see p. 214) but can occur with a B_{12} deficiency because B_{12} is necessary for the body's efficient utilization of folic acid. Megaloblastic anemia results in irritability, weakness, lack of energy, sleeping difficulties, and loss of facial color, because the folic acid is needed to generate mature red blood cells.

PEOPLE WHO MAY BENEFIT FROM SUPPLEMENTATION

Vegetarians

A vegetarian who consumes milk or other dairy products or eggs will receive adequate amounts of B_{12}. A vegan (one who avoids all animal-derived foods) usually gets little B_{12} in the diet. In actual practice, B_{12} deficiency is not that common among vegetarians, possibly because the deficiency takes years to develop due to the extensive storage of B_{12} in the liver. Also, the efficiency of your absorption system may improve when levels are low. Furthermore, eating fermented foods such as soy sauce or miso provides some B_{12}. Some cases of B_{12} deficiency have been observed in infants born of vegan mothers who did not take prenatal vitamins.

Strict vegetarians should take a regular B_{12} supplement to be on the safe side. This is most inexpensively and conveniently accomplished by purchasing a multivitamin that contains B_{12}. Vegetarians can rest assured that supplemental B_{12} is not obtained from animal products; it is prepared commercially as a by-product of the fermentation processes used in making some antibiotics.

Other Groups

Other groups of people who are likely to need a B_{12} supplement are pregnant or breast-feeding women and senior citizens who may not be getting proper nutrition or who lack stomach acid or intrinsic factor. If you lack stomach acid or intrinsic factor, you will need B_{12} shots to bypass the absorption problem. Some experts have suggested that seniors who develop psychosis should be evaluated for their B_{12} status before other treatments are given.

Extra B_{12} may also be needed by people with severe illnesses, who must be sure that they have enough of the vitamin to allow active tissue growth and healing, and by those who have had their stomachs surgically removed.

TOXICITY

Vitamin B_{12} is considered nontoxic. There is not enough cyanide in the cyanocobalamin doses used in medicine to cause any problem.

INTERACTIONS

Vitamin B_{12} can interact with para-aminosalicylic acid (PAS), used to treat tuberculosis; colchicine, used for gout; and the antibiotics chloramphenicol and neomycin. There were early reports of high doses of vitamin C causing B_{12} deficiencies, but this has not proved to be an important adverse interaction. People taking prescription or over-the-counter acid-blocking medications for ulcers or indigestion should be aware that the lack of acid could decrease B_{12} absorption, though this effect is not likely to be seen for several years. A supplement may be worthwhile.

THERAPEUTIC USES

The only recognized therapeutic use for vitamin B_{12} is to prevent and correct pernicious anemia. If the problem is due to a poor diet, the diet should be improved and a multivitamin supplement taken. This is a rare cause of B_{12} deficiency. More common is a deficiency due to poor absorption caused by the lack of effective intrinsic factor or of stomach acid. Here, injections of B_{12} are needed, usually once a month. Occasionally very large (1,000 mcg) oral doses are used. This sometimes works because a little (about 1 percent) is absorbed by simple diffusion. It should be noted here that when B_{12} is given to correct pernicious anemia due to faulty vitamin absorption mechanisms, the treatment must be continued for life.

We strongly discourage the use of "shotgun" antianemia therapies that combine a number of factors (iron, B_{12}, folate, and so on), unless prescribed by a doctor. If you are anemic, you need a professional evaluation to find out why. It could be due to unseen blood loss, iron deficiency, folate deficiency, B_{12} deficiency, or other diseases such as cancer. The problem needs to be pinpointed and the appropriate treatment given. Taking high doses of folate-containing preparations can actually hide the obvious symptoms of B_{12} deficiency by making the diagnosis difficult. Supplemental high-dose folate will stimulate red blood cell production, so you feel better, but the nerve damage due to B_{12} deficiency will progress unchecked. The amount of folate in most multivitamins is too low to mask B_{12} symptoms, however.

UNSUBSTANTIATED CLAIMS

Lack of Energy

It has been the unfortunate practice of some doctors to administer monthly B_{12} injections for tiredness, undiagnosed anemia, and other vague symptoms. The usual dose is 1,000 mcg, ten times the usually recommended injectable dose, and about six months' worth of B_{12}. This practice is costly, unnecessary, and potentially dangerous because it exposes the patient to the possibility of reactions to the injection. Allergic reactions to B_{12} injection can involve itching, redness, and swelling; in rare cases the reaction may be more severe. If supplements are needed and your intestinal absorption mechanism is intact, take B_{12} by mouth in liquid or pill form.

Other Uses

B_{12} will not improve resistance to infection and disease, increase appetite, or promote growth. Nor will it improve memory or the ability to learn.

AVAILABILITY

Vitamin B_{12} is available without a prescription as cyanocobalamin tablets in strengths from 25 mcg to 1,000 mcg. Cyanocobalamin injections are available in strengths ranging from 100 to 1,000 mcg/ml, but they require a doctor's prescription. Hydroxycobalamin also requires a prescription and is available only as an injection (1,000 mcg/ml). A nasal gel form of B_{12} is also commercially available, containing 400 mcg per dose. Most multivitamins that contain B_{12} have about 6 mcg per tablet.

VITAMIN C (ASCORBIC ACID)

Despite the long history of experience and research with vitamin C, dating back several centuries to the search for the cause of scurvy among sailors on long voyages, we still have much to learn about how it works in the human body. We know that humans are one of the few creatures on earth that don't make their own vitamin C, but we don't know why.

Professor Linus Pauling proposed that humans' inability to make ascorbic acid and the decrease in C content of our diet over the years, particularly as early humans shifted from an all-vegetarian diet to a partly meat diet, has placed us at risk for getting less vitamin C than we need for optimum health. Some vitamin C advocates are quick to point out that animals that make their own vitamin C produce the human equivalent of 10 to 20 g per day. The average human diet, on the other hand, contains only 30 mg per day. They also point to apes, which get an average of 5 g of vitamin C a day in the wild.

This theory is disputed by many nutritional experts, who

claim that humans' diet was probably never strictly vegetarian and has always contained both meat and vegetables. Conventional wisdom tells us that if the ability to make vitamin C had been needed in our species' early history, it would have been carried down to today's humans through our genes. Some evidence indicates that animals make their own vitamin C in large amounts because they use it up much faster than we do. Perhaps humans are more efficient than most members of the animal kingdom in that we efficiently absorb and can store small amounts of vitamin C. Why carry the machinery to make vitamin C when you can let plants do it for you? Both sides of this debate are pure speculation, and no one can conclusively prove any of these points. Nevertheless, as knowledge of the importance of antioxidants in the diet grows, increasing vitamin C intake seems like a good idea (see Chapter 7).

FUNCTION

Vitamin C is a modified sugar molecule that is water soluble. One of the important functions of vitamin C is to serve as a water-soluble antioxidant and free-radical scavenger (see Chapter 7). It is one of the compounds in the body that protects us from oxidative free-radical damage.

It is also known that vitamin C is necessary in the synthesis of hydroxyproline and hydroxylysine. These hydroxylated amino acids are building blocks of collagen, the main supporting component in connective tissue, which is the tissue that holds us together. Some types of connective tissue are cartilage, tendons, and fibers. A lack of vitamin C causes defects in the formation of mucous membranes and interferes with the normal healing of wounds. Without sufficient vitamin C, the tissue that surrounds and supports capillaries (the smallest blood vessels) breaks down, and the capillaries themselves then break from lack of support. This results in black-and-blue bruise marks as blood leaks into tissue and clots there. The hallmark of scurvy, the vitamin C deficiency disease, is a lack of collagen synthesis.

Vitamin C also stimulates the adrenal glands to manufacture cortisone and other body hormones involved in helping us cope with stresses of daily life. Vitamin C levels are high in the adrenal glands. Vitamin C is known to participate in the hydroxylation of a chemical called dopamine in the adrenal gland to form the neurotransmitter norepinephrine. Norepinephrine is essential to life because it affects many parts of the central nervous system and all of our major organs. Another important chemical in the body whose synthesis is dependent on vitamin C is carnitine. Carnitine is needed to move sugars into the mitochondria of the cells so that they can be metabolized to yield energy.

Vitamin C increases the amount of iron absorbed from nonmeat sources through the intestines by chemically reducing and chelating the iron. To be effective, the vitamin C must be taken at the same time as the iron. If you have iron-deficiency anemia, taking the iron tablet simultaneously with 100 to 200 mg of vitamin C will increase absorption by 30 to 40 percent. The vitamin C is involved in the conversion of folic acid to its active form, dihydrofolic acid, in the body. In fact, one of the features of vitamin C deficiency is an anemia similar to the kind found in people deficient in folic acid. Small amounts of ascorbic acid are also needed to break down cholesterol in the blood.

White blood cells contain relatively large amounts of vitamin C, and it seems to be key to the ability of these cells to attack and engulf invading bacteria. Immune function is diminished in vitamin C deficiency. Deficient individuals are more susceptible to viral and bacterial infections. Interferon production by cells is stimulated by vitamin C, which may account for its importance in the defense against viruses. In addition, vitamin C is involved in the manufacture of a group of enzymes that are essential to the body's ability to break down drugs and other chemicals the body considers foreign.

DAILY REQUIREMENTS

Only about 10 mg a day of ascorbic acid is enough to protect against scurvy, which is the disease resulting from a deficiency of vitamin C. Nevertheless, the average adult RDA for ascorbic acid has been set at 60 mg to provide an extra margin of safety during times of illness and stress. In the United States it is estimated that 20 to 30 percent of adults consume less than the RDA value. A current controversy is whether levels of vitamin C over the RDA value are needed for optimal health. Given the importance of this vitamin as a water-soluble antioxidant we believe that higher levels would be beneficial (see Chapter 7). In considering what intakes might be optimal, it is important to note that 200 mg will provide about 80 percent of complete saturation of blood. Because vitamin C is "pumped" into cells by an enzymatic process, blood cells and body tissues are completely saturated at this dose. Doses of 500 mg to 1,000 mg will saturate blood. Vitamin C intakes of RDA amounts (30 mg–90 mg) will not saturate. Thus if you believe that for optimum health, you want to saturate your body with vitamin C, you will need to take in more than 200 mg per day. If five portions of fruits and vegetables were consumed each day, as recommended by nutrition authorities, vitamin C intake would be in the 100 to 300 mg per day range. Researchers at the National Institutes of Health note that 100 mg to 200 mg of vitamin C daily will benefit most healthy Americans. Intakes higher than 300 mg will be difficult to achieve without taking supplements.

DIETARY SOURCES

Fruits, potatoes, and green vegetables are the best natural sources of this vitamin. There is little vitamin C in meats, cereals, grains, and the foods we normally think of as being loaded with B vitamins. Interestingly, the richest sources of vitamin C are not the citrus fruits, as we have been led to believe, but rose hips, broccoli, Brussels sprouts, and green peppers. Additional good sources are listed in the accompanying table.

Vitamin C is chemically unstable and therefore presents some problems in terms of storage and processing. Drying fruits and vegetables destroys much of their vitamin C content. In one experiment, up to 54 percent of the vitamin was destroyed by drying. Vitamin C also breaks down after exposure to light and air. In addition, long storage of fruits and vegetables allows the vitamin to be broken down by natural enzymes. Another problem unique to ascorbic acid is that if fruits and vegetables are picked before they reach their fully ripened state, they will not have produced their full quota of vitamin C.

Freezing does not destroy the vitamin C content of foods. A typical cup of freshly squeezed orange juice contains 100 mg of ascorbic acid, while a cup of juice reconstituted from frozen concentrate contains about 120 mg of the vitamin, probably because of a special effort to concentrate ascorbic acid during the quick freezing process and the fact that vitamin C is most stable in an acid medium, such as fruit juice. However, the vitamin in frozen orange juice can be broken down by oxygen as soon as the juice is reconstituted and warmed to refrigeration temperatures.

VITAMIN C (ASCORBIC ACID) CONTENT OF SELECTED FOODS
(Average adult RDA is 60 mg)

FOOD	APPROXIMATE CONTENT (MG PER 3 OZ)
Bananas	8.5
Black currants	220.0
Broccoli	110.5
Brussels sprouts	119.0
Cabbage	30.0
Grapefruit	34.0
Green peppers	93.5
Guava	226.0
Lemons	31.0
Liver (calf's)	30.0
Milk	1.5
Oranges	42.5
Orange juice	51.0
Potatoes	21.3
Radishes	21.6
Rose hips	1,000.0
Spinach	76.5
Strawberries	51.3
Tomatoes	21.3
Watercress	72.0

Estimates of actual cooking losses range between 30 and 60 percent, although some procedures, such as blanching vegetables and then cooking them in iron or copper pots, can result in the destruction of almost all of the vitamin C. In summary, the vitamin C content of foods is highly variable. For optimal C content, consume fresh, uncooked fruits and vegetables and drink reconstituted frozen juices.

DEFICIENCIES

The disease associated with vitamin C deficiency is scurvy, which was common in sailors (who had little access to fresh foods during long voyages) in the days before vitamin C was known. Also hard hit were people in northern climates who did not have access to fresh fruits and vegetables during the long winter months. Now our ability to transport fresh food over great distances has dramatically decreased the amount of scurvy worldwide. Nevertheless, marginal vitamin C deficiencies still exist in some people, even in Westernized countries. It takes several months of a vitamin-C-deficient diet before scurvy develops. However, marginal deficiencies can develop sooner.

Deficiency Symptoms

Our basic descriptions of the symptoms of scurvy come from the logs Jacques Cartier kept during long sea voyages. Cartier's log, written in 1535, graphically tells how severe the disease can be: "Unknown sickness began to spread itself amongst us at the strangest sort that was ever heard or seen; inasmuch that some did lose all their strength and could not stand upon their feet; then did their legs swell, their sinews shrunk and became black as coal. Others also their skins spotted with spots of blood, of a purple colour. It ascended up their ankles, knees, thighs, shoulders, arms and neck. The mouth became stinking; their gums so rotten that the flesh came away to the roots of their teeth, which at last did fall out." The latter symptom is a result of periodontal disease, which can be caused by vitamin C deficiency as well as other factors.

Some symptoms of marginal deficiency are fatigue, shortness of breath, digestive difficulties, bleeding gums, easy bruising, swollen or painful bone joints, nosebleeds, anemia (weakness, tiredness, loss of color), more frequent infections, and slow wound healing. Some nutrition experts claim that people deficient in C who are at risk for heart attacks or strokes are more likely to develop one of these serious problems because of blood vessel weakness.

Vitamin C can be measured directly in the blood. The symptoms of scurvy start to appear when the blood level falls below 1 mg for every 100 ml of blood. The vitamin can also be measured in white blood cells. These levels are often taken as a better representation of the amount of vitamin C in body tissues because they are not as subject to variation as the blood level.

PEOPLE WHO MAY BENEFIT FROM SUPPLEMENTATION

Senior Citizens

Marginal C deficiencies have been found in seniors, particularly those living in nursing homes or other health care facilities. The reasons for this deficiency seem to be inattention to diet, the loss of appetite, and in some cases difficulty digesting foods rich in vitamin C, many of which are also high in roughage. On the basis of this information, we suggest that all people over age sixty-five take a daily multivitamin containing at least 60 mg of ascorbic acid. Of course, this does not eliminate the need for a balanced diet, including vitamin C–rich foods, but it does provide a measure of protection against possible deficiencies.

Other Groups

Pregnant women should supplement their daily vitamin C intake because of the demands by the fetus's developing bones, teeth, and connective tissue. Breast-feeding women also need supplemental C because they must supply enough vitamin C in their milk to support their baby's rapid growth. Smokers, women who take oral contraceptives, and people under any kind of stress (including those with infections or other medical illness or injury, those undergoing surgery, or those experiencing psychological stress) should supplement their daily intake of vitamin C, but the amount does not have to exceed 500 mg per day.

TOXICITY

Vitamin C is considered nontoxic in doses less than 1 g per day. Over 1 g, less is known about long-term consumption. However, large-scale clinical trials involving thousands of volunteers who received between 1 and 30 g of vitamin C per day revealed very few problems. Since the 1970s large doses of vitamin C have been consumed by millions in the United States with very few reports of adverse effects. As discussed later, the body is saturated at about 500 mg per day, and higher doses are simply eliminated in the urine.

There are scattered reports of a variety of adverse reactions to vitamin C, including upset stomach and diarrhea, but these are rare. Because vitamin C is metabolized in the body to oxalic acid, which is relatively insoluble in urine, high doses of C have the potential to contribute to the formation of kidney stones. High doses can also block the body's ability to eliminate urate, which could be deposited in joints, causing gout. The significance of these risks is controversial, but if you have bladder problems, kidney stones, or gout, we suggest not using large (over 200 mg) amounts of vitamin C because of potential problems associated with crystal deposits.

Patients with iron overload conditions should avoid large amounts of vitamin C because it will increase iron absorption. Hemolysis (the bursting of red blood cells) has been reported in patients having glucose-6-phosphate dehydrogenase (G6PD) deficiency. This deficiency makes patients susceptible to hemolysis from taking many common drugs. These patients need to avoid high-dose vitamin C.

Sudden stoppages of large doses of vitamin C have been reported to result in deficiency symptoms. This is called rebound scurvy; it is considered a very rare event and is not well documented. This is also true of infants born of mothers who consumed megadoses of vitamin C. They have developed deficiency symptoms soon after birth, probably because their body tissues had become used to very large amounts of vitamin C in the blood circulating from their mother. High doses of any vitamin or mineral should be avoided during pregnancy because the risks are simply not known.

INTERACTIONS

Vitamin C can interfere with certain urine and blood tests for sugar and for the test for occult blood in the stool. See Part 6, "Vitamin, Mineral, and Herbal Drug Interactions."

THERAPEUTIC USES

Vitamin C supplements may be given to counteract any of the standard symptoms of vitamin C deficiency reviewed earlier in this profile. However, such symptoms will not be alleviated by vitamin C unless they are, in fact, caused by vitamin deficiency.

Antioxidant Uses

The important role of vitamin C as a water-soluble antioxidant and free-radical scavenger is discussed in Chapter 7. Low dietary vitamin C intake has been associated with increased risk for cancer, especially cancer of the stomach, throat, intestines, and lungs. Low intake also increases the risk for heart disease, high blood pressure, and cataracts.

Wound Healing

Vitamin C is often given after surgery to speed the healing of surgical wounds. Vitamin C has an important role in the synthesis of new connective tissue, and controlled studies have shown that supplements speed up healing of bedsores and experimentally administered cuts in the mouth. Not all studies show benefit, however. We suggest that supplements be used following any significant injury or surgery in order to ensure ample vitamin C to help speed the healing process. Doses of 250 to 500 mg per day are sufficient for this effect.

UNSUBSTANTIATED CLAIMS

Prevention and Cure of the Common Cold

The claim that vitamin C will cure or prevent the common cold is of obvious interest to everyone. This is not a new idea, but it was popularized in 1970 with the publication of *Vitamin C and the Common Cold,* by Dr. Linus Pauling. Incredibly, surveys have shown that as many as half the American people have, at some time, taken extra vitamin C to prevent or treat the common cold, an illness responsible for billions of dollars' worth of lost time and productivity each year. Advocates of this treatment claim that between 1 and 5 g a day of ascorbic acid will prevent the common cold and that still higher doses are useful in treating cold symptoms, if you are unlucky enough to get sick in spite of the prevention regimen.

What is the evidence? Vitamin C advocates usually cite the results of studies conducted in the 1940s and 1950s, but most of these early studies are technically incorrect and have been criticized for that reason. The publication of Linus Pauling's book and the increased popularity of vitamin C have sparked careful evaluations by a number of reputable investigators. At least ten careful, technically correct studies have appeared in the literature since 1970. What emerges from these investigations is a picture far less optimistic than that presented by advocates. In these large, controlled studies, Vitamin C does not seem to have much of an effect in preventing the cold but has a small effect in decreasing its severity.

One study worth noting was conducted using school-age twins as subjects. One twin from each pair was given vitamin C (adjusted for age, but in the range suggested by advocates), while the other was given a placebo with the same appearance and taste of the vitamin C. As the twins lived in the same household, they were exposed to all the same factors, such as diet and contact with others, that could potentially influence a cold. Technically, this was a nearly ideal experiment. The results of this study were similar to those reported by other investigators: The children taking vitamin C had somewhat less severe colds, but the number of colds was essentially the same as experienced by those taking the placebo.

Despite the evidence from the large clinical trials, many claim to benefit from taking vitamin C during the winter months. Probably everyone has friends and coworkers who swear by vitamin C and claim, "I never get a cold while I take vitamin C." It is difficult to evaluate these claims of success. The evidence shows otherwise. There may be a subset of the population that strongly benefits, but their response does not show up in the large trials. On the basis of the evidence, you might expect a mild reduction in cold symptoms, although the high doses usually suggested do not seem to be necessary. Studies have been conducted in which a dose of between 80 and 200 mg per day was sufficient to produce this effect (a glass of orange juice contains 100 to 125 mg). It is possible that a small number of people are deficient in vitamin C or need unusually large amounts. Taking extra vitamin C will help these few people. We believe that a saturation-level dose of vitamin C (200 to 500 mg per day) is enough to provide excellent antioxidant and free-radical-scavenging activities and will optimize the immune system to fight infections such as the common cold.

Cancer

In the 1970s there was some enthusiasm for using very high doses of vitamin C in the treatment of cancer. Interest has waned, however, as the results from several trials did not show benefit. Now most attention is focused on the antioxidant properties of vitamin C and the connection between supplementation with antioxidants and protection against cancer. As discussed in Chapter 7, vitamin C is an important link in the antioxidant sequence, but vitamin E may be the most important antioxidant vitamin with respect to cancer and heart disease prevention. Consumption of fruits and vegetables high in vitamin C is protective, and this is the best step you can take to decrease risks. Additionally, we recommend daily consumption of 200 to 500 mg of vitamin C to optimize antioxidant and free-radical protection.

Detoxifying Alcoholics and Drug Abusers

There are a small number of unverified reports attesting to the usefulness of enormous doses of ascorbic acid, in some cases given by injection, in drying out alcoholics and detoxifying people addicted to narcotics and tranquilizers. People treated with vitamin C are given massive doses (up to 85 g a day) and are supposed to experience fewer of the adverse effects normally associated with drug withdrawal: cramps, nausea, generalized discomfort. This application of vitamin C should be considered unproven, although future research may shed some light on a possible role for this vitamin in this regard.

Cholesterol and Lipid Lowering

The story of vitamin C and blood lipids is riddled with conflicting information. While there is agreement that ascorbic acid will lower blood cholesterol in vitamin-deficient patients, it does not necessarily follow that cholesterol levels in other people will be affected. In fact, studies have shown that people with high blood cholesterol who are otherwise healthy are not affected by vitamin C. There are better drugs to lower cholesterol.

AVAILABILITY

A stroll down the vitamin aisle of your local pharmacy, health food, or vitamin store will soon make you aware that ascorbic acid is available in just about every possible dosage form (tablet, capsule, liquid, syrup, natural, synthetic, crystals, chewable, timed-release, wafers) and strengths (25 mg to 1,500 mg). The combination of vitamin C with bioflavonoids improves vitamin C absorption somewhat, but these products are more expensive, and at doses of over 500 mg per day, the small extra amount absorbed is probably not important. Timed-release products are poorly absorbed. Synthetic vitamin C tablets are fine and are inexpensive. We suggest you follow the guidelines laid out in Chapter 6 for product selection.

VITAMIN H (BIOTIN)

Though it is one of the less-publicized vitamins, biotin actually plays an important role in the metabolism of carbohydrates and fats. Biotin deficiencies are extremely rare in humans because biotin is found in almost all living things and is made in our own gastrointestinal tract by microorganisms that are normally present. The only known way to develop a biotin deficiency is to eat large amounts of raw egg whites, because they contain a substance called avidin, which prevents biotin from being absorbed into the blood. Symptoms of this deficiency are therefore collectively called egg white injury.

FUNCTION

Biotin serves as a catalyst in a chemical reaction called carbon dioxide fixation, which attaches carbon dioxide to other molecules. The first step in carbon dioxide fixation is binding to biotin. Then the carbon dioxide molecule is attached to the appropriate acceptor site on another molecule. Biotin's role in the process makes it an important ingredient in carbohydrate metabolism. The formation of an important intermediate factor in the energy-yielding citric-acid cycle (also known as the Krebs cycle) is dependent on a biotin-containing enzyme. Also, biotin is needed for the synthesis of fat from carbohydrate and the metabolism of fatty acids with an odd number of carbon atoms.

DAILY REQUIREMENTS

The Food and Nutrition Board of the National Academy of Sciences has determined that 30 to 100 mcg per day is an estimated safe and adequate level for daily intake among adults. There is no assigned RDA value for biotin. Infants require only 10 to 15 mcg per day.

DIETARY SOURCES

Rich dietary sources of biotin include liver, soybeans, sunflower seeds, butter, eggs, nuts, and several vegetables; other good sources are listed in the accompanying table. Biotin is reasonably stable in normal food processing and cooking. Some losses occur due to air oxidation when foods are cooked.

BIOTIN CONTENT OF SELECTED FOODS
(The estimated safe and adequate daily intake is 100 mcg)

FOOD	APPROXIMATE CONTENT (MCG PER 3 OZ)
Almonds	15.0
Beans	14.5
Bran	12.0
Brewer's yeast	80.0
Butter	85.0
Cashew nuts	25.5
Cauliflower	15.0
Chickpeas	27.2
Clams	17.0
Eggs	17.0
Green peas	9.0
Lentils	13.0

FOOD	APPROXIMATE CONTENT (MCG PER 3 OZ)
Liver (calf's)	102.0
Mackerel	17.0
Mushrooms	13.6
Peanuts	34.0
Pecans	25.5
Rice	60.0
Salmon	13.0
Sardines	20.0
Soybeans	161.5
Split peas	70.0
Sunflower seeds	60.0
Tuna	25.5
Walnuts	34.0

DEFICIENCIES

Natural biotin deficiency is rare. However, deficiency symptoms have been observed in a small number of people whose total nutritional requirements were being provided by intravenous feeding and no vitamins were provided in the intravenous solution. Biotin deficiency has also been produced by feeding volunteers large numbers of raw eggs. Biotin exists in foods as a protein complex and needs to be hydrolyzed (broken down) by proteolytic enzymes to release the free biotin before absorption. A special enzyme called biotinidase is involved in the release of free biotin. A few people lack this enzyme and develop deficiencies until they take biotin supplements.

Deficiency Symptoms

Symptoms noted among test volunteers were nausea, loss of appetite, numbness, muscle pains, rashes, depression, anemia, and high blood cholesterol. One of the most complete descriptions of biotin deficiency was reported on a woman who developed symptoms of biotin deficiency after surgery to remove a large section of diseased intestine. The woman developed a rash, lost her body hair, had a "waxy" appearance, and was tired all the time. But all her symptoms showed remarkable improvement after only a few weeks of treatment with 10 mg per day of biotin by injection.

A very severe kind of infant seborrheic dermatitis called Leiner's disease has, in some cases, responded to biotin treatment. How this rare but serious condition relates to biotin deficiency is uncertain.

A small number of rare inborn errors of metabolism due to poor binding of biotin to necessary enzymes can be treated by giving massive amounts of the vitamin. Detection of biotin deficiency can be made from blood samples using the ability of biotin to displace radioactive biotin bound to avidin. It can also be measured directly by chromatographic techniques.

TOXICITY

Biotin is considered nontoxic.

THERAPEUTIC USES

There are no recognized therapeutic uses for biotin except to treat rare genetic errors leading to failure to bind biotin to biotin-dependent enzymes.

UNSUBSTANTIATED CLAIMS

Biotin has been promoted as a treatment for baldness but this use is not supported by good evidence.

AVAILABILITY

Biotin is often a component of multivitamin products. These products usually contain 30–60 mcg biotin per dose.

FOLIC ACID

Folic acid was given its name because it was first isolated from green leafy vegetables. (In Latin, *folium* means "foliage" or "leaf.") Folic acid works closely with vitamin B_{12} and is vital to the creation of healthy red blood cells and for cell division. Folic acid deficiency can lead to megaloblastic anemia, named for the improperly formed red blood cells characteristic of the disease.

Folic acid is the simple form of the vitamin found in vitamin products. The term *folate* refers to all compounds with folic acid activity, including the many reduced, methylated, and conjugated forms of the vitamin found in different foods. All forms of folate have equivalent vitamin activity and are interchangeable. Most use the term *folic acid* to indicate all forms of the vitamin and we will also in this book. Folic acid requirements and food concentrations are expressed as folate equivalents. New evidence places folic acid as one of the most important vitamins needed for good health.

FUNCTION

Folic acid acts together with vitamin B_{12} in reactions that are critical to the process of normal cell division and are required for the synthesis of RNA and DNA, the architects of every body cell and body function. At least six active folic acid derivatives are used in this process, which is particularly important in the areas of bone marrow tissue where blood cells are manufactured. Basically, folic acid is reduced to tetrahydrofolic acid and then picks up a methyl group which, in turn, participates in complex enzymatic reactions that form the nucleic acids needed to make DNA and RNA.

For cells to divide, they need to replicate DNA and RNA and thus need ample folate. The most rapidly dividing cells in the body are the bone marrow cells, which form red blood cells. Thus folate deficiency leads to anemia; it is especially problematic in children, in whom normal growth can be slowed by insufficient folate.

Vitamin B_{12} is also involved in the body's system to regenerate folate, so that it can pick up another methyl group and work again in the synthesis of DNA and RNA; thus a deficiency of B_{12} can lead to a folate deficiency and the associated anemia. Both folic acid and vitamin B_{12} are involved in converting homocysteine to the amino acid, methionine.

Homocysteine is considered undesirable because high blood levels of it have been associated with heart disease and stroke.

DAILY REQUIREMENTS

The minimum requirement of folate for normal adults has been scientifically estimated at 50 mcg per day, but the average adult RDA is set at 200 mcg for males and 180 mcg for females. Since folate is needed for cell division, it follows that folate needs are increased during periods of injury or illness and during pregnancy. The RDA value for pregnancy is 400 mcg.

DIETARY SOURCES

Green leafy vegetables are a good source of this vitamin, as its name implies, but liver and many beans and seeds contain even more folate. There is relatively little absorbable folate in fruits and lean meats.

Cow's milk and human milk contain more than enough folate to prevent vitamin deficiency in infants, but goat's milk is very low in folate. Infants fed goat's milk will need extra folate to prevent deficiency from developing. Additional sources of folate are listed in the accompanying table.

FOLATE CONTENT OF SELECTED FOODS
(Average adult RDA is 400 mcg)

FOOD	APPROXIMATE CONTENT (MCG PER 3 OZ)
Almonds	42.5
Asparagus	102.0
Bananas	25.5
Barley	17.9
Beans	255.0
Bran	40.0
Brazil nuts	42.5
Brewer's yeast	1,500.0
Broccoli	180.0
Brussels sprouts	142.5
Cashew nuts	21.2
Chickpeas	349.0
Coconut	25.5

FOOD	APPROXIMATE CONTENT (MCG PER 3 OZ)
Collard greens	85.0
Corn	51.0
Cottage cheese	25.5
Eggs	70.0
Greens	51.0
Hazelnuts	60.0
Kale	60.0
Lentils	289.0
Liver (calf's)	247.0
Milk	6.0
Orange juice	54.0
Peanuts	51.0
Peas	110.0
Pecans	25.5
Rice (white)	14.0
Soybeans	595.0
Spinach	68.0
Split peas	196.0
Sprouts	119.0
Sunflower seeds	85.0
Vegetable greens	51.0
Walnuts	51.0
Wheat	187.0
Wheat germ	264.0

Folate is one of the least stable vitamins in cooking and processing, particularly in vegetables and dairy products. It has been estimated that more than 90 percent of folate content may be lost from vegetables when they are cooked. Additional losses occur when the cooking water is discarded, because folate is very water-soluble. It is very important to eat some fresh uncooked vegetables on a daily basis so that food folate is available for absorption; surveys have revealed that many Americans have a marginally low folate intake. Folate absorption is dependent on the presence of adequate amounts of vitamin C, and signs of folate deficiency (anemia) are also seen with vitamin C deficiency. This interdependence among vitamins is why we recommend use of a balanced multivitamin product when vitamin supplementation is needed.

DEFICIENCIES

Since folate is essential for cell division and reproduction, organs and tissues that divide rapidly are severely affected by folate deficiency. Bone marrow, which produces blood cells, is a good example. Folate deficiency causes the bone marrow to become less efficient in making new blood cells and produces a type of anemia called megaloblastic anemia. The differentiation between megaloblastic and other types of anemia, such as iron-deficiency or pernicious anemia, can only be made by your doctor on the basis of information gleaned from laboratory analyses of your blood.

Because fetuses grow so rapidly, a lack of folate early in pregnancy can result in birth defects.

Studies have shown that people eating a folate-deficient diet take between three and five months to show signs of deficiency; as is the case with other water-soluble vitamins, the body maintains limited stores of folate to provide a reserve during periods of low intake.

Deficiency Symptoms

People with folate deficiency experience many of the same symptoms as those with other forms of anemia: irritability, weakness, lack of energy, sleeping difficulties, and loss of facial color. Nerve damage does not develop as it does in B_{12} deficiency.

Folate levels can be measured directly in the blood. Normal concentrations range from 4 to 20 nanograms per milliliter. Anything less than 4 ng/ml is considered a deficiency. Changes in the process of making red blood cells become apparent within a week or two after folate levels reach deficiency levels, and symptoms can develop anytime thereafter.

PEOPLE WHO MAY BENEFIT FROM SUPPLEMENTATION

Alcoholics

Alcoholics are often folate-deficient because they don't eat very much or very well and because of the fact that alcohol interferes with body reactions that prepare folate for reuse.

Women Who Are Pregnant or Who May Become Pregnant

Pregnant women need at least 400 mcg per day because of the rapidly growing fetus in their womb. Nursing mothers also need the same amount because they must supply enough folate in their milk to support their baby's rapid growth. Folate deficiency is the most common cause of anemia during pregnancy. More of this vitamin is needed, and it is relatively difficult to eat enough food to get at least 400 mcg daily. Pregnant women should take a daily prenatal vitamin containing at least 400 mcg (0.4 mg) of folate.

One of the most important recent findings is an association of low folate intake during the early stages of pregnancy with two fetal neural tube defects, spina bifida and anencephaly. This was first demonstrated in England, where women who had given birth to an infant with a neural tube defect were given folate supplements prior to a second pregnancy and subsequently had a dramatically lower rate of these birth defects in their second children. Subsequently, studies in Hungary and in the United States showed a reduction in neural tube defects in first-time pregnancies among women taking a supplement containing folate. (There is some evidence that low folate is associated with other birth defects as well.) Red blood cell folate levels that were found to be protective against birth defects can be achieved with folate intakes of at least 400 mcg per day.

Good multivitamin supplements contain 400 mcg per tablet. It has been estimated that if women regularly took 400 to 500 mcg per day of folate, neural tube defects could be reduced by as much as 70 percent. But the timing of the supplementation is important. The neural tube closes about twenty-six or twenty-seven days after conception—about twelve or thirteen days after the first missed menstrual period. Therefore it is essential that the mother have adequate folate in her system when she becomes pregnant.

We recommend that sexually active women of childbearing age take a daily multivitamin supplement with 400 to 800 mcg of folate per tablet, and try to eat well. If you do become pregnant, folate levels will be sufficient to minimize the risk of neural tube birth defects in your baby.

Women Taking Oral Contraceptives

Birth control pills tend to lower folate levels in the body, and we recommend that all women on oral contraceptives take a folate-containing multivitamin supplement.

People with or at Risk for Heart Disease or Vascular Disease

As discussed earlier, folate is needed to convert homocysteine to methionine. Elevated blood homocysteine has recently been established as a very important risk factor for heart attacks. In fact, it rivals high cholesterol and smoking as risk factors for atherosclerosis, strokes, and heart disease. An increased risk for clots in the deep veins of the legs is also associated with elevated homocysteine. It seems that homocysteine might increase the oxidation of LDL cholesterol (see Chapter 7 on antioxidant vitamins) and promote atherosclerosis.

Three vitamins are involved in metabolizing homocysteine. Vitamin B_{12} and folate convert homocysteine to methionine, as discussed earlier. Vitamin B_6 (pyridoxine) catalyzes the conversion of homocysteine to cystathionine and then to cysteine, a harmless amino acid. Studies of patients with high blood levels of homocysteine have revealed that the amounts of B_{12}, B_6, and folate found in multivitamin supplements are probably sufficient to normalize elevated homocysteine levels. Women who received high amounts of folate and B_{12} from either supplements or diet were found to have reduced incidence of heart disease, compared to women taking in low levels of these vitamins. Folate is the most important vitamin in reducing homocysteine levels, but B_{12} and B_6 also help.

We believe the research findings associating homocysteine with increased risk of heart disease and stroke have profound implications with respect to vitamin supplementation. Since good multivitamin supplements are inexpensive, nontoxic, and have enough of the three vitamins to lower homocysteine levels, their use can be now recommended for all. Of course a wholesome, balanced diet is most important, but the ingestion of a multivitamin is inexpensive insurance for an adequate intake of B_{12}, B_6, and folate.

Other Groups

Since adequate folate is necessary for normal cell division, there has been interest for some time in the connection between low intake of folate and cervical, colon, and possibly other types of cancers. The strongest link is with cervical cancer. It seems that folate may help prevent cervical cancer but will not arrest precancerous lesions. The protective properties of folate in cervical cancer, birth defects, and heart disease suggest that all women should make sure their folate intake is adequate. We suggest multivitamin supplementation.

The evidence linking low folate to a risk of heart disease, stroke, and birth defects has convinced the U.S. Food and Drug Administration to mandate supplementation of flour, beginning in 1998, with 140 mcg of folate per 100 g of flour. Some are concerned that this level might mask symptoms of B_{12} deficiency, while others think that higher fortification levels are needed. We believe that the benefits of this program far outweigh the risks. This, plus greater attention to a balanced diet and the use of multivitamin supplements will go far in improving the health of our citizens.

TOXICITY

Folate is considered nontoxic in humans. Daily doses as large as 15 mg have been well tolerated. However, large amounts of folate may counteract the effects of phenytoin, primidone, and phenobarbital, used to counteract seizures; and pyrimethamine and trimethoprim, used to treat infection.

INTERACTIONS

Folate can interact with chloramphenicol (Chloromycetin), pyrimethamine (Daraprim), and phenytoin. See Part 6, "Vitamin, Mineral, and Herbal Drug Interactions."

THERAPEUTIC USES

We strongly discourage self-treating any anemia with folate, iron, or other supplements. You must have a professional evaluation to determine why you are anemic. Anemia could be due to unseen blood loss, iron deficiency, folate deficiency, B_{12} deficiency, or another problem such as bowel disease or cancer. The cause needs to be identified and the appropriate treatment provided.

FOLATE RESEARCH HAS LED TO THE DISCOVERY OF VALUABLE DRUGS

Research into the role of folate in body metabolism has led to the development of some lifesaving drugs. A folate inhibitor, methotrexate, has become one of our most important anticancer drugs. Rapidly dividing cancer cells need lots of folate and other nutrients.Methotrexate has a selective effect on these cells and, by antagonizing folate metabolism, dramatically slows their growth. Knowledge of the folate cycle has led to the further sophistication of methotrexate treatment. In a procedure known as leucovorin rescue, cancer patients are given what might ordinarily be lethal doses of methotrexate and then given calcium leucovorin, an intermediate in the folate cycle that bypasses the blockade created by methotrexate. Interestingly, normal cells are rescued by leucovorin before cancer cells.

In another research development, trimethoprim, a selective inhibitor of the enzyme that allows bacteria to convert folic acid to its active form, has been discovered to be a useful antibacterial medicine, because it inhibits the bacteria's ability to make folic acid. Trimethoprim is usually prescribed together with a sulfa drug, and the two agents work together to produce a greater effect than either could if they were used alone. These medications have few side effects because they don't usually affect human enzymes that change folic acid to its active form. Some drugs to treat parasitic infections work in the same way. Research will, as time passes, produce even more medicines that exert their effects through the folic acid cycle.

UNSUBSTANTIATED CLAIMS

We cannot recommend that you take this vitamin to treat pain or skin blemishes. Folate will also not improve lactation, increase resistance to infection, protect against internal parasites or food poisoning, prevent canker sores, or delay the onset of gray hair.

AVAILABILITY

Folic acid tablets in strengths of 400 mcg (0.4 mg) and 800 mcg (0.8 mg) may be purchased without a prescription. Tablets of 1,000 mcg (1 mg) are sold by prescription only, as are injections of folic acid. Folic acid is also included as an ingredient in many vitamin combinations, where the same basic rules apply. Vitamin products with more than 800 mcg of folic acid can be obtained only by prescription (as in many prenatal vitamins, for example).

Many multivitamin preparations contain no folic acid. Using one of these products is unwise, for folate is one of the most important vitamins for both men and women and, as discussed above, low levels are associated with heart and vascular disease and with cervical abnormalities. Low folate during pregnancy is associated with birth defects. If you believe you need a vitamin, make sure you buy one that contains at least 400 mcg of folate.

9

FAT-SOLUBLE VITAMINS

VITAMIN A

Historically, vitamin A has been most well known as a cure for night blindness. In fact, night blindness is a symptom of vitamin A deficiency, which can be alleviated by taking sufficient amounts of that vitamin. Symptoms of night blindness were first recognized in ancient Egypt around 1500 B.C. Although at the time the problem was not linked to a dietary deficiency of any kind, the symptoms were treated by placing roasted or fried liver over the eyes. Later, Hippocrates suggested eating beef liver, a rich source of vitamin A, as a cure for night blindness. Today we know that vitamin A serves several other important functions in the body, and chemical derivatives of vitamin A have important medical benefits, particularly in the area of treatment of skin conditions and in cancer treatment. We also know that vitamin A deficiencies lead to a higher risk for some cancers, including lung cancer in smokers.

Several compounds with similar chemical structures in nature have vitamin A activity. In animal tissues, retinol, retinal, and retinoic acid are the active forms. In animal-derived foods, most vitamin A exists as retinol or retinal. Vitamin A from plants is in the form of carotenoids. Carotenoids are considered "provitamins" because they must be metabolized in the body before they can act as a vitamin. Alone, however, they may serve as free-radical scavengers and quenchers of singlet oxygen. There are many carotenoids in plants, but not all have vitamin A activity. Beta carotene is the most common, and it has the most potent vitamin A activity.

All compounds with vitamin A activity are fat-soluble; like all fats, they are absorbed from the intestinal tract with the help of bile.

FUNCTION

Vitamin A is essential to a variety of biochemical and physiological processes in the body. In many of these processes, the vitamin must undergo a minor chemical change to allow it to participate in that function. Vitamin A, as retinal (retinol is easily oxidized to retinal), is a part of the pigment called rhodopsin, found in the retina of the eye. Rhodospin is sensitive to small amounts of light and is essential for night vision because it allows us to discern objects in very low light. To function in this way, the retina of the eye must contain a large concentration of vitamin A.

Retinoic acid is present in very small amounts, yet it has an important function in promoting cell growth and cell differentiation. Skin cells and the cornea of the eye are especially affected by vitamin A deficiency. The skin turns rough and scaly, and hair follicles become obstructed. Vitamin A, as retinoic acid, probably plays an important role in preventing cancer because of its ability to regulate cell division and differentiation.

Vitamin A, as retinol, is needed for reproduction. Rats deprived of vitamin A cannot reproduce. Retinoic acid will not cure the infertility.

Vitamin A is also important in maintaining a normal immune system. Vitamin A deficiency results in an increased susceptibility to infections, and it has been called the "anti-infective vitamin." In recent years it has been recognized that measles occurring in vitamin A–deficient children is very severe, often resulting in death. A program started by the World Health Organization gives occasional high oral doses of vitamin A to children in certain developing countries that have a high death rate from measles and other infections. The association between very severe measles requiring hospitalization and low vitamin A status has been made even in the United States, and a call has been made to pay more attention to vitamin A intake in children. Some have suggested that all hospitalized children with measles be given a high-dose vitamin A supplement.

Beta carotene, the most potent plant-derived precursor of retinol, retinal, and retinoic acid, has a biological activity of its own. It is an excellent free-radical scavenger, and it neutralizes reactive singlet oxygen. However, other plant carotenoids may be even more important in protecting us against the damaging effects of oxygen (see Chapter 7 on antioxidant vitamins).

DAILY REQUIREMENTS

The strength of vitamin A can be expressed in terms of a measure of biological activity, international units (IU), or as retinol equivalents (RE), which indicate the amount of retinol to which the substance can be converted in the body. The use of IU is older and has been mostly replaced in nutrition tables by the use of RE values. Commercial vitamin products, however, still use the old IU system and the older U.S. RDA values, which are in IU. To convert between systems, simply remember that 1 RE of vitamin A equals 3.3 IU.

The adult RDA for vitamin A is 1,000 RE for men and 800 RE for women. Pregnant or breast-feeding women need an additional 200 and 400 RE, respectively. The U.S. RDA value for adults is 5,000 IU. The RDA for infants and children is smaller than that for adults (375–700 RE), but when compared on a pound-for-pound basis, it is considerably larger because of the need for vitamin A in normal processes of growth and development.

Small amounts of vitamin E will increase the capacity of all body tissues, including the retina and liver, to store vitamin A. For this reason, people who must take vitamin A to correct a deficiency state should also take a modest amount of vitamin E. Most comprehensive multivitamin formulas have enough vitamin E in them to satisfy this need for the vitamin.

We should point out that there is no need for a person in good health to take a vitamin A supplement by itself. A daily multivitamin with about 5,000 IU of A is more than sufficient for the average person, because the vitamin A received in the diet must also be taken into account.

DIETARY SOURCES

It is easy to recall which foods are rich in vitamin A if you remember that retinols dissolve in fat and carotenes are found in yellow plant pigments. Some rich animal sources of vitamin A are liver (the storage depot for vitamin A in all animals), whole milk, cream, and butter. Additional good sources are listed in the accompanying table. Four ounces of beef liver has more than a seven-day supply of vitamin A, and fish liver has even more. Cod liver oil was commonly used as a source of this vitamin and of vitamin D before purified vitamin A was available. A single teaspoon of cod liver oil will fulfill the adult RDA (5,000 IU). High concentrations of carotene are found in dark green vegetables, where the green of chlorophyll usually covers the yellow-to-orange carotenoid color, and yellow-orange vegetables such as carrots, pumpkin, and squash. Other sources are listed in the accompanying table.

VITAMIN A CONTENT OF SELECTED FOODS
(Average adult RDA is 900 RE, or 4,500 IU)

FOOD	APPROXIMATE CONTENT (IU PER 3 OZ)
Apricots	2,430
Asparagus	810
Butter	2,520
Broccoli	3,150
Cantaloupe	3,060
Carrots	9,000
Cheese	1,170
Cherries	900
Chicken	190
Cod	163
Corn	360
Crab	1,980
Cucumbers	175
Eggs	1,080
Endive	3,000
Green beans	540
Green peppers	380
Herring	135
Kumquats	540
Halibut	765
Lettuce (iceberg)	900
Lettuce (romaine)	1,700

FOOD	APPROXIMATE CONTENT (IU PER 3 OZ)
Liver (beef)	33,300
Lobster	828
Mackerel	400
Mango	1,620
Milk (low-fat)*	155
Milk (whole)	200
Nectarine	1,440
Okra	470
Oranges	180
Oysters	280
Papaya	1,530
Peaches	1,170
Persimmons	2,430
Pimentos	2,070
Pistachios	205
Pumpkin	6,300
Soybeans	630
Spinach	7,200
Sprouts	495
Squash (summer)	360
Squash (winter)	3,600
Swordfish	1,890
Tomatoes	800
Walnuts	270
Watermelon	475
Whitefish	1,800

*Normally, vitamin A is found in the milk fat, which is completely or partially removed from skim and low-fat milk, respectively. If the milk you buy is supplemented with vitamin A (not all are), it also has 200 IU in 3 oz.

Carotene is converted to retinol in the wall of the small intestine as it is being absorbed into the blood. The process of conversion continues only as long as retinol is needed. Once the need for retinol has been satisfied, the conversion process stops, so high doses of beta carotene do not result in toxic levels of retinal.

Vitamin A is sensitive to oxygen. Thus, prolonged heating in the presence of air will destroy the vitamin A activity of any food. To minimize this loss while cooking your food, place a lid on the pot or pan used to boil such vegetables as squash or carrots, and use a small pot with just enough water to cover the vegetables. Acid also destroys A, but most food sources of this vitamin are nonacidic, so this is not a practical problem.

DEFICIENCIES

About 15 percent of Americans, mostly infants and children, get less than the RDA value for vitamin A. Fortunately, the average person has about a two-year supply of vitamin A in their liver, so you have to eat a vitamin A–deficient diet for many months before symptoms will develop.

Deficiency Symptoms

Mild vitamin A deficiency may be easily overlooked. Dry, rough skin is common. Sometimes the skin can crack and may even become infected. The infection develops because cracks and rough areas in the skin leave openings for microorganisms to enter and because vitamin A is needed for a strong immune response.

The most recognizable sign of vitamin A deficiency is night blindness (difficulty seeing at night or in low light). This is followed by further damage to the cornea in the form of a condition called xerophthalmia. If left untreated, severe vitamin A deficiency can lead to permanent blindness. Vitamin A deficiency is the leading worldwide cause of blindness in childhood and is an enormous problem in many developing countries.

People who are deficient in vitamin A have an increased susceptibility to respiratory infections because of changes in the cells that line the respiratory tract. Because of their depressed immune response, deficient children develop more severe forms of common childhood diseases. And as mentioned earlier, measles can be lethal in a vitamin A–deficient child.

Other possible effects of vitamin A deficiency include slow growth, thickening of bone, kidney stones that originate with changes in some of the cells that line the kidney tubules, diarrhea, and reduced production of steroid hormones in the body. Steroids are produced by the adrenal gland and are a part of your natural response to stress and your immune function. Failure to make these important hormones will leave your immune system in a less-than-ideal state. Damage to hearing, taste, and smell, nerve damage, and reduced sweat gland function may also occur.

It is possible to measure vitamin A in your blood, but the results of this test are difficult to interpret because of the large amounts that are stored in the liver. Repeatedly low blood values are a direct indication of a severe vitamin deficiency that demands immediate attention.

TOXICITY

Adults may develop symptoms of vitamin A toxicity after taking more than 50,000 IU a day for long periods of time or after taking a single dose of 300,000 IU or more. Infants given 7,500 to 15,000 RE (25,000–50,000 IU) of vitamin A for thirty days have developed toxicity symptoms. In children, vitamin A toxicity has usually been caused by an overzealous parent giving excessive quantities of supplemental vitamin A. Infants and children who are given 6,000 RE (20,000 IU) of vitamin A a day and who are not deficient are likely to develop overdose symptoms after several months.

Vitamin A overdose is characterized by vomiting, fatigue, swelling due to fluid accumulation, hydrocephalus (water on the brain), and headache (caused by excess fluid in the skull, resulting in increased pressure on the brain). Vitamin A overdose has, in some cases, been misdiagnosed as a brain tumor. Other symptoms of overdose are liver and lymph gland enlargement, difficulty sleeping, joint pains, constipation, and rough skin. The effects of an overdose of vitamin A will usually reverse themselves after you stop taking the vitamin.

Since the body will convert as much carotenoid to retinol as it needs, it is possible to have excess unconverted carotene in the blood. A very high concentration of unconverted carotenoids in the blood is known as hypercarotenosis and can cause a yellow discoloration of the skin. This condition has been confused with jaundice, but the two are not related. Hypercarotenosis is unsightly but usually not dangerous.

Toxicity and Pregnant Women

Pregnant women taking excess vitamin A risk bearing a child with birth defects because of the action of the vitamin on the developing fetus. Some of the possible defects are urinary tract malformations, hydrocephalus, and bone deformities. If you are pregnant, do not exceed your doctor's recommendation for any vitamin or drug, including vitamin A. Current recommendations are to take no more than 10,000 IU per day during pregnancy, and prenatal vitamins contain no more than this amount. But vitamin supplements containing up to 50,000 IU per capsule are readily available, so be careful when selecting a product.

INTERACTIONS

Vitamin A can interact with corticosteroid-type drugs, oral contraceptives, calcium, zinc, and mineral oil. It can also interfere with certain blood tests. See Part 6, "Vitamin, Mineral, and Herbal Drug Interactions," for details.

THERAPEUTIC USES

Vitamin A supplements may be given to counteract any of the standard symptoms of vitamin A deficiency reviewed earlier in the profile. However, such symptoms will not be alleviated by vitamin A unless they are, in fact, caused by vitamin deficiency.

Antioxidant Uses

Plant carotenoids are excellent free-radical scavengers and quenchers of singlet oxygen. As such, they play a role in protecting our cells against oxidative damage and presumably help protect us from a number of chronic diseases linked to free-radical damage. This subject is discussed in Chapter 7, on antioxidant vitamins.

Measles

As discussed earlier, measles can be life-threatening if the child is deficient in vitamin A. It has been recommended that the vitamin A status of all seriously ill patients with measles be checked and a high-dose supplement given if needed. A program of providing vitamin A supplements to children in some developing countries has lowered the infant death rate due to infections.

Cancer Prevention

Animals deficient in vitamin A get cancer more often and their tumors spread more quickly than animals without this deficiency. There is evidence that the same thing holds true for people: Those who are deficient in vitamin A may be at an increased risk of developing cancer, and individuals who do get the disease may find that their cancer spreads more quickly. Low vitamin A intake from vegetables is directly related to an increase in cancer of the lung, bladder, and larynx. However, it is not known whether the protective effect of vitamin A can be attributed to beta carotene, other plant carotenoids, retinol, or some other component of green and yellow vegetables (see Chapter 7 on antioxidant vitamins). Our best advice is to eat plenty of vegetables, as high vegetable intake is consistently associated with a lower risk of cancer.

Retinoic acid is the form of vitamin A required for normal cell differentiation and thus cancer prevention. Unfortunately, it is metabolized too quickly and is too toxic in high doses to be practical for therapeutic use in cancer treatment. Other synthetic derivatives of retinoic acid (called, as a group, retinoids) show some promise and are under investigation.

Treatment of Acne

One of the symptoms of vitamin A deficiency is an acnelike condition. This observation led to the use of vitamin A capsules as an acne treatment in the 1950s and 1960s and consequently to the discovery that high doses of vitamin A are toxic. After several decades of using vitamin A capsules to treat acne, the consensus is that the treatment is only marginally effective and carries a significant risk of toxicity.

In the 1970s retinoic acid applied to the skin became popular as an acne treatment, and it is still used today. Topical retinoic acid appears to reduce the plugging of sebaceous (oil-producing) glands. Plugged sebaceous glands can become infected and turn into pimples. Retinoic acid also mildly irritates the skin and causes peeling, which also helps to free plugged sebaceous glands.

Retinoic acid cream or lotion is not the ideal treatment. It can take months for the treatment to begin working, and it is irritating to the skin. In the search for more potent and less toxic retinoic acid derivatives, researchers have discovered several that can be taken by mouth without the usual adverse effects. Isotretinoin, or 13-cis-retinoic acid, has been of some benefit to people who suffer from the most severe form of acne and who have not responded to other forms of treatment. These retinoic acid derivatives are strong teratogens (they cause birth defects), and patients on the drug must take steps to make sure they do not get pregnant.

Treatment of Psoriasis

Several retinoic acid derivatives are used with some success to treat psoriasis. These drugs are available only by prescription and carry a significant risk for causing birth defects if taken during pregnancy.

UNSUBSTANTIATED CLAIMS

We cannot recommend that you take this vitamin to treat alcoholism, allergies, angina pectoris, arteriosclerosis, arthritis, asthma, bad breath, broken bones, bronchitis, canker sores, cataracts, colitis, the common cold, constipation, cystitis, diabetes, diarrhea, double vision, ear infections, emphysema, epilepsy, eyestrain, fever, flu, gout, hair problems, hay fever, headache, heart attack, heart failure, hemorrhoids, hemophilia, hepatitis, infertility, jaundice, kidney stones, learning disabilities, liver cirrhosis, meningitis, mononucleosis, muscular dystrophy, nail problems, osteomalacia, prostate trouble, psychosis, sinusitis, stroke, swollen glands, thyroid disease, tuberculosis, vaginitis, varicose veins, or worms.

AVAILABILITY

Despite its toxicity, vitamin A can be obtained in any strength without a prescription. Attempts by the FDA to attempt to limit the doses that can be purchased without a prescription have been met with fierce opposition by nutritionally oriented consumer groups.

We do not recommend taking more than 10,000 IU a day unless you are under the guidance of a licensed health care professional who is expert in therapy with vitamin A. This is especially true if you are or might become pregnant. *Do not take vitamin A doses over 10,000 IU per day if you are pregnant or if there is any chance you may become pregnant.*

VITAMIN D

You can satisfy your vitamin D requirement simply by being out in the sun. That's why vitamin D is commonly called the "sunshine vitamin." Until the discovery of vitamin D in 1924, many urban children suffered from rickets, a crippling bone disease resulting from insufficient calcium. Some thought that rickets was caused by a lack of sunshine and fresh air, while others felt a dietary factor was responsible for this problem. By 1920 it was shown that both notions were true, and that either cod liver oil, which contains large amounts of both vitamins A and D, or exposure to sunlight would prevent or cure the disease.

The term *vitamin D* describes two dietary substances with the ability to increase the absorption of calcium into the bloodstream from the intestine. The first substance, now called vitamin D_3 or cholecalciferol, is made in the body from cholesterol that has been exposed to the ultraviolet rays of direct sunlight. Electric lights do not give off the kind of light needed to convert cholesterol to vitamin D_3; you must be exposed directly to the sun. Sitting behind a window on a sunny day also doesn't work because the glass absorbs ultraviolet rays. The second form, called vitamin D_2, or ergocalciferol, is made in the laboratory by exposing ergosterol, a fatty substance found in plants, to ultraviolet light. Vitamin D_2 is the form often used for food fortification. Both D_2 and D_3 are equally potent; your body can use either form.

FUNCTION

Vitamin D is best described as a regulator of calcium levels in the body. In fact, vitamin D is so important to calcium function that many researchers consider it a hormone, not a vitamin. The two most important ways that vitamin D functions to maintain normal calcium levels are the absorption of calcium through the intestines into the bloodstream and the mobilization of calcium from bone, where 95 percent of body calcium is stored. For vitamin D to affect calcium absorption, it must be converted in the liver to 25-hydroxycholecalciferol and then by the kidney to 1,25-dihydroxycholecalciferol. The latter form is called calcitriol, and it is this activated form of the vitamin that induces the formation of a specific calcium-binding protein in the intestinal cells. By an independent mechanism, calcitriol also stimulates absorption of phosphate from the intestine. In addition, vitamin D exerts a direct effect on the kidneys to prevent the release of calcium and phosphates from the body via the urine.

Vitamin D, as calcitriol, is a key to maintaining calcium blood levels. Because of the critical importance of blood and tissue calcium for nerve function, muscle contraction, blood clotting, and other functions, the calcium level is under tight control, and vitamin D is involved in that control. If blood calcium levels drop and little dietary calcium is available, vitamin D (along with parathyroid hormone) is involved in stimulating the release of calcium from bone to bring the blood calcium back to normal. This makes your bones more brittle and easier to break. You can see the importance of taking in enough calcium in the diet so that bone loss does not occur.

Both the vitamin D that you convert in the skin after exposure to sunlight and that which you get from your diet must be converted to calcitriol, and both the liver and kidneys are involved in this process. Liver disease does not impede the conversion, but kidney failure is serious because less-than-optimal amounts of calcitriol are then produced, leading to calcium deficiency symptoms. The kidney damage seen in some diabetics may result in bone loss by this mechanism, and calcitriol is often given to stabilize calcium levels.

There is interest in the role vitamin D plays in the development of cancer. The vitamin has been shown to have inhibitory effects in animal models of several human cancers, but it remains to be seen whether some therapeutic advantage for vitamin D can be found in human cancer treatment and prevention.

DAILY REQUIREMENTS

Vitamin D is measured either in units based on biological activity (IU) or as micrograms (mcg) of cholecalciferol. Ten mcg of cholecalciferol is equal to 400 IU of vitamin D activity. As with vitamin A, most nutritional tables express requirements as mcg of cholecalciferol, but the vitamin products still use the IU value. One hundred IU of vitamin D per day is probably all that is needed to prevent deficiency symptoms, but 400 IU is the value recommended as the RDA for most people. Few people need to take more than that, and people who live in the Sunbelt and expose themselves to the sun probably don't need to take any vitamin D in their diets. On the average, we make 6 IU of vitamin D every hour for every square inch of skin exposed to the sun. This varies because people whose skin color is darker make less vitamin D. People with a very dark skin color make about 4 IU per square inch per hour because less light penetrates the skin to the layer where the conversion is carried out. In the winter, it has been estimated that 2–3 hours of exposure of the face to the sun would be needed to achieve synthesis of the RDA value. So for most people, dietary intake of supplements of preformed vitamin are important.

DIETARY SOURCES

While sunshine provides enough vitamin D for people who live in warm and sunny climates, those who live in northern areas with fewer days of sunshine and extended periods of cloud cover and darkness have to depend on dietary sources of vitamin D. Unfortunately, vitamin D is present in limited concentrations in most of the foods we eat. In order to prevent rickets, many countries, including the United States and Canada, have fortified common food items with vitamin D. Milk is one of our major dietary sources of vitamin D because it is fortified with irradiated ergosterol to provide vitamin D activity equivalent to 400 IU (10 mcg) per quart. Fortified margarine is also very high in vitamin D. Vitamin D is chemically stable and survives the usual modes of food processing. Additional food sources are listed in the accompanying table.

VITAMIN D CONTENT OF SELECTED FOODS
(Average adult RDA is 400 IU, or 10 mcg)

FOOD	APPROXIMATE CONTENT (IU PER 3 OZ)
Butter	36
Cheese	27
Cod liver oil	10,000
Eggs	45
Liver	45
Margarine (fortified)	270
Milk (fortified)	36
Milk (human)	6
Mushrooms	135
Salmon	360
Sardines	450
Shrimp	135
Sunflower seeds	83
Tuna	225

DEFICIENCIES

When a growing child is deficient in vitamin D, he or she develops rickets, a disease in which newly formed bone lacks calcium. Vitamin D–deficient adults may develop osteomalacia, or adult rickets. Osteomalacia is most likely to occur during times of increased calcium need, such as pregnancy. It also occurs in some elderly people and people with kidney failure. Until recently, people with kidney failure had to take enormous amounts of vitamin D_2 to maintain normal calcium levels, and frequently even this was not enough. Now the active form of vitamin D, calcitriol, which does not have to be converted in the body, is available on a prescription-only basis.

Deficiency Symptoms

In rickets, soft, defective bone is especially likely to form at sites of active growth. This results in bent, bowed legs, late tooth development, weak muscles, and listlessness. In osteomalacia, there is a generalized loss of calcium from bones throughout the body, leaving large areas of porous, brittle bone without calcium to strengthen the matrix. Osteomalacia must be distinguished from osteoporosis, in which calcium is also lost from bones, but the losses are not general in nature. They are isolated in specific locations in the skeleton, for example the hip, and are associated with the drop in estrogen after menopause.

TOXICITY

Vitamin D can be toxic if you take too much. It should never be taken in daily doses larger than 400 IU per day, except if prescribed by your doctor to treat a specific condition. In adults, single doses of 150,000 IU or more are toxic, and daily doses of 2,000 IU or more taken on a regular basis can lead to abnormally high blood calcium levels. Infants taking more than 400 IU every day may experience toxicity symptoms: weakness, tiredness, headache, nausea and vomiting, loss of appetite, constipation or diarrhea, excessive thirst and urination, protein in the urine, high blood pressure, high blood cholesterol, premature atherosclerosis, mental retardation, and slower-than-normal growth. In addition, calcium may be deposited in vital tissues, leading to serious consequences such as liver damage and kidney failure.

INTERACTIONS

Phenytoin and barbiturates (taken to control seizures) can stimulate the metabolism of vitamin D to inactive forms and lead to vitamin D deficiencies. See Part 6, "Vitamin, Mineral, and Herbal Drug Interactions."

THERAPEUTIC USES

Vitamin D supplements may be given to counteract the symptoms of vitamin D deficiency reviewed earlier in this profile.

However, such symptoms will not be alleviated by vitamin D unless they are, in fact, caused by vitamin deficiency.

In addition to the prevention and treatment of the deficiency diseases rickets and osteomalacia, vitamin D may be prescribed for people whose parathyroid gland is not properly functioning. The parathyroid is involved in the regulation of calcium use by the body. When the blood calcium is low, the parathyroid releases a hormone that stimulates the kidneys to convert vitamin D to its active form, calcitriol, which in turn stimulates the absorption of more calcium through the intestines and the removal of some calcium from bones. The process continues until the imbalance is corrected. An improperly functioning parathyroid will not stimulate the conversion of vitamin D to calcitriol. Plain vitamin D may be used to treat this condition, but people often do not respond even to larger doses of the vitamin. Other vitamin D derivatives, dihydrotachysterol (DHT) or calcitriol (Rocaltrol), are more effective and are used as the treatment for people who do not respond to plain vitamin D.

Conditions associated with low blood levels of phosphate, such as Fanconi's syndrome, are treated with vitamin D as well. Vitamin D can help to restore normal phosphate levels by increasing absorption from the intestine.

There is some interest in the use of derivatives of vitamin D to treat psoriasis. A topical synthetic compound with a chemical structure similar to calcitriol called calcipotriene is available as a prescription ointment (Devonex) and is helpful for some.

Vitamin D, along with calcium, is frequently recommended to help stop the bone loss of osteoporosis. A supplement with 400 IU of vitamin D and 1 to 2 g of calcium is appropriate and has been shown to help slow down the loss of bone mass and decrease fractures due to weak bones in elderly women. Giving the active form of the vitamin, calcitriol, may work better if bone loss is severe. The best advice is to try to build and maintain bone mass with exercise and good dietary calcium and vitamin intakes prior to menopause. At menopause, calcium supplements with vitamin D are a good idea.

UNSUBSTANTIATED CLAIMS

We cannot recommend that you take this vitamin for acne, aging symptoms, alcoholism, allergies, arthritis, backache, bedsores, broken bones, bronchitis, burns, cancer, canker sores, carbuncles, cataracts, the common cold, constipation, cystic fibrosis, cystitis, diabetes, eczema, emphysema, epilepsy, eyestrain, fatigue, fever, gallstones, glaucoma, herpes simplex, herpes zoster, high cholesterol, jaundice, leg cramps, liver cirrhosis, meningitis, osteoporosis, pyorrhea, rheumatic fever, sciatica, sleeplessness, stress, tuberculosis, vaginitis, or worms.

AVAILABILITY

Vitamin D, at a dose of 400 IU, is an ingredient of virtually every multivitamin formula. Pure vitamin D products are available in strengths of 400 IU to 1,000 IU per tablet. Ergocalciferol drops, capsules, tablets, and injection dosage forms are also available.

VITAMIN E

No other vitamin has attracted as much attention from both basic scientists and clinical scientists over the past decade as vitamin E. Interest grew as researchers learned that oxidative damage to vital tissues plays an important role in the development of many chronic diseases and in the aging process. The presence of vitamin E in cell membranes helps protect the cell because it serves as a fat-soluble free-radical scavenger and antioxidant. It works hand in hand with the other antioxidant vitamins and compounds in the body. Chapter 7 explains the role of antioxidant vitamins and evidence for their usefulness in maintaining good health. This section summarizes the properties of vitamin E.

FUNCTION

Vitamin E sits in cell membranes, and its primary function is as a biological antioxidant and cell membrane protector. Oxygen is life-giving, but it can also be harmful. One of the most potentially damaging reactions involving oxygen is with unsaturated fatty acids. Free radicals generated during normal metabolic reactions in which oxygen is involved can react with unsaturated fatty acids in cell membranes to form substances called organic peroxides. Organic peroxides are toxic to cells because they can take part in a chain reaction with other neighboring fatty acids, eventually destroying the cell. Without vitamin E and other antioxidant vitamins, oxygen can, in effect, convert fluidlike unsaturated fatty acids to inactive solids, rendering them unable to function. The body has several other antioxidants and free-radical-scavenging compounds that back up and complement the action of vitamin E. For example, vitamin C is needed to regenerate vitamin E after it has been inactivated by picking up a free radical.

There is ample research on this role for vitamin E. For instance, people who eat more polyunsaturated fat in their diet need more vitamin E to prevent cellular damage. Relatively little vitamin E in the diet may lead to the deposition of oxidized fats in tissues. That is not to say that vitamin E can stop the aging process; it cannot. But it is possible that vitamin E deficiency may speed the aging of essential tissues. Unless free radicals are quenched, they can react with blood fats, setting up an inflammatory process associated with atherosclerosis that leads to the formation of blood clots, and possibly heart attack. A free-radical attack on the cell nucleus can result in mutations that could lead to cancer. Low vitamin E intake has been associated with a higher risk of heart disease and cancer. Thus vitamin E's main function is unlike most other vitamins in that it does not participate in biochemical reactions. Rather, vitamin E simply acts as a sponge to soak up damaging free radicals.

DAILY REQUIREMENTS

The strength of vitamin E was originally based on measures of biological activity and expressed in international units (IU), and different forms of the vitamin have slightly different IU equivalents.

In human nutrition, the most important form of vitamin E is alpha tocopherol, and the natural form of this substance is d-alpha tocopherol. It has a strength of 1.5 IU per mg. Synthetic alpha tocopherol, dl-alpha tocopherol, comes in two types: dl-alpha tocopheryl acetate (with an acetate group to stabilize the vitamin E) has a strength of 1 IU per mg, and dl-alpha tocopherol (without the acetate) has a strength of 1.1 IU per mg. In 1980 the RDA for vitamin E was changed from IUs to d-alpha tocopherol equivalents (TE). One TE is equivalent to 1 mg of d-alpha tocopherol and also to 1.5 IU. Vitamin products still use IU to express the amount of contained vitamin E. Nutrition tables have switched to TE values, however.

Based on early studies, an RDA of 30 IU of vitamin E per day was set in 1968. In 1974 the National Research Council reduced the RDA to 10 TE (15 IU) for adult males and 8 TE (12 IU) for adult females on the basis of dietary surveys that revealed that most diets contained between 10 and 15 IU per day. The RDA value has not been altered since 1974. Since there were no obvious signs of vitamin E deficiency in the United States, it was assumed that the previous recommendation was too high. This decision was extremely controversial. On one hand, there was no evidence that 15 IU per day would not satisfy human needs for the vitamin. On the other hand, emerging knowledge of the important role vitamin E plays in removing damaging free-radical compounds in the cells suggests to many (including us) that more, not less, vitamin E is needed for optimal health. Since vitamin E is nontoxic, it is not unreasonable to push for higher intakes. This controversy is still not settled. While it would be difficult to get more than 30 IU from food, it seems prudent to increase our consumption of whole grains and unprocessed foods to increase vitamin E intake. Vitamin E supplements may be warranted as discussed in Chapter 7, "Antioxidant Vitamins."

DIETARY SOURCES

The tocopherols are made by plants, probably as protection against oxidation of their vital fatty acids. Animals pick up their tocopherols from plant sources and use them as protection from the adverse effects of oxygen. There are more than six tocopherols found in plants, but alpha-tocopherol is the most potent. Unlike vitamins A and D, which are stored only in body fat and the liver, vitamin E is found in all body tissues in the cell membranes, so it is present in meats, but in rather low amounts. Over 60 percent of the dietary vitamin E consumed in the United States comes from plants, especially from corn or cottonseed oil (in margarine), green vegetables, and wheat germ. Other good sources are listed in the accompanying table.

VITAMIN E CONTENT OF SELECTED FOODS
(Average adult RDA is 10 TE, or 15 IU)

FOOD	APPROXIMATE CONTENT (IU PER 3 OZ.)
Almonds	13.5
Almond oil	5.8
Apricot oil	19.0
Brazil nuts	5.9
Cabbage	6.4
Cashew nuts	4.6
Corn oil	19.0
Cottonseed oil	40.0
Hazelnuts	19.0
Margarine	16.2
Peanuts	6.3
Peanut oil	14.4
Safflower nuts	31.5
Sunflower seeds	28.0
Walnuts	20.0
Wheat germ	144.0
Whole wheat flour	27.0

Vitamin E is destroyed in the presence of oxygen and heat. Thus the vitamin E content of foods varies widely depending on how they were handled during processing and storage. Prolonged freezing of vitamin E–containing foods will destroy vitamin E content unless care is taken to prevent exposure to air. Eating uncooked fresh fruits and vegetables will help increase vitamin E intake.

DEFICIENCIES

Most vitamin E deficiency signs and symptoms are related to oxidative damage to cell components. One perplexing point is that while a vitamin E–deficient diet is life-threatening to animals, humans are not affected as severely. Vitamin E–deficient animals develop sterility, liver damage, muscular dystrophy, heart degeneration, and anemia, but no such vitamin E deficiency symptoms exist for humans. Part of the reason for the difference may be that vitamin E is widespread in our diets and that we have some reserves stored in our body fat.

A true human vitamin E deficiency state was not discovered until the 1960s, when a group of premature infants was accidentally given formula with no vitamin E. The infants became anemic and developed edema (swelling) that responded to vitamin E treatments. In Illinois, a group of volunteers was given a diet with low levels of vitamin E. These studies showed that red blood cells from normal individuals survived longer than cells from those who were vitamin E–deficient. There were no other obvious deficiency signs in the volunteers. The findings of this study, which originally set out to determine how much vitamin E would be needed to return the volunteers' red blood cells to normal, led to the 1968 recommendation by the Food and Nutrition Board to set the RDA at 30 IU of vitamin E.

Patients who have a problem absorbing and digesting dietary fats may with time develop a vitamin E deficiency. People with bile problems (bile is involved in fat absorption) have difficulty absorbing fats, as do premature infants and cystic fibrosis patients. After several years (less time for infants), signs of nerve damage begin to appear, leading to loss of reflexes, loss of sensation, muscle weakness, problems with eye movement, and difficulty with balance and coordination. If the vitamin E deficiency is not corrected, the damage may be irreversible.

Because of the high susceptibility of the red blood cell membranes to oxygen damage, hemolysis (bursting of red cells) may occur in people deficient in vitamin E. Patients with inherited conditions that predispose them to oxidative stress, such as glucose-6-phosphate dehydrogenase (G6PD) deficiency, are prone to vitamin E deficiency. Iron is a pro-oxidant that can place an increased demand on vitamin E stores. Patients taking an iron-containing product or those who have trouble eliminating iron from their body should take vitamin E supplements.

TOXICITY

There are no major side effects associated with vitamin E; it is remarkably nontoxic.

One of the best evaluations of vitamin E toxicity was conducted at the National Institutes of Health. Twenty-eight institute employees voluntarily took doses ranging between 100 and

800 IU a day for an average of three years. A battery of tests designed to uncover possible toxic effects was performed on each volunteer, and none was found. There are a few reports in the medical literature describing possible stomach upset, diarrhea, dizziness, and increased blood-clotting time with high doses of the vitamin, but most agree that vitamin E is nontoxic in doses below 800 IU per day.

INTERACTIONS

Vitamin E facilitates the absorption, tissue storage, and utilization of vitamin A. People who must take vitamin A to correct a deficiency should also take vitamin E. However, in huge doses (greater than 2,000 IU), vitamin E can actually slow the absorption of vitamins A and K from the gastrointestinal tract.

Vitamin E can also inhibit formation of the active forms of vitamin K, thereby inhibiting the ability of blood to clot. It can also inhibit the ability of blood platelets to aggregate. This may be beneficial, for less-sticky platelets theoretically confer a reduction in the risk of stroke, blood clots in the lungs, and heart attacks.

Vitamin E supplements should probably not be used in doses larger than 50 IU per day by people taking anticoagulant drugs, aspirin or similar drugs with an effect on platelets, or those with blood-clotting disorders.

See Part 6, "Vitamin, Mineral, and Herbal Drug Interactions."

THERAPEUTIC USES

Vitamin E is perhaps the most important of the protective antioxidant and free-radical-scavenging compounds in the body. It has a clear role in protecting the body against the damaging effects of oxygen. Higher intakes lower the risk for heart disease and cancer. This aspect of vitamin E is covered in Chapter 7, "Antioxidant Vitamins." Below are listed some other uses for vitamin E based on the ability of this vitamin to act as a fat-soluble free-radical scavenger and antioxidant.

- *Reduce environmental hazards such as ozone, nitrogen dioxide, and cigarette smoke.* Increasing levels of pollutants in our atmosphere can lead to adverse health effects because these components are reactive and cause free-radical oxidative damage. Some suggest that people who live in areas with air pollution problems should increase their intake of antioxidant vitamins, especially vitamin E. We agree.

- *Reduce cardiac toxicity of the anticancer drugs daunorubicin and doxorubicin.* These drugs are toxic to the heart muscle because they promote the formation of free-radical intermediates. Vitamin E supplements have been shown to reduce this damage.

- *Treat hemolytic anemia associated with hereditary deficiencies of the enzymes known as G6PD and glutathione peroxidase.* Both of these conditions can lead to excess oxidation and consequent damage to body tissues. Vitamin E supplements have been shown to reduce breakdown of red blood cells in people with these disorders.

- *Relieve PMS symptoms.* There are several small studies indicating that a supplement of 400 IU per day of vitamin E may reduce some symptoms of premenstrual syndrome. Vitamin E can modulate prostaglandin synthesis through its antioxidant action, and this may be a possible mechanism of action here.

- *Relieve intermittent severe leg muscle pains (intermittent claudication).* Intermittent claudication is characterized by attacks of lameness and pain brought on by walking. The pain comes from arteriosclerosis in the blood vessels of the legs; the reduced blood flow means that the calf and buttock muscles receive insufficient oxygen. Several studies have evaluated the usefulness of vitamin E in this condition by measuring the exercise tolerance of patients receiving the vitamin compared with patients who received traditional treatment and others receiving no treatment at all. By all criteria, vitamin E in doses over 400 IU per day was shown to be of some benefit after six months of continuous use.

- *Relieve nighttime leg cramps.* There is limited evidence that vitamin E might offer some benefit to those who suffer from this annoying affliction, but controlled studies on the effectiveness of vitamin E for this problem are lacking. One study showed that a dose of 400 IU, taken before bed, was effective in reducing the frequency and severity of attacks.

- *Speed healing of wounds and clearing of scars.* Although this use of vitamin E has not been thoroughly tested, many people claim to have experienced great benefit from applying vitamin E creams or the oil from vitamin E capsules directly to wounds and scars. Vitamin E cream is a cosmetically elegant, more expensive way of applying the vitamin to your skin than simply using the oil from a vitamin E capsule, which can be removed by puncturing the capsule with a pin and squeezing the oil out. Either form of the vitamin should be applied to the wound or scar two or three times a day. Presumably vitamin E is working as an antioxidant and free-radical scavenger in preventing further damage to the tender new tissue being formed during the healing process, although this has not been proven. If so, the vitamin would presumably work best when applied to a wound that has closed and is starting to heal. There are few adverse effects to this remedy, as long as you don't rub the cream or oil directly into an open wound. If you have a stubborn wound that is not healing as fast as you would like, this controversial treatment may be worth a try. But you should remember that a sore that doesn't heal may be a warning sign of cancer or another serious medical problem, so get medical attention if you have any doubts.
- *Decrease platelet aggregation.* Aggregation of blood platelets is part of the process of blood clot formation, but an increased tendency to platelet aggregation is dangerous because of the risk for the formation of unwanted clots, leading to strokes and heart attacks. Vitamin E can decrease the aggregation of platelets in doses of greater than 200 IU per day. While this is generally beneficial, you should not take vitamin E if you have blood-clotting problems or are taking "blood thinners" such as warfarin.
- *Alleviate deficiencies in cystic fibrosis patients.* Individuals with cystic fibrosis do not absorb fats, and they show deficiencies of the fat-soluble vitamins, especially vitamin E. Doses of 200 IU per day or more are needed.
- *Reduce risk of cataracts.* Studies have shown that people who take vitamin E supplements have a lower risk of

cataract formation. Lipid peroxidation may be part of the process of the formation of cataracts. More studies are needed to define the optimal doses and the extent of their benefit, but vitamin E supplements may be beneficial for this and many other degenerative conditions in the elderly.

· *Benefit people who engage in heavy exercise.* Vitamin E has long been used by athletes in the hope of improved performance. Strenuous exercise has been shown to result in increased lipid peroxidation and free-radical damage in muscle tissue. Most studies on vitamin E and exercise have been done in animals; careful studies on student athletes in England and on members of a college swimming team in Louisiana have shown that vitamin E did not help, but studies with high-altitude mountain climbers indicated that vitamin E supplements have some benefits compared to placebo. More work is needed in this area.

· *Reduce tardive dyskinesia.* Tardive dyskinesia is a side effect of antipsychotic drugs. It is characterized by involuntary head movements and may be a consequence of free-radical damage to nerves. Small studies have shown that vitamin E in very high doses (1,600 IU per day) helps reduce these movements.

· *Protect premature infants.* Premature infants have a low capacity for protection against oxidative damage. Vitamin E is sometimes supplemented to prevent damage to their lungs and eyes. Earlier use of a vitamin E injection product resulted in some deaths associated with the product, and most supplementation now is given orally.

· *Prevent cancers, heart disease, atherosclerosis, and decreased immune function.* The application of vitamin E supplements in the prevention of these diseases is considered in Chapter 7, "Antioxidant Vitamins."

· *Slow the progression of Alzheimer's disease.* A well-designed study showed that high-dose vitamin E (2,000 IU per day for three years) slowed the progression of Alzheimer's as well as did a drug called selegiline, a standard treatment. While this study does not represent a major breakthrough, this benign vitamin may help people with Alzheimer's and their families. Further study may reveal other uses in mental degeneration.

UNSUBSTANTIATED CLAIMS

Treatment of cystic breast disease

Noncancerous breast lumps affect millions of American women. Early studies indicating benefit with vitamin E have not been substantiated.

Treatment of angina

While vitamin E has a role in the prevention of heart disease and the prevention of further heart attacks after the first, it does not seem to be of help in treating angina.

Improvement of sexual function

Sorry—despite its reputation, vitamin E will not do anything for your sexual prowess. A Canadian evaluation could not demonstrate any effect of vitamin E on the sexual activities of couples when compared with a group receiving a placebo.

Vitamin E has also been promoted for other uses for which its value has not been proven. We cannot recommend that you take this vitamin to treat acne, allergies, anemia, arthritis, athlete's foot, backache, baldness, bedsores, boils, bronchitis, bursitis, colitis, the common cold, constipation, cystitis, dandruff, diabetes, emphysema, eyestrain, fatigue, fluid retention, gallstones, gout, hay fever, headache, hemorrhoids, impetigo, impotence, infertility, kidney stones, loss of vision, measles, Meniere's disease, menstrual cramps, mental illness, multiple sclerosis, muscular dystrophy, nephritis, night blindness, obesity, osteoporosis, Parkinson's disease, phlebitis, prostatitis, sciatica, sinusitis, sunburn, thyroid disease, ulcers, vaginitis, or warts.

AVAILABILITY

Another controversial point about vitamin E is the merit of using the natural form, d-alpha tocopherol, versus either of the synthetic forms, dl-alpha tocopherol or dl-alpha tocopheryl acetate. Most common vitamin products contain synthetic vitamin E. However, the natural d-alpha tocopherol seems to bind better with one of the proteins that help move vitamin E into and within the cell. The implications of this observation are that with equal amounts of synthetic or natural vitamin E, the natural would be better-utilized. Since generic natural vitamin E is readily available and not much more expensive than the synthetic kind, we recommend purchase of the natural product. But be careful: Some brands have *Nature* or *Natural* as part of the brand name, thus giving the consumer the impression that the vitamin E in the bottle is the natural kind. But unless the product label says it is d-alpha tocopherol, the vitamin E is synthetic. The "semisynthetic" d-alpha tocopheryl acetate is recommended also. The acetate group confers stability to the molecule and is readily removed by enzymes in the intestine, thereby releasing the d-alpha tocopherol.

Recently some vitamin E products have appeared on the shelves labeled as all natural vitamin E, but close examination of the label reveals that the capsules contain a mixture of natural d-alpha tocopherol and synthetic dl-alpha tocopherol. These products are basically mislabeled and should be avoided. If you want to take the all natural vitamin E, demand a product that is 100 percent d-alpha tocopherol. Some natural vitamin E products contain "mixed tocopherols." These products contain a mixture of tocopherols obtained from the plant source (usually soybeans). As far as we know, 400 IU of mixed natural tocopherols is as beneficial as 400 IU of d-alpha tocopherol. The knowledgeable consumer can make a good choice in purchasing dietary supplements, but it will require careful scrutiny of the label. When in doubt, ask your pharmacist for assistance.

Another product is micronized or emulsified vitamin E. These products are water-soluble because the vitamin has been dispersed into fine droplets in water. For those with fat-absorption problems, it may be worthwhile to use these water-soluble products because they do not need to be absorbed like fats. But if you have no problem with fat absorption, the cheaper vitamin E oil capsules will work well.

Capsules and tablets of vitamin E are available without a prescription in strengths ranging from 200 to 1,000 IU. The concentration in multivitamin products is usually 30 IU. Vitamin E ointments, lotions, and creams are also available without a prescription. The usual concentration of vitamin E in these products is 30 IU per gram.

VITAMIN K

You cannot form a blood clot without vitamin K. This fact was discovered by a Danish doctor experimenting with the diet of chickens who bled spontaneously. He named this vitamin after the Danish word *koagulation*. The term *vitamin K* refers to a series of compounds with similar chemical structures. The most important and useful vitamin K compound found in plants is called phytonadione or phylloquinone (vitamin K_1). Phylloquinone is the chemical name but the "generic" drug name is phytonadione. The latter name will be used on vitamin labels.

Bacteria found in our intestinal tract make a group of compounds known as menaquinones (vitamin K_2). Menaquinones provide some of our daily vitamin K requirement. Vitamin K_3, called menadione, can be chemically produced in the laboratory. All of the forms of vitamin K dissolve in body fat, and some people who have trouble absorbing dietary fat into their bodies must take a vitamin K supplement. Injectable and water-soluble forms of vitamin K have been developed to help these people.

FUNCTION

Blood clotting is a complex process involving at least eleven factors; all eleven factors are necessary for a clot to form. Vitamin K is needed to make the active form of the factors II, VII, IX, and X, and this is the vitamin's main function. Some research suggests that vitamin K also plays a role in the formation of bones and other proteins whose function is not well understood. Its major function is in making blood-clotting factors.

DAILY REQUIREMENTS

The Food and Nutrition Board of the National Academy of Sciences have estimated infants' need for this vitamin at about 5 mcg per day for babies up to six months and 10 mcg per day from age six months to one year. Children's requirements vary with age, from 15 to 30 mcg per day. The RDA value for adult males is 80 mcg per day and for females it is 65 mcg per day. Bacteria normally found in our intestines provide about half of

our daily requirement of vitamin K, and the rest is provided via
dietary means.

The average diet provides at least ten times the amount of vitamin K thought to be necessary for efficient blood clotting. The
only exception to this rule is the newborn infant. Infants are born
without vitamin K–making bacteria in their intestines. Newborns in most countries are routinely given 500 to 1,000 mcg of
vitamin K by intramuscular injection immediately after birth
to prevent a gradual decline in clotting factors over the days
following birth and to prevent possible bleeding. A second
dose may have to be given if the mother had been taking anticoagulant or anticonvulsant medicines or if the infant develops a
bleeding tendency. Clotting factors begin to rise to normal levels
after about a week, when the appropriate bacteria take up resi-
dence in the intestine, but the amount of vitamin K produced in
the gut varies depending on whether the infant is formula-fed
(higher) or breast-fed (lower).

DIETARY SOURCES

Vitamin K is found in a variety of plants and other food sources.
Brussels sprouts, spinach, cabbage, cauliflower, soybeans, cheddar, and Camembert cheeses are particularly rich sources. Additional good sources are listed in the accompanying table.

Vitamin K is relatively stable under normal storage and
cooking processes.

VITAMIN K CONTENT OF SELECTED FOODS
(Estimated safe and adequate intake for adults is 70–150 mcg per day)

FOOD	APPROXIMATE CONTENT (MCG PER 3 OZ)
Alfalfa	470
Asparagus	50
Bran	62
Broccoli	180
Brussels sprouts	1,350
Cabbage	225
Camembert cheese	14,500

FOOD	APPROXIMATE CONTENT (MCG PER 3 OZ)
Cauliflower	250
Cheddar cheese	20,000
Coffee beans	35
Green tea	640
Lettuce	116
Liver (beef)	81
Oats	440
Peas	40
Potatoes	72
Soybeans	270
Spinach	300
Turnip greens	585
Watercress	54

DEFICIENCIES

Infants who were not given vitamin K at birth are may have a bleeding tendency during their first five months of life. Diarrhea or antibiotics that kill bacteria in the intestine can make matters worse for infants with an already inadequate intake of vitamin K. Breast-fed infants are more likely to develop a bleeding tendency than bottle-fed babies because breast milk contains only a little vitamin K. Also, the intestinal bacteria of infants who are exclusively breast-fed apparently lack the ability to make as much vitamin K as the formula-fed infants' bacteria do. Formulas with cow's milk do contain sufficient amounts of vitamin K. For these reasons, most recommend an injection of vitamin K at birth.

Vitamin K deficiency is rare in adults and usually occurs only in people who do not have enough bile to absorb this fat-soluble vitamin; this group must receive supplemental K by injection. Long-term antibiotic therapy, which may destroy vitamin K–producing bacteria in the gut, may lead to a deficiency when coupled with a poor diet.

Deficiency Symptoms

People with a vitamin K deficiency may experience nosebleeds, blood in the urine, stomach bleeding, and many small black-and-blue marks on the skin. It is not uncommon for a person with vitamin K deficiency to vomit blood.

TOXICITY

Large quantities of vitamin K are not stored in the body, despite the fact that it is fat-soluble. Phytonadione is now the only form of vitamin K available in tablet or injection form; it is relatively free of adverse effects when given by mouth or by intramuscular or subcutaneous injection. Serious allergic reactions have been documented with intravenous administration of phytonadione, however, and this route is not recommended.

INTERACTIONS

Vitamin K can interact with oral anticoagulant drugs to decrease their effect. Therefore, if you are taking anticoagulant drugs, you should avoid foods high in vitamin K.

THERAPEUTIC USES

Because of its interaction with anticoagulant drugs, vitamin K is sometimes given as an antidote to these drugs. It is also used therapeutically in cases of prolonged intravenous feeding and in situations where antibiotics are administered to kill all micro-organisms in the intestines.

UNSUBSTANTIATED CLAIMS

We cannot recommend that you take this vitamin to treat alcoholism, cancer, cirrhosis, cystic fibrosis, gallstones, hepatitis, jaundice, or ulcers. It also will not delay aging.

AVAILABILITY

Most vitamin K products are available on a prescription-only basis because it is unusual to be deficient in this vitamin. You should not try to self-medicate clotting disorders.

Part 3

MINERAL PROFILES

10

ESSENTIAL MINERALS

CALCIUM

Every schoolchild has heard that calcium helps build strong bones and teeth. What isn't often appreciated is the critical importance of this mineral in the blood and the body's complex mechanism for ensuring that blood calcium levels remain constant at all times, even if bones must be weakened in the process of providing necessary calcium.

FUNCTION

Calcium, together with phosphorous and magnesium, is a primary ingredient of your bones, the skeletal framework that keeps you upright and mobile. Your bones and teeth contain more than 99 percent of the body's supply of calcium, yet the remaining 1 percent plays a critical role in many other important functions. Calcium is needed for normal blood clotting, blood vessel and heart function, muscle contraction, nerve function, and the storage and release of body hormones.

Bone is a dynamic tissue that undergoes constant breakdown and rebuilding. Bone formation is greater than breakdown in growing children and is balanced in healthy adults. Breakdown exceeds rebuilding in women after menopause and in *all* older adults. Each year a portion of your skeleton is remodeled; that is, it is reabsorbed and replaced by new bone. Unfortunately, less and less bone is remodeled as we get older.

If you receive between 500 and 2,000 mg a day of calcium from food and other sources, your body will absorb what it needs for day-to-day function, send some to be stored in bone, and eliminate the rest through the urine. If your average daily intake drops below these levels for any length of time, calcium will be withdrawn from bone storage sites to maintain normal body function.

The amount of calcium absorbed into the blood varies with age. Infants absorb 60 percent of all the calcium they eat. Calcium absorption declines after infancy and rises again during puberty, a furious period of growth; it remains at about 25 percent through young adulthood. In pregnant women absorption rises during the final six months of pregnancy, when fetal skeleton formation is occurring. This is true for pregnant women of any age. Calcium absorption gradually declines with age (about 0.2 percent a year) in postmenopausal women and older women and men.

Some differences in calcium absorption exist between people of different racial backgrounds. African-Americans absorb about the same amount as Caucasians, but they release less calcium from their bodies through the kidneys. The result is that African-Americans have thicker, stronger bones and suffer fewer bone fractures.

Experts agree that regular physical activity is important in determining the quantity and quality of bone. Exercise determines the strength, shape, and amount of bone, though the exact way that this is regulated is still not well understood. Regular activity builds strong bones and should be considered an integral part of any nutritional program.

Blood calcium levels are controlled by a complex hormone system involving vitamin D, parathyroid hormone, and calcitonin, a hormone normally produced by the thyroid gland.

Vitamin D regulates the absorption of calcium in the intestines by activating a transport system responsible for moving it across intestinal walls into the bloodstream. When blood calcium levels are low, vitamin D causes the kidney to reduce the amount of calcium it allows to pass out of the body and also stimulates the removal of calcium from bone storage sites. But vitamin D must be activated to perform these functions, and this is taken care of by parathyroid hormone. This hormone is also largely responsible for controlling the delicate balance between blood calcium and phosphorous levels; if calcium is high, phosphorous is excreted, and vice versa. Calcitonin is the final participant in calcium metabolism. Its function opposes parathyroid hormone. Calcitonin stops calcium from moving out of bone into the bloodstream. Calcitonin from various sources may be prescribed by a doctor to help control hypercalcemia (very high blood levels of calcium) that may be associated with cancer or some other conditions.

DAILY REQUIREMENTS

Unfortunately, evaluating calcium status is difficult because there is no single blood or other test that reflects calcium nutrition. Measuring your blood calcium level is not helpful because calcium levels are tightly managed by the body. Ideally, people should take enough calcium every day to reduce osteoporosis and bone fractures to a minimum. The information on exactly how much calcium each person should take is generally not available, but some have tried to measure bone mineral density and bone mineral content, measures of the amount of calcium in a particular area, in an attempt to arrive at reasonable recommendations for daily calcium intake.

Adequate Daily Intakes of Calcium

GROUP	AGE	ADEQUATE DAILY INTAKE (AI)
Infants (boys and girls)	0 to 6 months	210 mg
	6 to 12 months	270 mg
Children (boys and girls)	1 to 3 years	500 mg
	4 to 8 years	800 mg
	9 to 18 years	1,300 mg
Adults (men and women)	19 to 50 years	1,000 mg
	51 years and older	1,200 mg
Pregnant women and nursing mothers	14 to 18 years	1,300 mg
	19 to 50 years	1,000 mg

The latest Food and Nutrition Board recommendations for calcium intake do not include an RDA because the experts who serve on that board feel we do not know enough to determine an exact RDA. Instead, the board has established an Adequate Intake (AI) for all ages, beginning at birth. It has also established a Tolerable Upper Limit (UL) of calcium intake for people, beyond which some people can develop kidney stones or other problems. There is no known UL for infants up to one year. The

UL for children age one year and older and adults of all ages, including pregnant women and nursing mothers, is 2,500 mg a day.

DIETARY SOURCES

Most of the calcium in our diet comes from milk and milk products. Cheese and yogurt are particularly good calcium sources because most of their calcium is calcium caseinate, a highly concentrated form of calcium that the body finds particularly easy to use. Other good sources of calcium are listed in the accompanying table. It must be emphasized that palatable forms of calcium can easily be obtained from common foods. Many calcium supplements are difficult for people to take because they don't taste good and may be hard to swallow.

CALCIUM CONTENT OF SELECTED FOODS
(Adult AI is 1,000 mg to 1,300 mg)

FOOD	APPROXIMATE CONTENT (MG PER 3 OZ)
Almonds	214
Brazil nuts	171
Bread (whole wheat)	91
Carob	315
Caviar	252
Cheddar cheese	682
Dates (pitted)	53
Eggs	49
Figs (dried)	114
Haddock (fried)	41
Ice cream	112
Kelp	990
Milk	107
Molasses, light	150
Parmesan cheese	1,036
Prunes (dried)	80
Pistachio nuts	117
Raisins	56
Rhubarb	87

FOOD	APPROXIMATE CONTENT (MG PER 3 OZ)
Salmon	135
Sardines	315
Seaweed	1,710
Sesame seeds	1,080
Soybeans	214
Sunflower seeds	108
Swiss cheese	841
Walnuts	85
Watercress	135
Yogurt	105

DEFICIENCIES

With a system as complex as the one that regulates body calcium, a malfunction can occur at several points; as a result, regulating body calcium is a problem for many people. Difficulties with the amount of calcium in the blood are usually not associated with the amount of calcium you take in every day. They are more likely to be associated with the hormones that regulate calcium. People who make too much or too little parathyroid hormone or calcitonin, individuals who don't take in or make enough vitamin D, and those whose kidneys and livers cannot activate vitamin D can have blood calcium levels that are too high or too low.

High-protein diets increase the amount of calcium loss because of the need for calcium by body systems that digest proteins. In addition, some foods (rhubarb and spinach, to name two) interfere with the absorption of calcium through the intestines because they contain lots of a chemical called oxalic acid. Calcium combines with oxalic acid to form an unabsorbable compound called calcium oxalate. Though dairy products are a good source of calcium, the phosphate they also contain can be a problem, because phosphate and calcium combine to form another unabsorbable form of calcium called calcium phosphate. People concerned about getting enough calcium from their diets should depend on a variety of different sources.

Some drugs, especially those used to treat epilepsy and other seizure disorders, speed the inactivation of vitamin D and can lead to calcium deficiency. People taking phenytoin or other seizure medicines should consider taking a modest vitamin D supplement. Children taking medicine for seizure control should also take in at least 800 to 1,200 mg of calcium per day.

Deficiency Symptoms

Calcium is found all over the body. It interacts with many other nutrients and is essential to the activity of every cell. As such, changes in calcium metabolism can cause a wide variety of problems.

Children with an insufficient supply of calcium in their blood develop a disease called rickets (a vitamin D deficiency can also cause this disease). In this condition, developing bones become deformed because they are too weak to support the weight of a growing child. Rickets is rare in the United States and other developed countries because the need for calcium was recognized some time ago and many foods have added calcium in them.

Some developing countries face a major problem in childhood nutrition and associated diseases, including rickets, with its characteristic bowed legs.

In adults, calcium and vitamin D deficiency can lead to osteomalacia, a disease in which bone becomes soft and gradually bends. In osteoporosis, calcium is gradually withdrawn from healthy bone and the bone becomes thin, weak, and unable to bear normal weight and stress. This makes people with osteoporosis susceptible to broken bones. Osteomalacia and osteoporosis are significant problems in all older adults, but especially so for older white women. While there is no cure as yet, important progress has been made in understanding how the complex system that regulates calcium and its associated elements works. Exercise, calcium, vitamin D, and estrogen supplements all have a place in treating and preventing osteoporosis.

Extremely low blood calcium can cause muscle contractions, throat spasms, and convulsive seizures. These conditions require treatment in a hospital with calcium, vitamin D, and other medicines. Correcting very low blood calcium is difficult because the problem usually lies with the underlying regulatory system.

PEOPLE WHO MAY BENEFIT FROM SUPPLEMENTATION

Menopausal Women

When estrogen levels go down, there are changes in the way that the body handles calcium. Less calcium is absorbed and more passes out of the body through the kidneys. For the first five years after menopause, women lose about 3 percent of their bone mass per year. Increasing calcium intake during this period does not prevent this loss of bone mass.

Lactose-Intolerant People

Lactose-intolerant people cannot consume milk and some other dairy products because of the high lactose content in these foods. About 25 percent of all American adults are lactose-intolerant and develop diarrhea and bloating if they consume a large dose of lactose. Lactose intolerance is highest in Asians (about 85 percent), moderate in African-Americans (about 50 percent), and lowest in Caucasians (10 percent). People with lactose intolerance are at risk of calcium deficiency because they tend to avoid dairy products, but these should be replaced with other calcium-containing foods or supplements.

Vegetarians

Vegetarians may have a problem getting enough calcium because they may avoid dairy products and because vegetarian diets can be high in oxalate and phytate, agents that reduce the absorption of calcium by combining with it in the gut. Vegetarian diets also may reduce the amount of calcium that passes through the kidneys. On balance, lacto-ovo-vegetarians and people who eat a wide variety of foods seem to have fairly similar dietary calcium intakes. At menopause, the lacto-ovo-vegetarians had more bone mass, but both lose bone at the same rate after menopause.

TOXICITY

The toxic effects of excess calcium usually arise from taking too much calcium from supplements, rather than from eating too many calcium-rich foods. The three most important toxic effects of excess calcium are kidney stones, milk-alkalai syndrome (given that name because it was most common in people combining milk and excessive antacid doses to treat ulcer symptoms), and the interaction of calcium and other nutrients.

Kidney Stones

Twelve percent of Americans develop a kidney stone at some time in their lives, and usually it has been assumed that kidney stones are largely a nutritional disease. Kidney stones are associated with excess calcium and with high intakes of oxalate, protein, and vegetable fiber. However, this issue is more complex because of the relationship between calcium and other nutrients (sodium, phosphorous, and magnesium), so ingesting high amounts of calcium may be only a part of the story in developing a kidney stone.

Milk-Alkalai Syndrome

The proper name for this condition is hypercalcemia and renal (kidney) insufficiency. This group of symptoms results from a severe clinical and metabolic change that affects virtually every body system. Since stomach ulcers are now rarely treated with very high doses of antacid, the occurrence of this syndrome has declined dramatically over the years.

INTERACTIONS

In addition to its relationship with phosphorous (see "Functions"), calcium can interact with zinc, digitalis drugs, tetracycline (an antibiotic), and vitamin C. It can also affect the results of some blood and urine tests. The release of sodium and calcium from the body is linked in the kidney; when the kidney releases sodium, it also releases calcium. Finally, caffeine has been associated with a moderate increase in hip fractures in women with a low calcium intake. For details, see Part 6, "Vitamin, Mineral, and Herbal Drug Interactions."

THERAPEUTIC USES

Calcium supplements may be taken to counteract any of the standard symptoms of calcium deficiency discussed earlier in this chapter. But these symptoms will not be relieved unless they are, in fact, caused by calcium deficiency and should be discussed thoroughly with your doctor.

In addition to preventing and treating rickets in children and osteoporosis and osteomalacia in adults, calcium may play an important role in regulating blood pressure. Studies have documented the fact that men taking a daily calcium supplement of 1,000 mg had a 9 percent reduction in blood pressure in the first few weeks of taking calcium. Women taking a similar supplement experienced an average 5.5 percent reduction in blood pressure. It is likely that the people who benefited most from taking calcium were already deficient. Their positive blood pressure response is probably a reflection of correcting that deficiency.

A related group of prescription medicines, the calcium channel blockers (nifedipine, verapamil, and others), lower blood pressure because they slow the movement of calcium out of the muscle cells that line our arteries and help control blood pressure. In effect, they may play a role similar to that of the calcium supplements mentioned above in that they raise blood calcium levels and help prevent these muscles from constricting. Do not start taking supplemental calcium for high blood pressure without first talking to your doctor.

UNSUBSTANTIATED CLAIMS

We cannot recommend taking calcium for allergies, anemia, arthritis, bone fractures, cataracts, celiac disease, colitis, the common cold, constipation, diabetes, diarrhea, dizziness, epilepsy, fever, hardening of the arteries, hemophilia, hemorrhoids, high blood pressure, insomnia, leg cramps, mental illnesses, Meniere's disease, nephritis, Parkinson's disease, tuberculosis, or worms.

AVAILABILITY

Calcium is never taken in its pure form. It is always combined with other chemicals, or "salts," because that is the way it is found in nature. Different calcium salts provide different amounts of pure calcium, and you must remember to always count the amount of pure calcium in the supplement, *not* the total amount of the calcium salt, which will be inevitably larger.

CALCIUM SALT	PERCENT CALCIUM	MG CALCIUM IN 1 G
Calcium carbonate	40.0	400
Calcium glubionate	6.5	65
Calcium gluconate	9.0	90
Calcium lactate	13.0	130
Dibasic calcium phosphate dihydrate	23.0	230

So, what's the most efficient way to take calcium? A gram of calcium carbonate (also known as chalk) is the winner, giving you 400 mg of calcium for every gram of calcium carbonate you eat. When choosing a calcium supplement, remember that you will have to take more of some supplements than others to get the amount of calcium you need.

Some people prefer to take their calcium as dolomite or bone meal tablets because of their high calcium content—dolomite is about 21 percent calcium (19 g in 3 oz), and bone meal is about 40 percent calcium (36 g in 3 oz). However, calcium carbonate still wins; it has more calcium than dolomite and is safer, too. Some samples of dolomite or bone meal products have been found to have too much lead in them. Bone meal is a by-product of meat processing, and it is possible for heavy metals to find their way into the diets of animals from which bone meal is obtained. Dolomite is a mixture of calcium and magnesium mined from the ground and may also contain traces of some heavy metals.

Bone meal and dolomite are two good examples of why natural is not always better. A highly purified form of calcium carbonate, such as Tums, is your best bet. Many popular products (Os-Cal and others) have calcium, phosphorous, vitamin D, and other minerals. They have been widely promoted as calcium supplements because of their ability to provide these three important ingredients in bone metabolism.

Calcium injections are commonly used in hospitals for a variety of purposes, most frequently to treat people whose blood calcium is so low that they have muscle spasms.

PHOSPHOROUS

Phosphorous is an essential ingredient of bone, second only to calcium. These two minerals are barometers for each other, and the body maintains a constant ratio between them. Every bone in your body contains both calcium and phosphorous in a ratio of 2:1. The same ratio is found in human breast milk.

FUNCTION

About 85 percent of the phosphorous in your body is located in bone, but phosphorous is an essential part of every body tissue. It is involved in virtually every important chemical reaction, including the body's utilization of fats, proteins, and carbohydrates (sugars). Phosphorous combines with fat to form phospholipids, which are part of the basic structure of every cell. It also combines with proteins and amino acids to play an important role in cell function. Finally, phosphorous and amino acids combine to assist in the body's basic process of generating energy.

About 70 percent of the phosphorous in our diet is absorbed into the blood through the intestine, a process that is aided by vitamin D. Unless a person is deficient in phosphorous, most absorbed phosphorous is eliminated from the body through the kidneys. In adults, between 55 percent and 70 percent of dietary phosphorous is absorbed into the blood. Infants absorb from 65 percent to 90 percent of the phosphorous they take in. The rest passes out of the body in the stool. Absorption automatically increases if you are phosphorous-deficient.

Phosphate, the most common form of phosphorous found in the body, is tightly controlled by biological mechanisms because of its importance to the body. The controls are nearly the same as those discussed earlier for calcium. The primary controller of phosphorous levels is parathyroid hormone, produced by the parathyroid gland. It controls phosphorous by increasing its elimination in the urine. This is different from parathyroid hormone's effect on calcium, where it acts to reduce excretion through the kidney. Thus the natural balance between calcium and phosphorous is maintained by the parathyroid gland. When calcium is high, phosphorous is low, and when calcium is low, phosphorous is high. Calcitonin, another hormone involved in calcium regulation, increases the excretion of phosphate in the urine.

DAILY REQUIREMENT

The most recent information from the Food and Nutrition Board, which sets nutrient requirements for Americans, established phosphate Adequate Intakes (AI) for some age groups and RDAs for other age groups, because there may be no way to directly measure a phosphorous or phosphate requirement. Previous phosphate requirements were related to calcium intake.

Phosphate RDAs

GROUP	AGE	DAILY RDA OR ADEQUATE INTAKE (AI)
Infants (boys and girls)	0–6 months	100 mg (AI)
	6–12 months	275 mg (AI)
Children (boys and girls)	1–3 years	460 mg (RDA)
	4–8 years	500 mg (RDA)
	9–18 years	1,250 mg (RDA)
Adults (men and women)	19 years and older	700 mg (RDA)
Pregnant women and nursing mothers	14–18 years	1,250 mg a day (RDA)
	19–50 years	700 mg a day (RDA)

DIETARY SOURCES

Phosphorous is found in most foods because it is a critical part of all living things. In fact, most people get more phosphorous in their diet than they need. Dairy products, meat, and fish are particularly rich sources. Phosphorous is also a component of many food additives and is found in soft drinks. The phosphorous in all plant seeds, such as nuts, beans, peas, and cereals, is not well absorbed because it is tied up with phytic acid, an unabsorbable material. Additional good sources are listed in the accompanying table.

PHOSPHOROUS CONTENT OF SELECTED FOODS
(Average adult RDA is 700 mg)

FOOD	APPROXIMATE CONTENT (MG PER 3 OZ)
Almonds	454
Barley	260
Bread (enriched white)	90
Bread (whole wheat)	244
Carob	72
Cheddar cheese	430
Cheese food (pasteurized process)	679
Chicken	260
Eggs	180
Flounder	306
Ice cream	104
Lamb	190
Liver (calf's)	432
Milk	84
Peaches (dried)	105
Peanuts	366
Peas	360
Pork	180
Potatoes	59
Pumpkin seeds	1,000
Rice	200
Sardines	520
Scallops	325
Soybeans	500
Sunflower seeds	756
Tuna	315
Turkey	188
Veal	207

DEFICIENCIES

Phosphorous deficiencies are relatively uncommon, since this mineral is found in virtually every animal and plant on earth. However, the long-term use of large quantities of antacids containing aluminum hydroxide can interfere with the body's absorption of phosphorous. As little as 1 oz of aluminum hydroxide gel three times a day for several weeks can affect phosphate levels. If you must use an aluminum hydroxide antacid, consider using a phosphate supplement or foods that add phosphate to your diet.

Deficiency Symptoms

Deficiency symptoms include bone pain, loss of appetite, weakness, and easily broken bones.

TOXICITY

Too much phosphorous can lead to increased calcium loss (remember that the balance is delicate). This may result in the formation of calcium deposits outside of bone (especially the kidney), loss of calcium from bone, and bone weakness. Calcium absorption may also be reduced. Toxicity is rare, except when the kidneys are diseased and unable to remove phosphate. Aluminum hydroxide antacids and a low-phosphate diet are prescribed for phosphate toxicity.

Infants, children, and adults tend to respond well to wide variations in calcium and phosphorous intake. However, newborns in their first month of life are unusually sensitive to phosphorous intakes greater than those found in human milk. That is one of the reasons why infants who are not nursed by their mothers are given prepared formula products. Very high phosphate intake during infancy can lead to unusual growth of the parathyroid gland, calcium formations outside of bone (especially in the kidney), and low levels of some calcium-regulating hormones.

The Tolerable Upper Limit (UL) for phosphorous, beyond which toxic effects are likely to occur, are:

GROUP	AGE	DAILY UL
Infants	0–12 months	Not possible to establish a value for this group
Children	1–8 years	3 g
	9–18 years	4 g
Adults	19–70 years	4 g
	Older than 70 years	3 g
Pregnant women	14–50 years	3.5 g
Nursing mothers	14–50 years	4 g

INTERACTIONS

Aluminum antacids reduce the amount of phosphorous absorbed because they combine to form aluminum phosphate, which is unabsorbable. For the interaction between phosphorous and calcium, see "Function," above.

THERAPEUTIC USES

Phosphorous supplements may be given to counteract any of the standard symptoms of phosphorous deficiency discussed earlier in this chapter. However, such symptoms will not be alleviated unless they are, in fact, caused by mineral deficiency.

In addition, sodium phosphate is used in both oral and rectal forms as a saline type of laxative (Fleet Enema, Fleet Phosphosoda) to draw water into the intestines, increasing intestinal contractions. Overuse of these products can lead to phosphorous toxicity.

AVAILABILITY

The best phosphate supplement is probably dibasic calcium phosphate, either with or without vitamin D (depending on your vitamin D status). We do not recommend bone meal because some samples have been shown by the FDA to be contaminated with lead. Lead poisoning is more dangerous than a marginal phosphate deficiency. Dibasic calcium is pure and inexpensive and provides ample calcium and phosphate.

MAGNESIUM

Popularly known as a basic ingredient of over-the-counter laxatives, magnesium is, in fact, one of the three important "bone minerals," along with calcium and phosphorous.

FUNCTION

The body contains about 25 g of magnesium. Of this, 50 percent to 60 percent is found in bone. The rest performs essential though less familiar functions. It is required for the normal operation of over three hundred enzyme systems in the human body. It is needed for vitamin D to work, and it is involved in regulating the flow of elements across cell membranes. Its most important function in that regard relates to its role in muscle relaxation. Calcium movement across cell membranes causes muscle contractions. When calcium leaves the cell and is replaced by magnesium, muscles relax. Magnesium is also essential to the process of transmitting nerve impulses across cell membranes.

Magnesium also takes part in the process by which sugar that has been stored in the liver as glycogen is converted to glucose, so it can be used by the body for energy. This function is specifically related to the transfer of energy via moving phosphate molecules inside the cell.

Between 15 percent and 30 percent of the magnesium you swallow is absorbed into the bloodstream; absorption goes up if you eat less magnesium and goes down if you eat more. Magnesium from food sources is better absorbed than supplemental magnesium. Magnesium passes out of your body through the kidneys. Excessive alcohol and some drugs, including diuretics, can cause the kidneys to release magnesium.

Many high-fiber foods bind their magnesium, reducing the amount absorbable from them. Most studies reveal no relationship between dietary calcium levels and the amount of magnesium absorbed into the body. A high-protein diet may improve magnesium absorption and retention.

DAILY REQUIREMENTS

Daily requirements increase in young children and teens because of their rapid growth. In adults, requirements vary, but they average 410 mg a day for men and 315 mg a day for women. The difference may be accounted for by dietary differences, differences in the rate of magnesium loss via perspiration, and other factors.

Magnesium RDAs

GROUP	AGE	DAILY RDA OR ADEQUATE INTAKE (AI)
Infants (boys and girls)	0–6 months	30 mg (AI)
	6–12 months	75 mg (AI)
Children (boys and girls)	1–3 years	80 mg (RDA)
	4–8 years	130 mg (RDA)
	9–13 years	240 mg (RDA)
Teens (boys)	14–18 years	410 mg (RDA)
Teens (girls)	14–18 years	360 mg (RDA)
Adults (men)	19–30 years	400 mg (RDA)
Adults (women)	19–30 years	310 mg (RDA)
Adults (men)	31 and older	420 mg (RDA)
Adults (women)	31 and older	320 mg (RDA)
Pregnant women	14–18 years	400 mg (RDA)
	19–30 years	350 mg (RDA)
	31–50 years	360 mg (RDA)
Nursing mothers	14–18 years	360 mg (RDA)
	19–30 years	310 mg (RDA)
	31–50 years	320 mg (RDA)

DIETARY SOURCES

Rich magnesium sources include molasses, nuts, fish, and whole grains. Additional good sources are listed in the following table.

MAGNESIUM CONTENT OF SELECTED FOODS
(Average adult RDA is 410 mg a day for men and 315 mg a day for women)

FOOD	APPROXIMATE CONTENT (MG PER 3 OZ)
Almonds	242
Barley	50
Beans (canned)	33
Bluefish	220
Bread (white)	23
Bread (whole wheat)	41
Carp	230
Cod	176
Cornmeal	92
Crab (steamed)	159
Figs (dried)	64
Flounder	177
Haddock	179
Halibut	191
Hazelnuts	135
Herring (fresh)	232
Lobster	166
Mackerel	217
Molasses (blackstrap)	370
Oat cereal (dry)	101
Oatmeal	130
Oats (rolled)	125
Ocean perch	192
Oysters	130
Peanuts	185
Pike	194
Pistachios	145
Prunes (dried)	37
Raisins	32
Rice	108
Salmon	170
Scallops	189
Shad	236
Shrimp	199
Snails	225

FOOD	APPROXIMATE CONTENT (MG PER 3 OZ)
Snapper	195
Soybeans	215
Spinach	52
Sunflower seeds	315
Swordfish	177
Tuna	75
Wheat germ	290
Yellow perch	163

Surveys of "typical" diets have shown that the current magnesium intake of boys and men age nine and older is about 325 mg per day. Some studies have indicated ethnic differences in magnesium intake, with blacks taking in less magnesium than Hispanics or whites. There is no evidence for a general magnesium deficiency among people with a lower daily intake.

DEFICIENCIES

Severe magnesium deficiency, usually accompanied by low blood calcium, is easily detectable by blood tests. Hyperexcitable nerve and muscle function is the first problem usually experienced by people who are magnesium-deficient. Body magnesium depletion is also associated with heart problems, including abnormal rhythms. People taking a digitalis heart medicine may be more sensitive to that medicine if they are magnesium-deficient.

The body has become very efficient at conserving magnesium because of its importance to regular daily life. When there is a magnesium shortage, excretion through the kidney is cut back substantially. Magnesium absorption through the intestines is sharply increased when a shortage exists. These protective mechanisms work so well that shortages are rare. Magnesium deficiencies have been reported in people with alcoholism, diabetes, chronic diarrhea, or damaged kidneys, and in people given intravenous feeding that is lacking in magnesium. Seniors are at a greater risk of magnesium deficiency than younger adults because their diets are likely to be magnesium-deficient and because magnesium absorption may decline with advancing age.

Deficiency Symptoms

Deficiency symptoms include muscle contraction, convulsions, tremors, confusion, and delirium.

TOXICITY

Toxicity from dietary sources of magnesium is unknown. When it does develop, toxicity may result from magnesium supplements. The exception is kidney failure, where excess magnesium is not eliminated from the body.

Signs of magnesium toxicity are muscle weakness, fatigue, low blood pressure, confusion, loss of reflexes, and depression of respiration and heart rates. Death is possible at very high levels. However, very large oral doses of magnesium are not likely to be toxic because, as discussed in "Therapeutic Uses," magnesium has a laxative effect when taken by mouth, and diarrhea resulting from a magnesium overdose would rid the body of excess magnesium remaining in the bowels. Nevertheless, people taking very large doses of magnesium can develop the symptoms mentioned above.

INTERACTIONS

Magnesium can interact with drugs used to relax muscles during surgery, oral anticoagulant drugs, and the tranquilizer chlorpromazine (Thorazine). See Part 6, "Vitamin, Mineral, and Herbal Drug Interactions."

THERAPEUTIC USES

Magnesium supplements may be given to counteract any of the standard symptoms of magnesium deficiency discussed earlier in this chapter. However, such symptoms will not be alleviated unless they are, in fact, caused by mineral deficiency.

Magnesium is frequently used as a laxative. Magnesium sulfate (Epsom salts), magnesium hydroxide (milk of magnesia, Haley's MO), and magnesium citrate are so-called saline laxatives that draw fluid from tissues and serum into the intestine. This causes the intestine to contract. In this process, up to 20 percent of the magnesium in these products may be absorbed into the bloodstream. Ordinarily this is not a problem, because the kidney takes care of any excess magnesium in the blood.

Magnesium plays an important role in bone and mineral metabolism and can influence bone function. Magnesium deficiency may be a risk factor for osteoporosis in postmenopausal women, but its exact role in this regard is not well understood.

Another therapeutic use of magnesium stems from its depressing effect on muscle action. Magnesium sulfate injections are sometimes used to block seizures that occur with a condition known as toxemia of pregnancy.

UNSUBSTANTIATED CLAIMS

Some people may take magnesium supplements because of the fact that atherosclerosis-related heart disease tends to occur at lower rates in places with hard water, that is, water with a high mineral content. Animals given low-magnesium diets developed atherosclerosis, high cholesterol, and high triglycerides. Unfortunately, evidence of this effect in humans is lacking. Accumulation of magnesium in the body may reduce complications and risk of death in people who have had a heart attack. Studies of intravenous magnesium given to people after a heart attack reduced the number of episodes of abnormal heart rhythms, a frequent reason for sudden death after a heart attack. There is no evidence that magnesium supplements will have a similar effect.

Magnesium may play an important role in maintaining normal blood pressure. People with low magnesium intake may have high blood pressure. Studies of magnesium supplementation in people with high blood pressure have yielded conflicting results; some say it will help people with hypertension, others say it doesn't. One study of people who increased their intake of fruits and vegetables, which are high in magnesium, showed that their blood pressure declined, but that could also have been due to the fact that their diet had substantially more potassium, an important factor in lowering blood pressure. The role of magnesium supplements in lowering blood pressure has not been established.

Magnesium is involved in glucose (sugar) use by the body, and studies have shown that people with low magnesium levels are resistant to insulin. Nevertheless, there is nothing to indicate that diabetes mellitus is the result of a magnesium deficiency or that magnesium supplements could be a treatment for diabetes or could improve glucose tolerance in people with diabetes.

AVAILABILITY

Magnesium sulfate, magnesium gluconate, and a magnesium-protein complex are all available for oral use without a prescription. Injectable magnesium sulfate products require a prescription. Dolomite, a magnesium and calcium carbonate complex mined from the ground, is used by some as a source of magnesium. As in the case of calcium, the FDA has found lead contamination in some of this material, and we do not recommend you use it regularly.

IODINE

Well known as an antiseptic for cuts, iodine is actually much more important to people because of its role in the proper functioning of the thyroid gland, the body's regulator of metabolism. Not having enough iodine in the diet results in an underactive thyroid gland or a goiter, a condition in which the thyroid becomes tremendously enlarged in an effort to compensate for the lack of iodine.

Goiter was once very common in the midwestern United States because of the low iodine content of locally produced foods—inland soils have a very low iodine content. But nowadays, several factors combine to make the incidence of goiter everywhere very small, despite iodine-poor regional soils.

The most important single factor is the addition of iodine to everyday table salt. Though the addition of iodine to salt is voluntary in America, most table salt consumed here is iodized, and all such products are clearly labeled. In addition, livestock used for meat production are usually given salt licks that contain iodine, increasing the iodine content of the meat in our diet. Some fertilizers also have added iodine, and this in turn finds its way into the food we eat.

FUNCTION

Over 80 percent of iodine in our bodies can be found in the thyroid gland. Iodine is necessary for the production of the thyroid hormones thyroxine and diiodothyronine. Since thyroid hormones are the "gas pedal" for body metabolism, the rate of metabolism and the amount of heat produced by the body are both directly affected by them. A low thyroid hormone level makes you feel sluggish and tired and may cause you to gain weight, since your body is working at a slower than usual pace. An abnormally high level of thyroid hormones is characterized by nervousness and hyperactivity.

DAILY REQUIREMENTS

Your daily need for iodine is in the range of 0.1 to 0.2 mg per day. Goiter is prevented by 0.05 to 0.075 mg a day. The RDA value for iodine in adults is 0.15 mg a day, increased to 0.175 mg a day during pregnancy and 0.2 mg a day for nursing mothers.

DIETARY SOURCES

Seafood and plants grown near the sea are the richest sources of iodine. Milk is also high in iodine because dairy cattle lick iodized salt blocks. Additional good sources are listed in the following table.

IODINE CONTENT OF SELECTED FOODS
(Average adult RDA is 150 mcg (0.15 mg)

FOOD	APPROXIMATE CONTENT (MCG PER 3 OZ)
Cantaloupe	18.0
Cod	126.0
Cod liver oil	755.0
Crab	28.0
Haddock	280.0
Halibut, broiled	41.4
Herring	47.0
Lobster	90.0
Oysters	44.0
Salmon, canned	46.0
Salt (iodized)	9,000.0
Salt (sea)	85.0
Sardines (canned)	33.0
Seaweed	55,800.0
Shrimp (boiled)	117.0
Sunflower seeds	63.0
Tuna (canned)	14.0
Turnip greens	42.0

DEFICIENCIES

Severe childhood iodine deficiency resulting in a failure to make enough thyroid hormone for daily functioning can cause slowed growth, delayed sexual development, mental retardation, and deafness. Infants who had severe iodine deficiency while in the womb may suffer from cretinism (short stature and feeble-mindedness).

Goiter is the classic iodine deficiency disease in adults. It is usually caused by an underconsumption of iodine, but it can also be caused by eating large quantities of raw foods containing substances called goitrogens. These chemicals inhibit thyroid synthesis. The condition is worse when iodine intake is low, and it may be relieved by taking an iodine supplement. Goitrogens are present in vegetables such as spinach, lettuce, turnips, beets, rutabaga, kale, and cassava, but are destroyed during cooking. Goitrogen-induced goiter is rare because raw forms of these vegetables are generally not eaten in huge quantity.

On the whole, we get plenty of iodine in our daily diet and there is no reason to be concerned about iodine deficiency, provided you use an iodized salt, are not eating huge amounts of goitrogenic vegetables, and do not have an underactive thyroid gland or hypothyroidism. There are a number of reasons why one might develop hypothyroidism but iodine deficiency is rarely the cause. There is generally no reason to take an iodine supplement.

TOXICITY

Doses of iodine under 3 mg (3,000 mcg) a day are considered nontoxic but can cause a rash, headache, difficulty breathing due to an accumulation of fluid in the lungs, and a metallic taste in the mouth.

Paradoxically, eating an excessive amount of iodine (over 20 mg or 20,000 mcg a day) can cause a form of goiter known as "iodine goiter." Excessive quantities of iodine can actually inhibit the release of thyroid hormone from the thyroid gland and lead to symptoms that are very similar to those of iodine deficiency. Iodine goiter is known in some parts of Japan where large amounts of seaweed are considered a food staple and iodine intake can be as high as 50 to 80 mg a day.

Generally, there is an upward trend in the iodine content of most diets. This is caused by the overuse of iodized salt, the use of iodine-containing antiseptics on dairy cows (traces of which find their way into milk), and the use of iodine compounds as bread dough conditioners in the baking industry. Some people are concerned about this upward trend, but average consumption is still far less than would be expected to have a toxic effect.

INTERACTIONS

Iodine can interact with lithium carbonate, taken for bipolar disorder (depression), and can interfere with some blood and urine tests. See Part 6, "Vitamin, Mineral, and Herbal Drug Interactions," for more information.

THERAPEUTIC USES

Iodine supplements may be given to counteract any of the standard symptoms of iodine deficiency discussed earlier in this chapter. However, such symptoms will not be alleviated unless they are, in fact, caused by mineral deficiency.

In addition to treating underactive thyroid and goiter, iodine supplements may also be given to slow thyroid function in people with overactive thyroid glands prior to surgery to remove the gland. This is done to temporarily inactivate the gland until surgery can be actually performed and the problem permanently remedied. Radioactive iodine may be given as a way of destroying the thyroid gland without surgery.

Aside from thyroid function, iodine is widely used as a medical antiseptic. Iodine complexes, such as 1 percent povidone-iodine, that release their mineral content slowly are superior for this purpose to plain iodine solutions such as tincture of iodine because they work for a longer period of time. Regardless of form, iodine's antiseptic effect is quite effective against virtually all bacteria and many viruses. Iodine's antiseptic property is also responsible for its use as a water sanitizer. Adding a small amount of iodine to water will kill any bacteria present, making it safe to drink. Adding 3 drops of tincture of iodine to a quart of water will make the water safe to drink in fifteen minutes' time without ruining the taste of the water.

UNSUBSTANTIATED CLAIMS

We cannot recommend that you take iodine to treat angina pains, arteriosclerosis, or arthritis. It will not restore vim and vigor or solve hair problems.

AVAILABILITY

Potassium iodide tablets are available in strengths of 50 to 300 mcg (0.05 to 0.3 mg), as is a highly concentrated solution of potassium iodide called SSKI. SSKI contains 5,000 mg per teaspoonful. The solution is prescribed in drop doses.

IRON

Iron, which is so essential for healthy blood, is the one mineral in which large segments of the American population are deficient.

Menstruating women are the largest single category of people who are iron-deficient. Surveys have shown that 10 to 30 percent of women studied were deficient. Among pregnant women, 10 to 60 percent were found to be deficient. Infants from two months to two years of age are also at risk.

Enriched flours have been fortified with iron as one way of combating this problem. There has been considerable interest in government regulation to require the fortification of more foods with iron.

FUNCTION

Sixty to 70 percent of all the iron in the body is stored in hemoglobin, carried in your red blood cells. Hemoglobin performs the vital function of carrying oxygen from your lungs to the rest of your body. Hemoglobin is also a component of myoglobin, an iron protein complex found in muscle tissues. This complex helps muscles get extra energy when they are hard at work. In addition, iron is important to the function of many enzymes involved in the body's energy generation system. Iron is stored in the spleen, bone marrow, and liver.

DAILY REQUIREMENT

The RDA for iron is 10 mg for adult men and 18 mg for adult women.

DIETARY SOURCES

Liver is the single richest iron source. Egg yolk, other meats, whole-grain products, nuts, and seafood also contain substantial amounts of iron. Wine contains some iron. Additional good sources are listed in the following table.

IRON CONTENT OF SELECTED FOODS
(Average RDA is 10 mg for men, 18 mg for women)

FOOD	APPROXIMATE CONTENT (MG PER 3 OZ)
Bacon	3.0
Beef	3.0
Bone meal	74.0
Bread (white, enriched)	2.3
Bread (whole wheat)	2.3
Cashews	3.5
Carrots (raw)	0.6
Caviar	10.8
Cheddar cheese	0.9
Chicken	1.5
Chickpeas	6.2
Currants (black)	1.0
Egg yolks	2.0
Figs (dried)	3.2
Green beans	1.4
Haddock	1.0
Lentils	6.0
Liver (calf's)	8.0
Loganberries	1.0
Lychees	1.5
Milk (whole)	0.0
Molasses (blackstrap)	8.1
Mussels	5.3
Oysters (canned)	5.0
Peanut butter	1.8
Pecans	2.2
Pistachios	6.5
Pears (dried)	1.1
Persimmon (native)	2.25
Pork	2.7
Prunes (dried)	3.2
Pumpkin seeds	10.0
Raisins	3.2
Seaweed	81.0
Sesame seeds	9.0

FOOD	APPROXIMATE CONTENT (MG PER 3 OZ)
Snails	3.2
Spinach	3.0
Veal	2.9
Walnuts	5.4
Wheat germ	8.5

Eating iron-rich foods is not as much help as one might think, because we absorb only a small amount of the iron found in foods. It has been estimated that, on average, only about 10 percent of food iron is absorbed into the blood. This can increase to about 20 percent if the body's iron stores are low. Unfortunately, these are only simplified estimates; in fact, the amount of iron you absorb depends on a number of different factors.

One major consideration is the nature of iron in the food. Iron that is bound to hemoglobin—the kind that is available in red meat and liver—is easily absorbed, and as much as 20 to 30 percent of that kind of iron may be available for absorption. Inorganic iron (not bound to hemoglobin) is poorly absorbed. Only about 5 percent of the inorganic iron found in plants is absorbed.

Compounding the complexity of calculating the amount of iron available in foods is the fact that other food substances can influence the amount of iron actually absorbed. For example, nutritionists talk about "highly available" and "poorly available" meals with respect to their iron content.

- Including meat in a meal will substantially increase the absorption of inorganic iron from vegetables eaten at the same meal.
- Taking 200 mg of vitamin C a day will increase the absorption of inorganic iron by as much as 25 to 50 percent.
- Iron absorption is *decreased* by tea, antacids, tofu and other soy proteins, and the tetracycline antibiotics.

The iron content of food, especially acidic foods, can also be dramatically increased by using iron cookware. The iron content of spaghetti sauce, for example, increases from 2.7 mg per ounce to about 80 mg per ounce if prepared in a cast-iron pot.

DEFICIENCIES

The disease associated with iron deficiency is called hypo-chromic microcytic anemia. In this condition, red blood cells become smaller than normal and pale in color because of the lack of iron in the hemoglobin. Deficiency symptoms are caused by poor oxygen delivery to tissues and include listlessness, heart palpitations on exertion, fatigue, irritability, a pale appearance, cracked lips and tongue, difficulty swallowing, and a general feeling of ill health.

Deficiency can be determined by examining your blood to look at the intensity of the color of your red blood cells or by measuring the total volume of your red blood cells (the hemat-ocrit test). Other tests involve measuring the content of iron-protein complexes in the blood and bone marrow.

A true iron-deficiency anemia responds fairly rapidly to an iron supplement, but the supplement must be continued for several months to replenish your body's iron stores. It is important to remember that anemia can be a symptom of another deficiency or of another, more serious illness. It can result from folic acid deficiency or a vitamin B_{12} deficiency as well as from a lack of iron. Anemia can also be a result of an adverse drug reaction or a reaction to an environmental toxin. Chronic bleeding, such as the kind that can occur from an ulcer or a tumor, would give the outward appearance of iron-deficiency anemia. Although taking iron may relieve some symptoms of the condition, it will not cure anything other than iron deficiency. Consult your doctor to determine the exact cause of your anemia, rather than trying to treat it yourself. A delay in getting the proper treatment could have dire consequences.

PEOPLE WHO MAY BENEFIT FROM SUPPLEMENTATION

Menstruating Women

During menstruation, blood loss accounts for substantial iron loss. The average menstruating woman loses about 0.7 mg of iron a day, but this is highly variable because of substantial differences in blood loss during menstruation. A woman with a heavy menstrual flow may lose as much as 2 mg of iron a day. Working with average figures, we all lose about 0.5 to 1 mg a day, and women have another 0.7 mg loss during menstruation, giving a total daily loss for menstruating women of about 1.7 mg. Since only about 10 percent of dietary iron is absorbed, the average woman would need to take in 17 mg of iron just to replace these losses. That is why the RDA for women is set at 18 mg. Unfortunately, the average 2,100-calorie diet provides only 13 mg of iron. Thus, an average woman eating an average diet can be expected to show signs of iron deficiency.

If you are in this category, you should modify your diet to include as many iron-rich foods as possible as well as items that would enhance iron absorption. The easiest way to do this is to make sure that you eat some meat and/or a vitamin C–containing fruit every day. Alternatively, you may consider an iron supplement.

Pregnant Women

Pregnancy creates a tremendous strain on iron stores. A growing fetus needs plenty of iron, and the mother's blood volume is substantially increased during pregnancy, which further increases the need for iron. Between mother and child, the demand for iron during pregnancy is increased to the point where it may be as much as 6 mg a day. This translates to 60 mg of dietary iron a day. Since it is almost impossible to get this much iron from your food every day, pregnant women need to take an iron supplement, and it is suggested that this supplement be continued for two or three months after giving birth to build your iron stores back up.

Iron needs during breast-feeding are not substantially different from those of non-pregnant women. While some iron is lost in breast milk, this is compensated for to some extent by the decreased menstrual blood flow experienced by nursing mothers.

Infants

If the mother is well nourished, the infant should have ample iron at birth, but there may be problems afterward. While breast milk has a small amount of iron and it is well absorbed by the nursing infant, cow's milk, cereals, and other baby foods usually consumed during the first two years of life are not good sources of iron. This puts the infant at risk of developing iron-deficiency anemia, because growing children need almost as much iron as adults.

Many nutritionists now feel that infants and children should receive an iron supplement during their first two years. Baby formulas, cereals, and vitamin preparations are available with supplemental iron. Infants should be screened for iron deficiency. Those who may be deficient should receive supplemental iron.

Vegetarians

Vegetarians need to be concerned about iron, but ample amounts of inorganic iron can be absorbed if you take enough vitamin C with iron-rich foods. Surveys of vegetarians have failed to reveal any serious problem with iron nutrition in this group of people despite the theoretical concern.

TOXICITY

Doses of iron over 1,000 mg can lead to iron toxicity. Symptoms include vomiting, diarrhea, weak pulse, exhaustion, and stomach cramps. If the amount of iron taken is high enough, the overdose victim can go into coma and eventually suffer cardiovascular collapse and death.

Swallowing iron-containing tablets is a frequent cause of iron overdose in children, because many supplement products are attractive in appearance and can be mistaken for candy. *Supplements containing iron, like all supplements, should be stored in a medicine cabinet out of the reach of children.*

INTERACTIONS

Iron can interact with allopurinol (for gout), antacids, the tetracycline antibiotics, the antibiotic chloramphenicol, cholestyramine resin (Questran—for high blood cholesterol), pancreatic extract (for enzyme replacement), penicillamine (for rheumatoid arthritis), vitamin C, vitamin E, calcium, copper, zinc, and claystarch (also interferes with the absorption of iron). See Part 6, "Vitamin, Mineral, and Herbal Drug Interactions," for more information.

UNSUBSTANTIATED CLAIMS

None.

AVAILABILITY

Ferrous sulfate tablets are inexpensive, and four 320 mg tablets will provide between 25 and 50 mg of absorbed iron. For most people, taking a ferrous sulfate tablet three or four times a day is more than adequate, and there are no real advantages to other, more expensive, iron supplements.

Sustained-release or timed-release iron products should be avoided because they deliver iron to the lower reaches of the intestine, where it is less efficiently absorbed. These products are beneficial only for someone who is having trouble with stomach irritation from ferrous sulfate. Iron also tends to be constipating, and some iron supplements combine ferrous sulfate with a stool softener to minimize this problem.

Since vitamin C increases the amount of iron absorbed, it is included in many iron supplements. Between 200 and 400 mg of vitamin C is needed for maximum iron absorption.

ZINC

Interest in zinc as a dietary supplement and nutritional agent has intensified over the years since reports of zinc deficiency syndromes were published in the medical literature. Interest in zinc has also grown because Western populations seem to have marginally low zinc intakes, and inadequate zinc has been associated with poor healing and slow growth rates in children.

FUNCTION

Zinc is an essential element of more than seventy body enzymes. Its most critical role is in the synthesis of DNA and RNA, needed for cell division, cell repair, and cell growth. It also plays a crucial role in bone growth and development and aiding in normal reproductive function. In addition, zinc seems to be involved with the activation of vitamin A in the eye and is thus a factor in normal night vision.

DAILY REQUIREMENTS

The RDA for zinc is 15 mg, increased to 20 mg for pregnant women and 25 mg for nursing mothers. Most diets are marginally low in zinc, supplying 10 to 15 mg, and do not come close to supplying the amount of zinc needed by pregnant or nursing women. For this reason, be sure to choose a prenatal vitamin that contains zinc—not all do.

DIETARY SOURCES

Since zinc is so important to life processes, it is present in all living systems but is richest in meat, poultry, liver, eggs, seafood (especially oysters), and whole grains. Other good sources are listed in the following table.

ZINC CONTENT OF SELECTED FOODS
(Average adult RDA is 15 mg)

FOOD	APPROXIMATE CONTENT (MG PER 3 OZ)
Bacon	4.5
Barley	2.5
Beef	2.7
Beets	2.5
Bone meal	3.3
Bread (white, enriched)	1.0
Bread (whole wheat)	2.5
Brewer's yeast	3.5
Cheddar cheese	0.8
Chicken	4.4
Cocoa	4.4
Coconut	2.7
Corn	2.8
Eggs	1.2
Herring	100.0

FOOD	APPROXIMATE CONTENT (MG PER 3 OZ)
Lamb	4.8
Maple syrup	6.8
Molasses (blackstrap)	7.2
Oysters	145.0
Pork	3.1
Sesame seeds	9.0
Soybeans	6.3
Sunflower seeds	5.9
Turkey	12.5
Walnuts	2.5
Wheat	2.9
Wheat germ	12.5
Yeast	9.0

Unfortunately, our ability to absorb dietary zinc is not uniform. The situation is similar to that discussed for iron in that the richest and best absorbed sources of zinc are meat products. The amount of zinc we absorb from other sources depends on several factors, including food combinations and the interaction of body chemicals. Do not take zinc supplements together with coffee, brown bread, or dairy products, especially milk, cheese, or other high-calcium foods.

Another important consideration in evaluating dietary sources of zinc is the fact that the milling process that produces white flour removes most of its zinc content. Whole-wheat flour has six times as much zinc as white flour but it may not be available to the body. So-called enriched bread and flour are enriched only with a few specific vitamins and iron—not zinc.

A varied diet, including substantial amounts of raw vegetables and whole-grain products, is the best way to ensure that your zinc needs are met. Variety is important because heavy reliance on any single food item for zinc (for example, high-fiber grains) may actually decrease zinc absorption, as discussed in the next section.

DEFICIENCIES

Human zinc deficiency was first noted in the 1960s in Egypt and other parts of the Middle East where unleavened whole wheat bread was a dietary staple. Phytic acid, found in whole wheat flour, forms an insoluble complex with zinc, making it unavailable for absorption from the gastrointestinal tract. Symptoms seen in Middle Eastern boys who were zinc-deficient were slowed growth, loss of appetite, loss of taste, diarrhea, skin rash, slowed sexual (gonadal) development, and enlargement of the spleen and liver.

Another disease, called *acrodermatitis enteropathica,* is associated with inefficient zinc absorption. People with this disease have diarrhea, muscle wasting, hair loss, and skin lesions.

Zinc levels seem to fall during stress situations, trauma, and infection, and when large doses of steroids are being taken. Alcohol, even in moderate amounts, can increase the urinary loss of zinc and can impair the body's ability to combine zinc into its proper enzyme combinations in the liver. In addition, excessive copper intake can worsen an existing zinc deficiency.

Zinc deficiency may be diagnosed by clinical symptoms or by a blood test to measure the amount of zinc in your blood. An enzyme in the blood called alkaline phosphatase depends upon zinc for its activity and may also be used as an index of zinc nutrition. Each test has it drawbacks, and there is disagreement over the most accurate way to test for zinc nutrition.

PEOPLE WHO MAY BENEFIT FROM SUPPLEMENTATION

Pregnant Women and Women Taking Oral Contraceptives

Women taking oral contraceptives may develop low zinc levels because of the action of the contraceptive hormones. Low zinc levels are also observed during pregnancy, probably due to hormone changes (mimicked by oral contraceptives), although the developing fetus draws heavily on the mother's zinc supply as well. Most pregnant women get only two-thirds of the zinc RDA from their diet. While the consequences of this are not clear, it is worrisome because some animal experiments have shown that zinc deficiency can result in birth defects and low-birthweight babies.

Vegetarians

Although some nutritionists have expressed concern that vegetarian diets might not provide enough zinc, surveys conducted in vegetarian volunteers have revealed adequate zinc levels. Soybean products, often used as a protein source in vegetarian diets, may be a factor in supplying zinc and enhancing absorption.

TOXICITY

Zinc can have some adverse effects, although it is not as toxic as some other minerals. Doses larger than 200 mg have caused vomiting in adults, and higher doses can lead to dehydration, stmach pains, poor muscle coordination, tiredness, and kidney failure. High-dose zinc supplements should be taken only for a short time and only for a specific purpose.

INTERACTIONS

High zinc intakes can decrease the absorption of iron and copper. Calcium interferes with zinc absorption. Zinc interferes with the absorption of the fluoroquinolone-type and tetracycline-type antibiotics. Some researchers have said that having high levels of zinc relative to copper predisposes you to coronary heart disease, but this theory is not universally accepted.

THERAPEUTIC USES

Zinc supplements may be given to counteract any of the standard symptoms of zinc deficiency discussed earlier in this chapter. However, such symptoms will not be alleviated unless they are, in fact, caused by mineral deficiency.

Zinc oxide ointment applied to the skin has been used for many years to aid in healing burns and other wounds. Studies of the effects of zinc supplements on the healing of surgical wounds and leg ulcers have shown that zinc seems to play a role in the later stages of wound healing, that is, after about ten days. Other studies in hospitalized patients who were marginally deficient in zinc showed that zinc supplements helped speed the rate of wound healing and restore the sense of taste. Doses used in these patients were high; they took about 220 mg of zinc sulfate three times a day, which provides about 130 mg of zinc. In most studies, the only people who benefited from zinc supplements were those who were already deficient in zinc.

Zinc supplements have been studied for their effect against the common cold. The theory is that high concentrations of zinc will kill common cold viruses. Because of zinc's toxicities, the only way you can get this much zinc in contact with the cold viruses that are causing your illness is to allow a zinc tablet or lozenge to dissolve in your mouth. In one study of zinc gluconate lozenges, sixty-five adults were asked to dissolve a lozenge containing 23 mg of zinc every two hours until cold symptoms had disappeared for six hours. The researchers found that seven people had no symptoms within twelve hours and fourteen had no symptoms after twenty-four hours. Zinc lozenges can help but you must begin early, continue taking lozenges until symptoms go away, and use a product that has enough zinc to do the job! Children should take half the adult dose.

The trick is beginning to take zinc as soon as the first symptom of a cold is felt and continue taking it three times a day for several days.

UNSUBSTANTIATED CLAIMS

Zinc supplements have been used for arthritis and various cancers, but the evidence for any effect here is weak.

AVAILABILITY

Zinc tablets come in two forms, each of which provides a different amount of zinc. Zinc sulfate is 23 percent zinc and comes in several strengths, from 66 to 200 mg. Zinc gluconate is only about 14 percent zinc and is available in strengths from 10 to 78 mg.

11

IMPORTANT TRACE MINERALS

CHROMIUM

Chromium—especially as chromium picolinate—is wildly popular and is being touted as a natural way to treat obesity, control blood sugar and blood fats, increase lean body mass, and improve overall energy. In addition, people have reported that use of chromium picolinate can improve your mood and help in the treatment of depression, improve your vision and the condition of your gums, treat skin conditions (acne and psoriasis), prevent insomnia, help you deal with addictive behavior, prevent osteoporosis, and help you to live longer.

Why chromium picolinate instead of another form of chromium? The absorption of chromium appears to be related to the form in which it is taken. In animal studies, chromium is more efficiently absorbed when it is combined with an organic substance to form a compound such as chromium nicotinate or chromium picolinate. It has been estimated that chromium picolinate is absorbed between four and fifteen times more efficiently than chromium from food sources. This is because chromium picolinate passes easily into fatty tissues; nonorganic forms of chromium, such as chromium chloride, do not.

The average diet is marginally low in chromium, and some researchers believe that chromium supplements may help diabetics control their disease and even prevent prediabetics from advancing to clinical disease.

FUNCTION

Studies of the function of chromium conducted during the 1950s showed that lab animals fed a diet deficient in chromium developed glucose intolerance. That is, they could not process sugar in a normal way and developed symptoms similar to those of diabetes, including poor tolerance to sugar, high blood fat levels, poor wound healing, and reduced resistance to infection. These problems were reversed when a small amount of chromium was added to the diet of the animals in this experiment. These studies suggested that an unknown dietary factor, labeled glucose tolerance factor (GTF), was needed to maintain normal metabolism in rats. Since then a number of studies have been conducted to try to determine the effect of various chromium-containing compounds on glucose metabolism in humans. The results of these studies varied: Three reported no effect, and twelve showed that chromium supplements improved glucose tolerance. The exact structure of GTF is still not known, but it has been suggested that GTF is really chromium picolinate.

DAILY REQUIREMENTS

Chromium enthusiasts recommend 50 mcg a day for infants and children up to one year, 100 mcg for children ages one to six, 200 mcg for children ages seven to ten, 300 to 400 mcg for teenagers, and 400 mcg a day for adults up to age sixty-five. People over age sixty-five, diabetics, people trying to lower their blood cholesterol level, and bodybuilders are advised to take 600 mcg a day. However, we do not believe that there is enough information to support these recommendations. An estimated safe and adequate range for daily chromium intake in adults is 50 to 200 mcg. A carbohydrate-rich diet needs more chromium to help utilize the glucose generated from those carbohydrates, but exact amounts are unknown.

DIETARY SOURCES

Accurate information on the chromium content of many foods is lacking. Oysters, eggs, whole grains, some condiments (black pepper and thyme), mushrooms, meat, cheese, and yeast are considered good sources of chromium. Brewer's yeast provides approximately 70 mcg per ounce and is the singe richest source of chromium. Chromium from brewer's yeast is also well absorbed. Wine and beer also contain about 0.3 mg per 3 oz. The refining and processing of foods probably accounts for a great deal of natural chromium loss. Less than 1 percent of dietary chromium is absorbed into the blood.

Typical American diets seem to provide between 50 and 80 mcg of chromium a day, an amount many experts think is marginally low. The average Japanese diet provides 100 to 200 mcg a day.

DEFICIENCIES

Chromium deficiency in animals has been produced only under experimental conditions. Deficiency symptoms are disturbances in the metabolism of fat, glucose, and protein; slowed growth; and reduced longevity.

Chromium deficiency in humans with deficiency symptoms similar to these produced in animals, has been seen only in people receiving long-term intravenous nutrition without protein supplementation. Additional evidence for human chromium deficiency comes from studies of patients with adult-onset diabetes, as discussed under "Therapeutic Uses."

TOXICITY

Chromium is considered to be relatively nontoxic in doses of 1,000 mg or less. Chronic exposure to chromium dust in industrial environments been associated with increased lung cancer rates. One animal study suggested that chromium picolinate may damage chromosomes.

THERAPEUTIC USES

Several studies report that diabetics have lower blood levels of chromium than nondiabetics. The body needs insulin to move glucose from the blood into individual cells, where it can be used to generate energy. It is believed that chromium increases the sensitivity of cells to the actions of insulin. In a chromium-deficient state, more insulin is needed to maintain normal glucose utilization in the body. Chromium has no effect on glucose itself; it works only with insulin to drive sugar into cells. This effect is similar to that of several new medicines for type 2 or adult-onset diabetes.

Studies of the effect of chromium picolinate on adult-onset (type 2) diabetes are generally small and have produced mixed results. The American Dietetic Association's guidelines on diabetic diets do not include a recommendation for supplemental chromium.

Body chromium levels decrease with age, while glucose tolerance time (the time it takes for the body to utilize a standard amount of glucose) increases with age. Increased glucose tolerance can be an indication that diabetes is developing. Reliable studies have shown that chromium supplements benefit some people with abnormal glucose metabolism. Usually doses between 180 and 1,000 mcg are used, and months of supplementation are necessary before an effect may be observed. A study of the effect of daily supplements of 1,000 mcg a day of chromium on 180 type-2 diabetics in Beijing, China, suggest that this level of chromium lowers blood sugar, glycosylated hemoglobin (a long-term measure of glucose metabolism), and blood cholesterol. Lower doses of chromium had a positive but less pronounced effect on the same measures.

The implication of these studies is that the people who benefit from chromium supplements did so because they were not getting enough chromium in their diet. The type of diabetic who would receive the most benefit from supplemental chromium and the extent of any possible benefit from chromium supplementation are both unknown. Chromium supplements should be taken by people with diabetes only under a physician's supervision. They may be helpful for some, but they should *never* be used as the sole treatment for diabetes.

Several researchers have examined the role of chromium in heart and blood vessel disease. Studies have found that people with coronary heart disease have less chromium in their blood than people without heart disease. Another study found that chromium supplements significantly raise blood levels of HDL cholesterol, the "good" cholesterol.

UNSUBSTANTIATED CLAIMS

Clinical studies of other uses of chromium picolinate—to treat obesity and high blood cholesterol, reduce body fat and increase lean body mass, improve overall energy and mood, help in the treatment of depression, improve vision, improve the condition of the gums, treat skin conditions such as acne and psoriasis, prevent insomnia, help control addictive behavior, prevent osteoporosis, and extend lifespan—are inconclusive. The studies were conducted in people of different ages, physical condition, and level of activity, and did not always include a control group for comparison. Also, the measurement techniques used varied from one investigator to another, and this makes it difficult to compare the results of different studies.

AVAILABILITY

Chromium picolinate is available in a dizzying variety of brands, forms, and strengths. It is absorbed much better than chromium chloride, which is available by prescription for use in intravenous nutrition solutions and without prescription as tablets and capsules for oral use. We believe that daily chromium supplementation should be kept below 1,000 mcg a day.

COPPER

Copper has received special attention because some people are concerned that our copper intake is inadequate and that copper supplements might help prevent some heart diseases. Others point to dietary surveys over more than twenty years that show we are taking in plenty of copper and that there are no signs of deficiency.

FUNCTION

Copper is a component of the enzyme superoxide dismutase (SOD). SOD is involved in regulating oxygen levels in tissues throughout the body. It has long been recognized that excess oxygen is bad for our bodies and may be a factor in heart attacks and strokes. Superoxide dismutase is an antioxidant that prevents this by using up excess oxygen molecules. Other antioxidants are vitamins E and C. See Chapter 7 for more information on antioxidants.

Copper is also a major component of ceruloplasmin, essential for the transport of iron in the blood. Copper also affects the release of iron from the intestines into the blood and is needed to recycle iron released from red blood cells that have died.

Finally, copper participates in the maintenance of body structure by helping to link collagen—the material that provides structure to all soft tissues—to connective tissue.

Like many other minerals, copper has an element that balances its effect in the body, molybdenum, and the levels of this mineral in the body rise as copper falls and fall as copper rises.

DAILY REQUIREMENTS

Adult requirements for copper are estimated to be 2 to 3 mg a day. No RDA for copper is published, but the U.S. RDA for adults and children age four and older is 2 mg.

DIETARY SOURCES

Shellfish and organ meats are the richest sources of copper, but fish and nonleafy vegetables also provide ample copper. Additional good sources are listed in the accompanying table.

COPPER CONTENT OF SELECTED FOODS
(Average adult requirement is 2 to 3 mg)

FOOD	APPROXIMATE CONTENT (MG PER 3 OZ)
Almonds	0.60
Applesauce	0.30
Avocadoes	0.35
Bacon	0.50
Bananas	0.45
Barley	0.63
Beets	0.20

FOOD	APPROXIMATE CONTENT (MG PER 3 OZ)
Brazil nuts	1.00
Bread (white)	0.20
Bread (whole wheat)	0.20
Brown sugar	0.27
Cashew nuts	0.70
Chicken	0.25
Coconut	0.35
Corn	0.40
Eggplant	0.27
Halibut	0.10
Hazelnuts	1.30
Honey	1.50
Kale	0.27
Lamb	0.22
Lentils	0.63
Liver (calf's)	3.50
Lobster	2.00
Molasses (blackstrap)	2.00
Mushrooms	5.40
Mussels	2.90
Oats	0.67
Oysters	3.10
Peanuts	0.65
Potatoes	0.13
Rice	0.35
Salmon	0.72
Seaweed	0.55
Shrimp	0.50
Spinach	0.80
Tuna	0.45
Turkey	0.16
Walnuts	0.80
Wheat germ	2.60

Refining and milling of food and grains removes most of their mineral content. Thus, the copper content of highly refined flour is low.

Nutritional surveys have indicated that most diets provide at least 2 mg of copper a day. This, together with the fact that as much as 0.5 mg a day of copper leaches into our water from copper pipes, suggests that copper nutrition is adequate. Some more recent surveys have indicted that some people's copper intake may be about 1 mg a day; also, the trend in modern plumbing is to move away from copper pipes because of their cost. This controversy is unresolved, but it would seem that the lack of general copper deficiency symptoms indicates that we should have little concern about the need for copper supplementation.

DEFICIENCIES

Copper deficiency is rare because the mineral is so widely distributed in our food. However, iron, calcium, and vitamin C have all been shown to decrease the amount of copper we absorb. In addition, excessive doses of zinc can worsen a copper deficiency.

People with chronic diarrhea, malabsorption diseases, severe malnutrition, or kidney diseases, those being fed intravenously without a copper supplement, and some people who have had extensive bowel surgery may develop symptoms of copper deficiency. Copper deficiency (and general malnutrition) has also been found in children fed a diet consisting mostly of milk (milk is not a particularly good source of copper).

Some people are born with a copper deficiency caused by enzyme defects or an inability to absorb sufficient copper. One of these diseases is albinism, where the body is unable to make melanin, its natural skin-coloring agent. The other is called Menke's syndrome and is characterized by slowed growth, degeneration of the central nervous system, and sparse, brittle hair. Intravenous copper has been given to these children but has not been successful in prolonging their lives. Death usually occurs within a year after symptoms begin to develop.

Anemia is a major symptom of copper deficiency. This is because copper is necessary for iron to be absorbed, transported, and utilized. In animal studies, copper deficiency results in the impairment of bone formation, hair or fur formation, and disorders of the blood vessels and heart, especially weakening and degeneration of the aorta.

In contrast to what is seen with other vitamins and minerals, oral contraceptive pills seem to increase copper levels, rather than to decrease them. Increased plasma copper levels are also noted during pregnancy and during acute and chronic infections and heart attacks. The significance of these observations is not known.

Hair analysis is sometimes used as a measure of copper nutrition because minerals are known to be stored in the hair, but this test is not reliable. Urine or blood plasma levels of copper should be used instead.

TOXICITY

Copper toxicity can result from taking 10 mg or more a day from any source, including foods or vitamin supplements. Symptoms of copper toxicity are nausea, vomiting, muscle aches, stomach pains, and surprisingly, hemolytic anemia. Wilson's disease, an inherited disease of copper metabolism, results in chronic copper toxicity. People with this condition slowly accumulate copper in their bodies from birth because of their inability to remove copper through the liver. The condition causes a progressive deterioration of mental function and loss of coordination. It also causes hemolytic anemia and liver damage and is fatal if untreated. Treatment involves restricted intake of copper-rich foods, medicines to prevent the absorption of copper that is ingested, and sometimes intravenous medicines that remove copper from the body.

INTERACTIONS

See the discussions under "Functions" and "Deficiencies."

THERAPEUTIC USES

There are no therapeutic uses for copper supplements, other than the relief of a copper deficiency.

UNSUBSTANTIATED CLAIMS

Heart Disease

One group of researchers believes that the amounts of zinc and copper in our bodies should be about equal to minimize the

risk of heart disease. This theory is based, in part, on four facts:
(1) high-fiber diets, which reduce the incidence of heart disease
by lowering cholesterol, are high in phytic acid, which decreases zinc absorption; (2) exercise, also known to reduce the
risk of heart disease, causes you to perspire, and perspiration
carries zinc with it; (3) copper deficiency can increase cholesterol levels; and (4) zinc inhibits copper utilization.

The copper/zinc ratio theory is very speculative, but it does
suggest caution for people who advocate routine zinc supplementation for wound healing and other purposes. It is better to eat a varied diet to achieve adequate mineral nutrition than to take extra
supplements that might upset the body's delicate balance.

Arthritis

Researchers have found that the fluid in arthritic joints contains a
higher-than-normal copper level. Nobody knows why this is so.
Some think that this is a sign of the body's response to arthritis.
Others think that this may be a part of the problem. Copper
bracelets have long been used to prevent and treat arthritis, and
they are endorsed by many professional athletes. But there is no
good evidence that they provide any benefit; the amount of copper
absorbed would be very low. It is true, however, that copper is an
important component of superoxide dismutase, a natural antioxidant that may have a protective effect against arthritis. Some
studies have looked at organic copper complexes for the treatment
of arthritis. Unfortunately these complexes are not stable in stomach acid and so, offer no advantage over other copper formulas.

Cancer Prevention

Animal studies showed that a dietary copper supplement was
protective against certain cancers. There is no direct proof that
copper supplements can protect people against cancer, but there
is a theoretical basis for believing that copper might help because of its role in SOD. Protecting cells from damage by excess
oxygen may be important in preventing cancer.

AVAILABILITY

Copper supplements are available as 2.5 mg tablets.

FLUORIDE

Fluoride is well known for its ability to reduce tooth decay and cavities. Applying or taking fluoride for this purpose is a therapeutic, not nutritional, use of this trace mineral. Supplementation of water supplies with fluoride has been routine in many U.S. cities since the 1950s and is now commonplace in many other countries as well. Adding fluoride to the water has decreased tooth cavities and decay by 40 percent to 70 percent with no discernible harm.

Fluoride is available naturally in the soil and in water supplies. It is presumed to be essential, though no deficiency conditions in humans are known.

FUNCTION

Fluoride is mainly found in teeth and bones, but its specific biochemical function in the body is not known. It makes the outer layer of teeth more resistant to attack by acids produced by bacteria in the mouth and makes those bacteria make less acid. Fluoride's ability to reduce the movement of other minerals out of tooth enamel strengthens the enamel and makes it more resistant to decay. Even the teeth of children who get fluoride before they erupt through the gum are protected. All teeth are protected where fluoride is present in saliva and dental plaque. In bone, fluoride can replace calcium, but the resulting bone is not as strong as bone formed with calcium.

DAILY REQUIREMENTS

Exact nutritional requirements for fluoride are not known. Daily intakes range from 0.5 to 1.5 mg in areas where the water is not fluoridated and 2 to 4 mg a day in areas where the water is fluoridated. Children whose water is not fluoridated or whose water does not have naturally high levels should receive supplemental fluoride of 1 mg a day in liquid or tablet form. This is particularly important for very young children because fluoride supplements become less effective after teeth have formed.

Adequate Daily Intakes of Fluoride

GROUP	AGE	ADEQUATE DAILY INTAKE
Infants	0–6 months	0.01 mg
Children (boys and girls)	6–12 months	0.50 mg
	1–3 years	0.7 mg
	4–8 years	1.1 mg
	9–13 years	2.0 mg
Boys	14–18 years	3.2 mg
Girls (including pregnant and nursing)	14–18 years	2.9 mg
Men	19 years and older	3.8 mg
Women (including pregnant and nursing)	19 years and older	3.1 mg

DIETARY SOURCES

The fluoride content of foods varies tremendously. It is relatively high where soils are rich and local vegetables are consumed, and where the drinking (and cooking) water is fluoridated. Seafood and tea are often good sources of fluoride. Half of all fluoride you swallow is absorbed into the bloodstream after about thirty minutes, and most of the fluoride in your body is stored in bone. Excess fluoride passes out of the body through your kidneys. Additional good sources of fluoride are listed in the accompanying table, but listed fluoride content is only approximate because of the variations in local fluoride content discussed above.

FLUORIDE CONTENT OF SELECTED FOODS

FOOD	APPROXIMATE CONTENT (MG PER 3 OZ)
Apples	0.80
Cod	0.70
Eggs	0.09
Kidneys	0.80
Liver (calf's)	0.13
Salmon	0.40
Sardines	1.00
Tea	0.30*

*Amount is in 8 oz of brewed tea

DEFICIENCIES

Under careful experimental conditions, the feeding of fluoride-free diets to mice and rats for extended periods of time led to reproductive and growth problems.

TOXICITY

Excess fluoride can be a problem. Adding more than two parts per million (ppm) of fluoride to the water supply can harm teeth and lead to the deposition of fluoride in bone joints. But most incidents of excess fluoride exposure are usually caused by drinking water from deep wells that have been through fluoride-containing rock. These wells can contain fluoride in amounts far greater than 2 ppm. Fluoride overdose can also occur from taking too many sodium fluoride tablets. Too much fluoride can lead to convulsions and respiratory and cardiac failure.

Children who receive more than 20 mg of fluoride a day over an extended period of time may develop fluoride toxicity, known as fluorosis. This results in discoloration, mottling, and weakening of the tooth enamel and permanent damage to the teeth. Dietary guidelines for fluoride issued by the Food and Nutrition Board of the Institute of Medicine say that infants up to six months should receive no more than 0.7 mg a day. Infants six months to one year should receive no more than 0.9 mg a day. Children between one and three years should receive no more than 1.3 mg. Children ages four to eight should receive no more than 2.2 mg daily. Adults, including pregnant women and nursing mothers, should receive no more than 10 mg a day.

THERAPEUTIC USES

The only proven use for fluoride is the prevention of tooth decay and cavities.

UNSUBSTANTIATED CLAIMS

Some studies have suggested that fluoride supplementation can help people with osteoporosis, while others failed to show that it is beneficial. More evaluation is needed.

AVAILABILITY

Most people get fluoride by using a fluoride-containing tooth-paste. On average, studies have shown that people swallow between 0.04 mg and 0.38 mg of fluoride per brushing. The amount increases substantially if a water rinse is not used after brushing.

Fluoride tablets are available in strengths from 0.25 to 1 mg; drops are available in strengths from 0.125 to 0.25 mg per drop, and as a mouth rinse. Tablets and drops are best taken after meals, but they should not be taken together with milk or dairy products, which interfere with fluoride absorption into the blood. Some researchers have said that caffeine increases the absorption of fluoride, but others have not been able to confirm this effect. Fluoride rinses and solutions for application to the teeth are used by dentists.

MANGANESE

Manganese is an "energy" mineral that has also been promoted for its antiaging property.

FUNCTION

Manganese is a part of many body enzymes needed in the process of generating energy; they could not function without manganese. Manganese is also a component of superoxide dismutase (SOD), a very important antioxidant.

DAILY REQUIREMENTS

There is no RDA for manganese, although 2.5 to 5 mg is considered a safe and adequate intake. The U.S. RDA value for manganese is 4 mg. Typical diets provide between 2 mg and 9 mg a day of this mineral.

DIETARY SOURCES

Nuts, whole grains, seeds, fruit, and vegetables are excellent manganese sources. Tea is surprisingly rich in manganese. Other good sources of manganese are listed in the accompanying table.

MANGANESE CONTENT OF SELECTED FOODS

FOOD	APPROXIMATE CONTENT (MG PER 3 OZ)
Almonds	1.70
Avocadoes	108.00
Bananas	0.60
Barley	3.00
Beets	0.55
Brazil nuts	2.80
Buckwheat	5.20
Chestnuts	3.40
Cloves	24.00
Coconut	1.20
Flour (whole wheat)	2.00
Ginger	8.00
Grapefruit	0.70
Green beans	0.30
Hazelnuts	3.80
Lettuce	0.70
Liver	0.30
Oatmeal	4.50
Parsley	0.85
Peanuts	1.30
Peas	1.80
Pecans	3.20
Rice	1.50
Seaweed	108.00
Spinach	0.75
Sunflower seeds	2.20
Tea	0.60
Watercress	1.80
Yams	0.45

DEFICIENCIES

Manganese deficiencies in animals have caused slowed growth, skeletal abnormalities, infertility, problems with sugar and protein metabolism, abnormal gait, and increased blood-clotting time. Human deficiencies of manganese are virtually unknown. This has happened only in intravenously fed hospitalized patients in cases of an accidental lack of mineral supplementation. Manganese deficiency results in weight loss, low blood cholesterol, rash, and hair color changes.

TOXICITY

Manganese toxicity has developed only in people who took too much supplemental manganese. It has not been seen in people who ate large amounts of manganese-rich foods. People exposed to manganese oxide dust at their workplace have developed psychiatric abnormalities and nervous system disorders that resemble Parkinson's disease. This nervous system damage is irreversible.

THERAPEUTIC USES

None.

UNSUBSTANTIATED CLAIMS

Manganese, like selenium, has been promoted for an antiaging effect because of its role in controlling oxygen levels in body tissues. It has also been promoted as a treatment for some psychiatric conditions (schizophrenia) and neurological illnesses, reproductive problems, osteoarthritis, diabetes, thyroid problems, multiple sclerosis, myasthenia gravis, dizziness, stress, fatigue, absent-mindedness, and irritability. Unfortunately, it doesn't work for these uses.

AVAILABILITY

Manganese is rarely taken alone, but is included as an ingredient in most vitamin/mineral combination products.

MOLYBDENUM

Most people are familiar with gout, but many may not realize that the little-known mineral molybdenum plays a major role in the cause and prevention of the painful ailment. Trace amounts of molybdenum can be found in all body tissues, and it is required for the proper functioning of several enzymes.

FUNCTION

Molybdenum is a component of the enzyme called xanthine (pronounced *zan*-theen) oxidase, involved in converting nucleic acids to uric acid, a body waste product eliminated via the urine. Too much molybdenum leads to too much xanthine oxidase. Too much xanthine oxidase means that too much uric acid will be produced. If this persists long enough and the amount of uric acid produced is too much for the kidneys to eliminate, uric acid crystals will be deposited in bone joints, leading to attacks of gout.

Molybdenum also functions on a seesaw basis with copper. Too much molybdenum means that copper levels will drop; excess copper means that molybdenum levels will drop.

DAILY REQUIREMENTS

Exact human molybdenum requirements are not known, but the usual diet provides between 90 and 350 mg of molybdenum a day. A safe and adequate range for daily molybdenum intake is considered to be between 150 and 500 mg.

DIETARY SOURCES

The amount of molybdenum in foods varies widely with the mineral content of the soil it grows in. There are significant concentrations of this mineral in meat, whole grains, and legumes.

DEFICIENCIES

Molybdenum deficiencies are very difficult to achieve, even in animals fed molybdenum-poor diets. The only clear sign of molybdenum deficiency is depressed xanthine oxidase activity, but some molybdenum-deprived animals have had slowed growth as well. Human molybdenum deficiencies are virtually unknown except in patients fed intravenously over long periods with a solution that did not contain molybdenum. The symptoms are rapid heartbeat, rapid breathing, night blindness, and irritability.

TOXICITY

Molybdenum is not considered toxic for most people, although Soviet researchers believe that excess molybdenum may cause a goutlike set of symptoms. In one area of Russia where the soil is unusually high in molybdenum, people average daily intakes of 5,000 to 10,000 mg a day and there is a an unusually high incidence of gout.

INTERACTIONS

See "Function" for a discussion of the interaction between copper and molybdenum.

THERAPEUTIC USES

None.

UNSUBSTANTIATED CLAIMS

Molybdenum has been promoted as protection against cancer primarily because of the discovery of an area of China that had an unusually low molybdenum content and an unusually high incidence of cancer of the esophagus. It has also been promoted for prevention of dental cavities, sexual impotence, and anemia. There is no evidence to support these claims.

AVAILABILITY

Molybdenum tablets or capsules are generally not available. It may be added to some vitamin and mineral supplement products, but is not necessary. There is no reason to take supplemental molybdenum.

SELENIUM

Selenium may be very important in human nutrition because this mineral may aid in preventing some cancers.

FUNCTION

Selenium is a component of one form of an important enzyme called glutathione peroxidase. This enzyme exists in fluid in and around all body cells and it inactivates substances called peroxides, which contain high levels of oxygen. Since excess oxygen can be toxic to body cells and cause tissue destruction, peroxides pose a threat to vital tissues and membranes, causing cancer or even death.

Glutathione peroxidase is thought to be our first line of defense against peroxidase damage. Vitamin E, located inside cell membranes, is a second line of defense against peroxide. Thus, selenium and vitamin E go hand in hand in their protective role for body tissues.

DAILY REQUIREMENTS

Human selenium requirements are not known with certainty. An estimated safe and adequate daily selenium intake is between 50 and 200 mcg. Since our daily requirement is not known and many vitamin/mineral supplements do not contain selenium, we are faced with a difficult challenge when it comes to choosing a selenium supplement. Because of possible toxicity concerns, you should keep your daily intake below 100 mcg. This, together with the selenium in your food, should be ample.

DIETARY SOURCES

The selenium content of food is highly variable because of the wide variability in selenium concentrations in the soil in which foods are grown. Seafoods, organ meats, and whole grains are considered to be good sources of selenium. Fruits and vegetables are considered to be selenium-poor. Food-refining processes, cooking, and discarding the water in which foods are cooked all contribute to our difficulty in getting enough selenium in our diet.

Dietary surveys indicate that daily average intake varies from 50 to 150 mcg a day.

DEFICIENCIES

Selenium deficiency has been well documented and studied in livestock and lab animals. Animal deficiencies cause a variety of serious and life-threatening conditions, including infertility, muscular dystrophy, exudative diathesis in fowl, pancreatic fibrosis in chicks, hepatosis in pigs, and unthriftiness or sickliness in cattle and sheep. These deficient states are much the same as those associated with vitamin E deficiency, and large doses of selenium will cure most, but not all, vitamin E deficiency symptoms. Since both selenium and vitamin E play a role in protecting against oxidative damage, it is not surprising that one can sometimes be substituted for the other.

Human selenium deficiency is almost unknown, even in areas of the country where livestock suffer selenium deficiency. Selenium deficiency has, however, been seen in a few people with alcoholic cirrhosis and a few people receiving long-term intravenous feeding without added selenium. They suffered from heart problems that responded to selenium supplements. There is also speculation that Keshan's disease, a fatal heart disease seen in children living in certain sections of China, may be related to selenium deficiency.

TOXICITY

Selenium toxicity in animals can lead to blindness, excess salivation, paralysis, and difficulty breathing. Interestingly, human selenium poisoning has *not* been reported to come from foods grown in the same areas where livestock are being poisoned by selenium. Selenium poisoning has, however, been reported in several Chinese villages where drought forced villagers to eat vegetables high in selenium. In these villages, daily intakes were found to be 3,000 to 7,000 mcg a day. Villagers suffered hair and nail loss and nervous system problems.

Epidemiological studies have also demonstrated a relationship between high selenium concentrations in water and dental cavities.

THERAPEUTIC USES

Animal studies have conclusively demonstrated that selenium deficiencies increase the number and growth rate of tumors when cancer-causing chemicals are administered. High selenium intake seems to exert a protective effect in these studies. Since the selenium-dependent enzyme glutathione peroxidase protects against cellular peroxidase damage, as discussed under "Function," it seems reasonable to assume peroxidase damage is somehow related to cancer.

The only evidence that selenium may protect against tumors in man is obtained from broad-based epidemiological studies. If one compares the selenium content of drinking water with cancer death rates in various parts of the country, or even beween countries, one finds the following relationship: Higher selenium levels are associated with a lower cancer rate. Other factors obviously enter into this and cancer is still a problem in high-selenium areas. It has been estimated that the risk for some cancers is twice as high in low-selenium areas than in high-selenium areas. High selenium concentrations can be found in parts of Wyoming, Alaska, Arkansas, Mississippi, South Dakota, and Colorado. Low selenium concentrations can be found in California, Ohio, Washington, Oregon, Pennsylvania, Indiana, and New York. Breast, colon, and lung cancers, our biggest killers, seem to be affected by selenium intake.

Zinc, cadmium, and copper counteract the effects of selenium in the body, and high intakes of these minerals may even counter the cancer-protective effects of selenium, though there are no human studies to support this claim. We believe it is better to take a mineral mixture balanced by Mother Nature—that is, the kind found in whole grains and seafood—than to fool with potent mineral supplements, at least until more is known.

The association of selenium deficiency with heart problems in humans has created interest in the therapeutic benefit of selenium supplements in heart disease. The answer to this proposition is not yet in.

UNSUBSTANTIATED CLAIMS

Selenium, like manganese, has been erroneously promoted for an antiaging effect because of its role in controlling oxygen levels. Other unsubstantiated claims include detoxifying heavy metals, drugs, alcohol, and cigarette smoke; improving skin problems; increasing male potency and sex drive; and arthritis treatment.

AVAILABILITY

Some vitamin/mineral supplement formulas contain selenium, and it is also available in tablet form.

12

MINOR TRACE MINERALS

Very little is known about the role of several trace minerals in human nutrition, but animal research has revealed a possible role for some of them. As of this writing, there is no reason to supplement any of these minerals on a regular basis.

Cadmium stimulates many enzyme systems, but none of them rely on cadmium alone; they are also stimulated by other minerals. Cadmium toxicity has been reported in industrial workers exposed to cadmium dust. They developed a disease called itai-itai, which causes breathing difficulties.

Cobalt has been identified with human deficiency symptoms. The deficiency symptoms are related to its role as a component of vitamin B_{12}. Cobalt toxicity can lead to thyroid overgrowth in infants.

Nickel may interact with iron, but its exact function is not known.

Silicon may play a role in the function of our connective tissue. This is where it is most common in the body, but its exact role is not known.

Vanadium is thought to play a role in the metabolism of our bones and teeth. Many claims have been made for vanadium, but none have been proven.

The functions of *tin* and *arsenic* in human nutrition are not known.

13

ELECTROLYTES: SODIUM AND POTASSIUM

Sodium and potassium are unlike other minerals, which are small amounts of inorganic material that participate in the body's metabolic reactions. Rather, sodium and potassium are considered electrolytes, whose most important function is maintaining the proper flow of water inside and outside of body cells. They are part of a delicate balancing mechanism that controls, among other things, blood pressure.

Athletes who lose excessive amounts of sodium through perspiration and people with high blood pressure or those at risk of high blood pressure need to be concerned about maintaining proper electrolyte balance.

FUNCTION

Sodium and potassium exist in and around cells as positively charged particles, known as ions. The water surrounding body cells contains thirty-one times as much sodium as potassium. Inside the cell, the ratio is reversed, with sixteen times as much potassium as sodium. Ions cannot exist in nature. They must be combined with another ion of equal but opposite charge. The most common negatively charged ion paired with both sodium and potassium is chloride. So the most common form of sodium found in nature is sodium chloride (common salt). Potassium also is most often found as potassium chloride.

Together, sodium and potassium provide the electrical potential necessary for cell membranes to be selective as to what they will or will not allow in or out of the cell. The flow of sodium and potassium into and out of cells is self-regulated to maintain the proper concentrations of each ion inside the cell. As electrolytes flow across the cell membrane, they carry water with them.

DAILY REQUIREMENTS

It is generally accepted that people need about 1,000 mg of sodium a day, which works out to about 2.5 grams of salt, though most Americans actually eat almost twice as much. Our daily potassium requirement is 2,000 to 6,000 mg.

DIETARY SOURCES

We all know of sources of salt in our diet; they are the highly processed foods we like so much, foods such as bacon, canned and instant soup, bouillon, potato chips, pretzels and other snack foods, canned goods, and ham. Additional high-sodium foods are listed in the following table.

Because of the American penchant for salty foods, a typical diet can contain anywhere from 3,000 mg to 7,000 mg of sodium. Low-sodium diets usually provide from 500 to 2,000 mg of sodium. Clearly, as experts have noted, most of us would do well to reduce our salt intake because of the beneficial effect it would have on lowering our blood pressure. This is especially true for people who already have high blood pressure and who are taking medicines to control their pressure, but it also holds true for everyone else.

The fact that the body has a natural balance between sodium and potassium means that you should pay attention to the amount of potassium in your diet. A good way to look at it is that substituting foods with a high potassium content for high-sodium foods will help to reduce the amount of sodium in the fluid outside body cells, lowering blood pressure and improving overall health. Low-sodium diets also help your body to conserve calcium, an important consideration if you are taking extra calcium for osteoporosis.

SODIUM AND POTASSIUM CONTENT OF SELECTED FOODS

FOOD	APPROXIMATE SODIUM CONTENT (MG PER 3 OZ)	APPROXIMATE POTASSIUM CONTENT (MG PER 3 OZ)
Apples (raw)	0.9	99
Bacon	919	3
Bananas	0.9	333
Beef (dried)	3,870	180
Beef (fresh ground)	42	405
Bread (white)	474	246
Bread (whole wheat)	456	95
Butter	888	21
Cabbage	13	93
Clams	909	180
Green beans (canned)	212	86
Green beans (fresh, cooked)	4	136
Grapefruit	0.9	122
Ham (cooked)	64	292
Margarine	888	21
Milk	45	130
Orange	0.9	180
Peas (fresh, cooked)	0.8	122
Potato	4	453
Raisins	24	687
Sardines (canned)	741	495
Squash	0.9	127
Tomatoes (canned)	117	424
Tomatoes (fresh)	3	366

Raw vegetables provide significant amounts of potassium, but their canned versions have lots of added salt and should be avoided. Clams, sardines, and lima beans are rich in sodium but also relatively high in potassium. Some good high-potassium foods are bananas, raisins, potatoes, tomatoes, apples, and oranges. Some other good sources of potassium can be found in the previous table.

DEFICIENCIES

While sodium deficiency can be associated with several diseases, it is found mainly in cases of overexertion, when sodium losses due to perspiration are excessive. Generally, a strenuous workout on the first hot day of the year is more likely to cause sodium depletion than continued exercise, even during hot weather. This is because the body is able to adjust its regulating mechanisms over time to protect itself from adverse conditions. Most people adapt to heat within a few days so that, even though exercise and perspiration may continue, less sodium is lost. Sodium chloride tablets (one or two 1 g tablets for the first few days) or a salt or sport electrolyte solution can be taken to prevent or relieve the condition.

Symptoms of sodium deficiency are muscle and stomach cramps, nausea, and fatigue. Occasionally, pregnant women on sodium-restricted diets develop symptoms of sodium deficiency.

Potassium deficiency usually develops for reasons other than a poor diet. Perhaps the most common reason for concern over potassium intake is the use of diuretic drugs that cause this electrolyte to be lost from the body through the urine. This phenomenon can be controlled to some extent by reducing the amount of sodium in the diet. Normally, the kidneys eliminate large amounts of sodium and some potassium along with water. If there is less sodium to be eliminated, more potassium will be retained.

Another common reason for potassium loss is prolonged diarrhea or vomiting. Fluids in the gut are potassium-rich, and prolonged losses of those fluids call for potassium replenishment. It is also possible, though unusual, to be potassium-deficient because of long-term intravenous therapy with fluids that are potassium-poor.

Symptoms of potassium deficiency include lethargy, poor reflexes, muscle cramps and spasms, weakness and, most important, abnormal heartbeat. If a person already has heart disease, potassium deficiency can make matters worse. Potassium deficiency can also make you more sensitive to digoxin, medicine used to treat heart failure and some abnormal heart rhythms. The symptoms of this problem would be the same as for a digitalis overdose: nausea, vomiting, loss of appetite, abnormal heart rhythms, and heart failure symptoms.

TOXICITY

Most health authorities agree that excess sodium increases your risk of high blood pressure. Of course, high blood pressure increases your risk of kidney and heart disease. So while salt is not the sole cause of kidney or heart disease, it is one factor we can control. The practice of salting foods leads to a pattern of increasing the desire for salty foods. This is especially true when salt is added to children's food. By sparing the salt shaker early in life, we can minimize the desire for salty foods later in life and minimize the potential for high blood pressure and kidney and heart disease.

Salt replacement products are designed to replace the sodium ion while keeping the salty taste people like. The usual approach taken in formulating a salt replacement is to substitute potassium salts for sodium, but this can produce a metallic taste. Newer products take advantage of a wider variety of replacement ions and do not seek to totally eliminate sodium from the product. This yields a better-tasting salt replacement product.

Excess potassium could accumulate if you ate more than 18 g a day, but this is highly unlikely. Potassium toxicity usually develops in people who take a potassium supplement (usually prescribed for people taking a diuretic drug) incorrectly. Potassium toxicity can also occur in people with kidney failure. Symptoms of potassium toxicity are similar to those of potassium deficiency: muscle weakness, pain, abnormal heartbeat, and even heart failure. Intravenous calcium (as calcium gluconate) or Kayexelate resin can be prescribed to fight potassium toxicity.

THERAPEUTIC USES

There is little reason for people to take either potassium or sodium, but they may be needed to counteract a deficiency symptom of either of these electrolytes or in situations where potassium or sodium replacement is medically necessary.

UNSUBSTANTIATED CLAIMS

None.

AVAILABILITY

Salt tablets (1 g each) may be purchased without a prescription. A great many potassium products are available by prescription. Some potassium replacement products can be purchased as food supplements, but neither sodium nor potassium supplements should be taken without your doctor's knowledge. Potassium tablets have caused damage to the stomach or intestine. This risk can be minimized by taking a timed-release potassium product.

Part 4

HERBAL MEDICINE PROFILES

14

TEN TOP HERBAL REMEDIES

Plants have been the main source of medicines since humans first walked the earth. A vast store of useful information on plant remedies was passed on orally from generation to generation. Late in the nineteenth century, an effort to identify and isolate the active ingredients in useful medicinal plants emerged, with the hope of developing drugs that were more potent and targeted. These efforts lead to the discovery of many plant-derived drugs still in use today. Some examples of useful natural products are the heart medication digoxin from the foxglove plant and the anticancer drug vincristine from the periwinkle plant. Over the years, however, the use of actual herbs and natural products derived from plants fell into decline, especially in North America. Federal drug regulations now demand sophisticated and expensive clinical trials to gain marketing approval. Since herbal drugs are not easily patented, pharmaceutical companies are generally less interested in funding the research necessary to bring a new herbal product into the American market as a Food and Drug Association (FDA) approved "over the counter" (OTC) drug or a prescription drug. Instead almost all herbal products in the United States are sold as "dietary supplements," a category only loosely regulated by the FDA.

Until 1994 herbal labels could not include information on their medical uses unless those statements were proven to the satisfaction of the FDA. In 1994 the Dietary Supplement Health Education Act (DSHEA) was passed by Congress under intense political pressure. DSHEA permits "structure and function claims" to appear on herbal product labels. A dietary supplement label under DSHEA is allowed to state that a product can "help," "strengthen," "support," or "assist" a natural function of the body. With a very few exceptions (for example, a vitamin treating a vitamin deficiency) a dietary supplement product label cannot state that a product will "treat," "cure," or "relieve" a disease or abnormality as this implies a therapeutic claim. For example, the label for a representative echinacea product states that the product "supports your body's natural resistance against infection" and "helps maintain health and well-being." It would be more useful if that label could also state that echinacea is used to prevent and treat the common cold and flu and should be taken at the first sign of the common cold or flu. But such specific information would be considered a "therapeutic claim" and not permitted under DSHEA. However, many manufacturers have pushed the limitations that DSHEA entails. For example, a ginseng label states that the product "enhances physical endurance." Recently the Federal Trade Commission has taken steps to enforce DSHEA and to demand evidence for advertising claims. The regulatory process is still in a state of flux with respect to dietary supplements.

Nevertheless, the past decade has seen a tremendous resurgence of interest in herbal drugs. This interest is sparked by research being done primarily in Europe that shows strong therapeutic value for some herbals. Another factor is the emerging view that a highly targeted and potent drug may not always be the ideal approach to treating nonfatal diseases. Most herbals can be considered "soft" drugs that deliver a mixture of complex chemicals that work together to produce a beneficial effect. This mixture would be difficult, if not impossible, to duplicate by chemical synthesis. Some herbals don't treat a specific condition but "strengthen" the body so that it resists disease better. Most practitioners of Western medicine do not appreciate these concepts. Meanwhile, consumers often self-medicate with herbals without professional advice and without the appropriate information on the product label. There are a number of herbal products that are safe and effective, and these should be recommended when needed, but some cautionary notes are warranted.

- Plants can be toxic. It is best to be very conservative with herbal drugs and take only herbals that have been used for a long time without problems. You should not assume that herbals sold in the United States have been scrutinized by the FDA.

- Since herbals are classified as "dietary supplements," it is difficult to remove them from the market unless serious problems develop in their use.
- Since anyone can introduce an herbal to the market as long as it is called a "dietary supplement" and no medical claims are made, consumers need to beware of new or untested herbal products.

Herbal experts believe that the United States should emulate the German herbal regulatory system. In this system, therapeutic claims can be made for herbals if there is "reasonable" evidence for efficacy and a long history of use without serious adverse effects. Large-scale clinical drug studies may not be needed for marketing approval of an herb in Germany. We believe that the current system of regulatory controls in place for herbals and dietary supplements should be strengthened, but strengthened in a way that will allow some therapeutic claims to be made by the manufacturer if there is "reasonable evidence" to support the claims. However, there should be no compromise on safety considerations.

Another huge problem is the general lack of quality control standards for herbal drugs. Quality control allows you to be confident that the product you buy contains the ingredients on the label. There is a great temptation for unscrupulous distributors to adulterate herbal products with cheaper plants because of high demand and the resulting short supply and high costs of popular herbals. For example, analyses have revealed that some commercially available ginseng products contain *no active ingredients* (ginsenosides). Other herbal products have been adulterated with synthetic chemicals.

Several herbal trade associations and the United States Pharmacopeia are working to develop standards for herbs. These steps are welcome. Our hope is that consumers may soon be able to buy herbal products produced to a national standard. Until changes are made in the regulation and labeling of herbals in the United States, we suggest the following for consumers wishing to take herbal products.

- Read objective information on any herb you take or are going to start taking. Several books by herbal experts that provide a critical appraisal of the usefulness of herbals are listed in the references. Avoid literature written by uncritical herbal enthusiasts.

- Take only herbal products that have a history of effective use for a given disease or condition.
- Avoid herbal fads until after objective evaluations are published. Herbal products can be dangerous, and little is known about the consequences of taking many herbs for a long time.
- Buy products from herbal product manufacturers with an excellent reputation. Avoid buying inexpensive generic herbal products until better standards exist for herbals. With the growing popularity of herbals, many large pharmaceutical manufacturers (such as Boehringer Ingelheim, Whitehall-Robins, Warner Lambert, and SK-Beecham) are introducing herbals in their line of drug products. While some would argue that this entry will crowd out smaller herbal entrepreneurs, these big companies have global reputations to uphold and have the analytical resources for the quality control efforts needed to produce a quality product.
- Purchase a "standardized" product or extract if available. The product should state the amount of the active ingredients or marker compounds per capsule or tablet on the label. The label should also list suggested uses, recommended doses, precautions for use (including any adverse reactions and drug interactions), and an expiration date. Beginning in 1999, all dietary supplements are required to have these elements on the label.
- Avoid products that contain multiple herbs or herbs plus vitamins or other compounds. If you want to assess the value of an herb or herbal product for your health, other ingredients will confuse your evaluation.
- Tell your health care providers, including your pharmacist, you are using an herbal product, so that the herbal product can be part of your drug profile and adverse drug/herbal interactions can be avoided. See the "Interaction" chart on p. 385.

In this chapter we discuss ten popular herbal products that we believe are safe and effective for the uses we describe. The products we discuss continue to be in the annual lists of the "top 20" herbal products sold, and their sales have been increasing each year. For example, the annual sales of ginkgo, St. John's wort, echinacea, and saw palmetto have each more then doubled in recent years. This popularity is due in part because there is reasonable evidence from clinical studies that these products can be effectively used by consumers. Below, we profile each herbal, discuss evidence of therapeutic uses, and recommend which product to select for optimum use.

CHAMOMILE

Chamomile is, like feverfew, a member of the daisy family (Asteraceae). It is a one- to two-foot-high plant with characteristic daisylike flowers, found wild in Europe and North America but now widely cultivated for both ornamental and commercial purposes. A related plant called Roman or English chamomile is sometimes used, but the most popular and best-studied chamomile is *Matricaria recutita*, known as German or Hungarian chamomile. The dried flower heads are used for medicinal purposes. A tea made by steeping a few teaspoonfuls of the dried flowers in hot water has long been popular for upset stomach, irritation and cramping of the gastrointestinal tract, and (when applied to the skin) to speed healing of rashes and skin disorders. There is evidence to support these uses.

EFFECTS

Chamomile flowers contain 0.3 to 2 percent of a volatile oil made up of compounds that have antispasmodic and anti-inflammatory activities. Other water-soluble compounds in the flowers probably contribute to the beneficial effects as well. Most scientific attention has centered on some unusual terpenoid compounds, some bioflavonoids, and another compound called matricin. Matricin is unstable and degrades to chamazulene, thought to be one of the most important active compounds in the dried flower heads. In the laboratory, chamazulene has been shown to be a potent inhibitor of free radicals and other reactions thought to be involved in inflammatory processes in the body. Some terpenes also have been shown to have anti-inflammatory activity. Other compounds in the plant have weak antimicrobial and antiviral properties. Thus this mix of phytochemicals together provide potentially effective therapy for irritation and inflammation on the skin and in the gastrointestinal tract.

EVIDENCE OF EFFICACY

Evidence to support the uses of chamomile preparations for stomach, intestinal, and skin irritations comes from a large number of animal and laboratory studies evaluating the various components in the plant. There are no recent large-scale, controlled human trials evaluating chamomile. Nevertheless, there is a long history of use, and ample evidence from laboratory studies points to chamomile's helpfulness as an anti-inflammatory and antispasmodic.

Based on the evaluation of all available data, the German commission that regulates herbals lists the uses of chamomile as treatment of inflammation of the skin and mucous membranes (when applied to the skin), treatment of inflammation and irritation of the respiratory tract (by inhalation of the vapor from the tea), and for complaints of the anal and genital areas (again when applied to the affected area). Taken internally, it is used for gastrointestinal spasms and inflammatory conditions of the gastrointestinal tract. Chamomile is also widely used as a mild relaxant and sedative. While these uses are not proven in human studies, chamomile is safe and seems to have mild benefits.

DANGERS

Chamomile is considered safe. The only important concern relates to the plant's potential to cause allergic reactions. The Asteraceae plant family contains several allergenic plants, including chrysanthemums and ragweed, and caution is advised if you have serious plant allergies. A few severe anaphylactic allergic reactions have been reported from drinking chamomile tea, and rashes (contact dermatitis) have been reported from topical uses.

RECOMMENDATIONS

Chamomile is usually taken as a tea three or four times a day for intestinal and stomach irritations. An infusion or proprietary extracts can be used as a mouthwash and gargle for oral and throat inflammation or can be applied directly to the skin. Avoid contact with the eyes. For the commercial extracts, follow the package directions. These uses are safe and have mild beneficial effects.

ECHINACEA

The most commonly cultivated species of echinacea (pronounced ek-i-nay-sha) is known botanically as *Echinacea purpurea*. The application of this herb in medicine is of American origin. Native Americans knew the beautiful purple coneflower as a valuable medicinal herb to "purify the blood." In the late 1800s the Lloyd brothers of Cincinnati first sold echinacea as an herbal product for treating infections. With the introduction of sulfa drugs in the 1930s and antibiotics in the 1940s, echinacea fell into disuse, though it has remained popular in Europe and is one of the leading pharmaceutical products in total sales, including the sales of conventional medications. In Germany, echinacea is listed for supportive use in colds and other upper respiratory infections.

Most commercially available echinacea products that have been tested for immune effects are standardized hydroalcoholic extracts of the plant or its juice. These products are, in effect, concentrates of the active principals of the plant. Less is known about the benefit of the whole dried herb.

The root or flowering tops of the plant contain a number of interesting compounds that have effects in stimulating the immune system and increasing the activities of the white blood cells that fight invading microorganisms. The water soluble polysaccharides in the plant seem to be important as immune stimulants but other chemicals such as cichoric acid and rutin probably are active also. Like so many of the botanicals, the exact compound or compounds in echinacea responsible for the therapeutic effects are not known.

EVIDENCE OF EFFICACY

Despite all of the interest and the popularity of echinacea as an agent to boost the immune system and to treat and prevent colds and flu, few studies have tested echinacea for these purposes. Most of the studies have examined the ability of extracts of echinacea to enhance indexes of the immune function, and the results indicate that they do. Nevertheless, the critical question of whether immune stimulation improves the body's ability to resist colds and flu is largely unanswered. One Swiss study tested a proprietary cold preparation with echinacea versus placebo on thirty-two adults. The investigators found that colds were a day shorter and less severe in the echinacea-treated group. Unfortunately, the product being tested also had 100 mg of vitamin C in it, so we cannot say for sure that the treatment success was due to the echinacea. Another study showed that 900 mg of echinacea significantly reduced flu symptoms compared to a placebo and a 450 mg dose of echinacea. A liquid extract of echinacea also was reported to reduce the length and severity of colds and flu over a two-month test period in 108 subjects.

Recent evidence suggests that taking echinacea every day to try and prevent colds or flu is not the best way to use this plant. The body may adapt to prolonged use of an immunostimulant so that it no longer works. A large German study of 300 volunteers found no benefit for use of a liquid extract of two types of echinacea twice a day for three months compared to use of a placebo for prevention of colds and flu. We believe that it is better to take echinacea at the first sign of the cold/flu and during the time symptoms are present. We are convinced that it works for many people when used in this way.

There is some evidence that echinacea treatment may decrease the recurrence rate of vaginal candida infections and that topical use might be useful for minor skin infections. Extracts of echinacea are also being tested in cancer patients to see if immune stimulation will improve survival times.

DANGERS

Echinacea and extracts of echinacea are considered nontoxic. Allergic reactions are possible, particularly if you are allergic to plants of the daisy family.

RECOMMENDATIONS

The extent to which echinacea might reduce the incidence and length of colds and flu is unknown; more studies are needed. As a whole, the literature points to echinacea's ability to enhance the immune system. The results from the few trials that have been reported indicate an ability to reduce both the incidence and severity of colds and flu. Taking echinacea in doses of 250 to 500 mg twice a day at the first sign of a cold or flu is worthwhile. Echinacea may have a future role as an adjunct to cancer and AIDS treatment.

Echinacea liquid extract (tincture) is preferred by us because it comes into direct contact with mouth and throat tissues, where local immunity is important in stopping the virus from attaching to tissues. Place the equivalent of 250 to 300 mg of extract of echinacea in a glass of water, swish it around in your mouth, and then swallow the liquid, three times a day. Capsules are readily available and can be opened and the content placed in juice or water and used like the liquid extract form in the mouth and throat. The crude dried herb in capsule form is also available, but the extract is more potent and is preferred. Chronic use is not advised unless recommended and monitored by a qualified health care professional.

FEVERFEW

Feverfew, *Tanacetum parthenium,* is a common, short bushy perennial plant that grows up to three feet tall and often can be found growing wild along roadsides. It is a member of the daisy family (Asteraceae) and has characteristic daisylike flowers with a yellow center and white outer leaves. It is now cultivated for medicinal use. The leaves, and sometimes the flowering tops, are used. The plant has long been used for a variety of medical problems including headache, fever (hence the common name), problems with menstruation and childbirth, stomach pain, and tooth pain. There was considerable attention in British newspapers during the late 1970s about the use of feverfew for the relief of migraine headaches. This led to scientific evaluation of plant components and to several human clinical trials.

EFFECTS

Feverfew contains relatively high concentrations of a compound called parthenolide, thought to be responsible for the plant's anti-inflammatory and antimigraine activity. Good-quality feverfew contains about 0.2 percent parthenolide. Laboratory studies have shown that parthenolide inhibits the release of a neurotransmitter called serotonin in blood platelets. The assumption is that parthenolide also blocks platelet serotonin release in the brain. This would be beneficial in preventing and treating migraine attacks because the release of platelet serotonin is thought to be part of the process involved in blood vessel dilation, which is characteristic of a migraine attack. Parthenolide may also help reduce migraine pain as well. Parthenolide can also inhibit an important enzyme called cyclooxygenase, which is involved in the synthesis of thromboxanes—mediators of inflammation in the body—so there is also interest in feverfew for the treatment of arthritis.

EVIDENCE OF EFFICACY

The limited research available to date indicates that feverfew is helpful in preventing and treating migraine headaches. This statement is based on the results of two scientifically conducted clinical trials reported in the 1980s and basic research on the physiological activities of parthenolide. Feverfew is listed as safe and effective by the Health Protection Branch of Health and Welfare, Canada, and is approved in the United Kingdom for migraine.

In the first trial, seventeen patients who had been taking feverfew for migraine continued taking feverfew (50 mg per day) or started on placebo capsules for six months. The nine placebo patients experienced a worsening in the frequency and severity of headaches, while the eight feverfew patients experienced no change in their migraines. In 1988 a larger, more conventional clinical trial was reported from the experiences of seventy-two volunteers. A one-month placebo phase was started, followed by a random assignment to placebo or feverfew (82 mg per day) for four months. After four months, the drugs were switched so that each volunteer had four months of placebo and four months of feverfew. Patients on feverfew had less frequent and milder migraine attacks. Even while still not having been told which drug they were taking, 59 percent of the patients could tell which one they were currently taking by the effect on their migraines. Seventeen percent could tell no difference. Feverfew had no special side effects.

A well-designed six-month clinical trial evaluating feverfew (70 to 86 mg per day) in the treatment of arthritis indicated no benefit compared to placebo.

DANGERS

Plants in the daisy family are well known for causing allergic reactions, so this is a potential side effect that must be kept in mind when taking feverfew. There have been some reports of mouth ulcers from chewing the leaves, but no allergic reactions or mouth ulcers were reported in the clinical trials using capsules of the dried leaves. Feverfew is generally regarded as having few side effects.

RECOMMENDATIONS

Migraine sufferers may benefit from a trial of feverfew. The clinical trials employed doses of between 50 and 82 mg per day, while Canadian health authorities have listed 150 mg per day of dried leaves containing 0.2 percent parthenolide as being safe and effective. We suggest taking a capsule or tablet product containing dried leaves with a labeled parthenolide concentration of at least 0.2 percent. Choose a name-brand, quality product. There have been reports of products with little to no parthenolide on the market. Taking 150 mg a day for at least six months is an adequate test to determine if you will benefit from this treatment.

GARLIC

Now here is a remarkable plant: a great culinary ingredient with medicinal benefits. We eat the perennial bulb of this three- to four-foot-high plant, which has been cultivated and used both as a condiment and for medicinal purposes since antiquity. From warding off vampires to treating infections, this little bulb has long been revered. Now proof is beginning to come in to support some of its folkloric uses.

The plant is a member of the lily family and is related to onions, shallots, and leeks. Garlic's botanical name is *Allium sativum*. You know what it looks and tastes like.

EFFECTS

The best evidence for a medical effect of garlic is in lowering blood cholesterol levels. Evidence for a benefit in preventing cancer and treating infections is preliminary. Other uses for which garlic has been promoted include its ability to lower blood pressure and its blood-thinning effect, but these lack scientific and clinical support at present.

Garlic has some very unusual organic compounds, the most important being a compound called alliin, the compound responsible for garlic's odor. Crushing and chewing the garlic releases an enzyme that causes alliin to be converted to allicin. Allicin and its breakdown products are the beneficial medicinal ingredients in garlic. When garlic is eaten, they are absorbed into the blood through mouth tissues.

It would be ideal to be able to mimic this situation when taking garlic pills. The challenge is to minimize the characteristic odor of garlic and still have effective levels of allicin and the other compounds thought to be therapeutically important. It seems to us that there are two options: Eat lots of garlic with your evening meal and/or take enteric-coated garlic powder tablets. If these tablets are made by drying garlic at low heat, they will still have alliin and the converting enzyme. Apparently, once alliin is released in the intestine and is acted upon by the enzyme, the resulting allicin and other breakdown products bind to food digestion products, minimizing the garlic odor.

EVIDENCE OF EFFICACY

Garlic is one of the best-studied herbals, but it is still not clear just how effective garlic therapy can be. Numerous animal studies show that garlic lowers high cholesterol, decreases signs of atherosclerosis, decreases excessive blood clotting, and reduces high blood pressure, all under experimental laboratory conditions. In humans, more than twenty-five clinical trials have been performed on the ability of garlic to lower blood lipids. Two large statistical analyses of the many separate clinical studies have concluded that garlic powder preparations lower cholesterol by about 12 percent. These same statistical analyses concluded that triglycerides, another undesirable blood fat, were also lowered by garlic doses of 600 to 900 mg per day. On the other hand, several recent well-conducted studies have found no effect of several months of garlic treatment on lowering excess blood cholesterol and other lipids. In these studies, the patients were placed on a low-fat diet and adherence to the diet was carefully controlled. Our assessment of the total evidence is that it is likely that there is overall benefit from taking garlic in cases of mild elevated blood lipids in patients consuming their usual diet. However, professional medical monitoring is needed to make sure garlic is having the desired effect.

There are fewer studies of the usefulness of garlic in lowering blood pressure. Nevertheless there seems to be a modest pressure reduction after a few months. For example, one trial of garlic studied forty-seven patients with mild hypertension. After twelve weeks of taking garlic, diastolic blood pressure in the garlic group was lowered from an average of 102 to 89, whereas the average pressure in the placebo group changed from 97 to 93 (nonsignificant).

What about other dosage forms of garlic and even raw cloves? Unfortunately, there is less information here. Small decreases (6 to 7 percent) in cholesterol have been obtained with an aged garlic extract (another way to eliminate the odor), and a small study found that eating one clove a day for four months reduced cholesterol and serum thromboxane (involved in unwanted blood clot formation). More work is needed to evaluate fresh garlic clove use, but the available results seem to indicate that culinary levels of fresh garlic taken daily could prove beneficial in preventing heart problems.

There is also interest in garlic as a cancer preventative. Some population studies, for example, show that groups consuming a lot of garlic (for example, in Italy and Spain) have a low prevalence of stomach cancer. Animal studies show that garlic consumption or consumption of allicin (but not alliin—see above discussion) reduces growth of some cancers. We don't know yet if the results from these animal studies are applicable to humans, but more study is certainly warranted.

Garlic has a long folkloric use in treating infections. Lab tests with garlic extracts and various other compounds from garlic show that they slow the growth of some pathogens. There is some evidence that putting garlic extracts on the skin might work against minor infections. The concentrations of garlic extracts that one can reach in blood and tissues with reasonable garlic intake are not enough to do the job, however; antibiotics will be needed for any significant infection.

DANGERS

Heartburn and odor are the major problems with eating garlic. Since garlic reduces the ability of blood to clot (useful in preventing heart attack and stroke), it is wise to avoid very high doses of garlic if you are taking other drugs that thin the blood. People at risk of bleeding problems should avoid garlic, except as a seasoning.

RECOMMENDATIONS

There are many unanswered questions about the medical usefulness of garlic. Product selection is the biggest unknown. As discussed earlier, the enzyme that converts alliin to allicin, its active form, must be preserved. Stomach acid and heat destroy this enzyme. Studies need to be done to determine the best form of garlic (fresh cloves, dried powder, or oil) for medical purposes and to determine if garlic treatment complements treatment with other drugs.

At the present time, we recommend liberal dietary garlic use. It tastes great and may offer several health benefits. If one has borderline high blood pressure or high blood cholesterol, garlic may be worth a try to bring values into the normal range. This should be done under a doctor's care because these conditions are dangerous and may need to be treated with established medicines. Garlic is a safe, effective, mild treatment, but don't expect it to fix seriously high blood pressure or high cholesterol.

If you want to take garlic for its therapeutic benefits, we recommend you eat lots of garlic and take a standardized (1.3 percent or greater alliin content) name-brand enteric-coated garlic powder tablet, at least until more is known about garlic's best dosage form.

GINGER

One of the world's important spices, ginger *(Zingiber officinale)* is, and has been since antiquity, consumed in significant quantities by many millions of people and is obviously a very safe herb. It is found naturally in tropical Asia but is now cultivated widely; Jamaica and China are big ginger producers. The plant is two to three feet in height with beautiful orchidlike flowers. The rhizomes (rootlike stems that send roots below and stems above) of this plant are of culinary and medicinal interest. You can buy fresh ginger rhizome or dried, powdered ginger in any supermarket. Both have a characteristically pungent taste and odor used to flavor foods and beverages (ginger ale, for example).

EFFECTS

In addition to its dietary uses, ginger has been known since ancient times as a digestive aid and as a way of relieving stomach gas and cramps. More recently, ginger has been used to prevent nausea and vomiting. The rhizomes contain a volatile oil that gives ginger its pungent odor, but the active compounds are thought to be the same as those responsible for the pungent taste, namely gingerol, shogaol, and chemically related compounds in the rhizome. These compounds have some interesting physiological activities under experimental conditions including the ability to inhibit platelet adhesion, decrease diarrhea, inhibit formation of stomach ulcers and intestinal tumors in laboratory animals, and block synthesis of prostaglandins. The latter are important mediators of inflammation and have many diverse activities in the body. The ability to reduce prostaglandin synthesis in the stomach and intestine might be the mechanism for ginger's antinausea effect.

EVIDENCE OF EFFICACY

The evidence is strongest for ginger's antinausea effect, yet even here the literature is not in full agreement. Of five placebo-controlled trials studying ginger for motion sickness, three said it worked and two said it did not. One study tested ginger versus placebo on eighty new naval cadets at sea. Vomiting and cold sweats were reduced compared to placebo, but nausea and dizziness or fainting were not. Another study placed thirty-six volunteers in a machine that spun them around. Those taking ginger were able to stay in the machine longer (336 seconds) than those receiving dimenhydrinate (also known as Dramamine) (216 seconds) or placebo (90 seconds). Yet another study done by a different group showed a significant antinausea effect for scopolamine (a prescription antinausea agent) but not for ginger compared to placebo.

There is also disagreement on ginger's ability to reduce postoperative nausea and vomiting. Several studies show that taking ginger before anesthesia reduces the number of episodes of nausea, while other studies were not able to demonstrate such an effect.

What can be concluded about ginger's ability to prevent nausea? In weighing the evidence, the German commission that regulates herbals determined that ginger is effective for indigestion and motion sickness at a dose of 2 to 4 g per day. We agree. There are very few nonprescription options for nausea. While its effectiveness has not been conclusively proven, ginger is nontoxic and worth trying if you suffer from motion sickness and nausea. We hope this spice will be studied in larger well-designed human studies.

One area of tremendous interest is whether ginger is safe and effective for nausea during the early stages of pregnancy. Currently there are no drugs approved for this purpose. One small study tested thirty pregnant women with particularly severe morning sickness. Patients received 250 mg of ginger or a placebo four times a day. About 70 percent preferred ginger to placebo and claimed some relief. One researcher has raised the question of ginger affecting testosterone binding in the fetus on the basis of ginger's ability to inhibit thromboxane syntheses, but this is speculative, and more recently one research group has reported that ginger does not affect thromboxane production in humans. Nevertheless, there is great concern about any drug used during the early months of pregnancy because of unknown risks for birth defects. With ginger, there is neither evidence of anything to worry about nor any evidence to establish its safety during pregnancy. Ginger proponents claim that its widespread use in foods without apparent harm to the fetus proves that it is safe, but most tread more cautiously due to a lack of hard information.

Neither the German commission nor the United States Pharmacopeia recommend that ginger be used medicinally during pregnancy. We also believe, however, that unremitting nausea during pregnancy is not without risk for the unborn. The expectant mother may not be able to eat, inadequately nourishing the fetus. Vomiting may also make her dehydrated, stressed, and subject to electrolyte imbalances. If nausea is serious and prolonged, the tiny risk of a problem for the fetus caused by ginger is probably smaller than the real risks of prolonged nausea and vomiting.

Many other uses have been suggested for ginger, such as a digestive aid, cough expectorant, or antiulcer agent, but there is little evidence to support them.

DANGERS

Ginger is considered nontoxic. Occasional allergic reactions have been noted from inhalation of the powder, and some people complain of heartburn.

RECOMMENDATIONS

Ginger is worth trying for the prevention and relief of motion sickness and nausea. Ginger may be worth a trial for severe and prolonged nausea and vomiting in early pregnancy, but no studies have been done to prove its safety, so talk to your doctor before taking anything.

Suggested doses for the prevention of nausea are 500 mg to 1 g of the dried powder taken thirty minutes to one hour before travel or surgical anesthesia. Repeat doses may be needed. For treatment of nausea, a total of 2 g of dried ginger per day in divided doses is appropriate.

GINKGO BILOBA

Ginkgo biloba is a commonly cultivated tree in many countries. The trees are long-lived (up to a thousand years) and have been estimated to have been growing on this planet for nearly 200 million years. The Ginkgo Petrified Forest State Park in Washington State, near the Columbia River, contains exposed petrified logs of trees that were growing millions of years ago. The tree is adaptable to an urban climate and is a common streetside tree in many large cities. Good examples are found near the White House and Washington Monument in Washington, D.C., and on the campus of the University of California, Berkeley. The fan-shaped leaves and the seeds from the fruit are mentioned in ancient Chinese pharmacopeias (drug compilations), and traditional Chinese medicine uses teas prepared from the leaves as remedies for asthma and bronchitis. Only since the 1950s, however, has a very valuable therapeutic property of the plant been discovered: its ability to improve blood circulation.

The development of ginkgo as a therapeutic agent is an excellent example of the value of a strong commercial interest in the product. A German firm developed an extract of the tree leaves that contained concentrations of compounds large enough to exert a beneficial effect on circulation. This company patented the extraction process and funded many of the better human studies to define the herbal's therapeutic usefulness.

EFFECTS

Ginkgo contains two types of compounds that contribute most of the beneficial effects on blood. One type, the bioflavonoids, was discussed briefly in conjunction with vitamin C. Bioflavonoids derived from citrus fruits have been used to improve capillary blood flow. There is some scientific evidence for this use, as these compounds seem to make capillaries less brittle and "leaky." Flavonoids also are strong antioxidants and stop blood platelets from sticking together (see Chapter 7). Ginkgo leaves contain several flavonoids of importance: quercetin, kaempferol, and isorhamnetin. Ginkgo flavonoids are linked to sugars, so they are called flavonoid glycosides. The commercial extracts that have been studied are standardized to contain 24 percent ginkgo flavonoid glycosides.

Terpenoids are the other important group of compounds in ginkgo. Terpenoids are very common in plants, but ginkgo has several unique diterpenes. Ginkgolide B blocks a platelet aggregating factor manufactured in the body. There is also evidence that the terpenoids may protect nerve cells and help in the nerve repair process as well as having a favorable effect on capillary circulation.

EVIDENCE OF EFFICACY

The standardized extract from the leaves of *Ginkgo biloba* is the best-studied herbal product available. There have been over forty clinical trials of ginkgo extract, and its effectiveness seems established for two conditions: poor blood flow to the brain (cerebrovascular insufficiency) and legs (peripheral circulatory problems). The signs of poor blood circulation in the brain include poor short-term memory, confusion, slow mental response times, dizziness, ringing in the ears, depression, mood swings, and anxiety. These signs are also often present in senile dementia and in early Alzheimer's disease. The relatively common condition known as intermittent claudication is a result of poor peripheral circulation. Characteristically, a person with intermittent claudication is unable to walk very far before cramping and pain in leg muscles become unbearable. Insufficient blood supply means that the lack of oxygen delivered to muscles in the legs results in pain, fatigue, and possible further injury.

Animal studies have clearly demonstrated that ginkgo extract improves blood flow to the brain and is a powerful antioxidant. In human studies, intravenously administered extract increased circulation in patients with poor blood flow. Several studies in older patients have shown ginkgo extract treatment to improve various test scores measuring memory and learning abilities. The doses used were 120 to 240 mg per day. It took three to six months for demonstrable improvements.

Recent studies conducted in Germany and the United States suggested ginkgo provides some benefit in early Alzheimer's disease and dementia. In the German study, 28 percent of people who took ginkgo responded, as compared with 10 percent who received placebo—a highly significant finding. In the U.S. study, treatment with 120 mg of the ginkgo extract for one year resulted in an overall delay in progression of the disease compared to placebo. While the benefits were modest, the treatment was well tolerated. Given that traditional medicines have little impact on the progression of Alzheimer's disease, a modest improvement with ginkgo is exciting. More studies to see if higher doses and longer treatment with ginkgo will be even more beneficial are clearly needed. It would be also of interest to evaluate a combination treatment of ginkgo and vitamin E, since vitamin E is an excellent antioxidant shown to have some benefit in Alzheimer's disease (see vitamin E section).

Treatment effects are easy to measure in people with intermittent claudication. You simply measure the distance patients can walk on a treadmill. Studies comparing ginkgo to placebo have shown ginkgo to have a significant benefit. A recent analysis of all published clinical studies concluded that ginkgo extract was useful for the treatment of peripheral artery disease. Doses of at least 120 mg of ginkgo per day for at least six months were tested. As with Alzheimer's disease and senile dementia, standard drug treatment of intermittent claudication is not very satisfactory, and ginkgo could play a valuable role in treatment.

Questions that should be addressed in future clinical studies include:

- Will ginkgo treatment improve memory and mental function in younger, disease-free individuals?
- Can ginkgo treatment delay Alzheimer's disease and senile dementia?
- What other circulatory diseases will respond to ginkgo treatment?
- Will the combination of ginkgo and other conventional drugs be synergistic in treatment?
- How much should you take and when should you take it?

DANGERS

The manufacturer of *Ginkgo biloba* extract claims that over seven thousand patients have taken its product under clinical study conditions without serious side effects. They list headache, gastrointestinal upset, and allergic reactions as possible side effects. Given the ability of some ginkgo components to inhibit platelet aggregation, one concern we have is the possibility that ginkgo treatment will result in hemorrhage. Indeed, there have been recent reports of hemorrhage with ginkgo use. Ginkgo was not absolutely established as the cause, but users must be aware of this uncommon but serious side effect. If you have a tendency to clot slowly, are taking a blood thinner such as Coumadin, or are taking aspirin or Ticlid to block platelet adhesion, it seems prudent to avoid ginkgo.

RECOMMENDATIONS

Ginkgo biloba extract is reported to be among the most-prescribed medicines in France and Germany, and its use is growing rapidly in North America. This ancient tree seems to be useful in circulatory disorders, but the true value of ginkgo preparations will be evident only after more study.

It is important to remember that ginkgo leaves probably don't contain enough of the active constituents to provide a therapeutic effect. All ginkgo studies showing benefit have tested a concentrated leaf extract. Commercially available extracts are usually a fifty-fold concentrate. If you want to take ginkgo to improve circulation, you should use a standardized extract of *Ginkgo biloba* leaves. As discussed earlier, it is better to buy an established, brand-name product, preferably the products based on the original German patent. In the United States, the label of these products will say "original standardized *Ginkgo biloba* extract" and "made using a patented process."

We believe that treatment with 120 mg to 240 mg of a standardized extract of *Ginkgo biloba* leaves containing 24% flavonoid glycosides and 6% terponoids for poor blood flow to the brain and intermittent claudication may be worthwhile. Treatment must be continued for at least three months before benefit will be noticed. Avoid taking other drugs that affect blood clotting while you are taking ginkgo.

GINSENG

There is great confusion about terminology for the medicinal herb ginseng, and it is important that you understand what you are purchasing.

- *Panax ginseng,* which has the common name Asian or Korean ginseng, is the best studied and best documented with respect to uses. If you wish to purchase ginseng, this is the one we recommend.
- American ginseng is *Panax quinquefolium,* Japanese ginseng is *Panax japonicum,* and Himalayan ginseng is *Panax pseudoginseng.* Note that these are all *Panax* species, part of the Araliaceae family.
- The herb called Siberian ginseng is not a *Panax* species but an *Eleutherococcus* species, a different plant altogether. It has different chemical constituents and should not be considered ginseng.

Panax ginseng can be found growing (now cultivated) in China, Korea, and Russia. In the United States, *Panax quinquefolium* grows wild in the hardwood forests of the eastern half of the United States and Canada. It is in high demand and has been overharvested to the point of being an endangered plant. Now ginseng harvesting is tightly regulated. Cultivation of the plant is important, but growth is slow and the grower must wait five to six years before the roots are considered ready for market. These difficulties make ginseng expensive; wild ginseng is exorbitantly expensive. The plant is a perennial, reaching a height of two feet. The feature that probably attracted early human healers to ginseng is the root system of the plant. The long taproots often have the appearance of a human with body (main root) and two legs (side roots). Sometimes a third large taproot gives the appearance of a phallus, reminiscent of the male human form, and this appearance has led to ginseng's mystique of being a virility enhancer.

To add to the confusion, numerous products are made from the roots. Red ginseng is Asian ginseng cured by steaming and drying. White ginseng is the unheated dried root. Various extracts of the root are also available, as well as root powders to be used for teas.

EFFECTS

Ginseng has been used as a sort of panacea for thousands of years in the Orient, particularly in China, Korea, and Japan. There it is believed to counteract fatigue and stress, increase resistance to disease, increase physical (including sexual) stamina, and improve mental functioning, among other health benefits. It probably cannot do all of these things. But can it do some of these things? Probably yes, to some extent.

Ginseng has been called an adaptogen, meaning it helps the body adapt to stress and disease and, in the process, will help "normalize" body functions. Ginseng cannot cure disease, but it is said to strengthen the body to help prevent and fight disease. These concepts are foreign to Western medicine, and until recently health providers considered ginseng to be an expensive Asian placebo. The only way to determine ginseng's properties is to subject it to the same kind of scientific evaluation as other drug substances.

The chemistry of ginseng is reasonably well understood. Ginsenosides, which have the most important physiological activity, are steroidlike molecules found in the roots. Good-quality roots contain 2 to 3 percent ginsenosides, and good-quality commercial standardized extracts contain at least 4 percent ginsenosides. Other compounds in the ginseng root that contribute to its activities include coumarins, flavinoids, and polysaccharides.

EVIDENCE OF EFFICACY

Animal studies have shown that ginseng can increase physical performance (treadmill time, for example), increase resistance to physical stress (cold temperatures), improve memory (in maze tests), enhance markers of immune function, and reduce the number and growth rate of some slow-growing tumors in mice. Ginsenosides can function as antioxidants and free-radical scavengers, decreasing heart tissue injury. They increase the release of nitric oxide, a mediator of blood vessel vasodilation, improving blood flow. These effects might explain ginseng's alleged ability to alleviate impotence.

But not all of these studies are well conducted and controlled, and the results of animal and tissue studies are not easily translated to humans. Nevertheless, several recent studies in humans indicate promise for ginseng in man. Unfortunately, not all of the human studies are scientifically valid, many studied a small number of patients or volunteers, and the studies were of short duration. Interestingly, almost none of these clinical studies was carried out in the United States or Canada.

A study from Korea, where ginseng use is widespread, involved nearly two thousand hospitalized patients. The investigators found that among people with and without cancer, ginseng users were more likely to be cancer free (75 percent versus 62 percent). Ginseng extract or dried powder seemed to be more protective than the fresh root or tea. Unfortunately, this study did not control for smoking and diet, factors known to influence cancer. Nevertheless, this finding and the findings of many animal studies are encouraging and justify further research on the role of ginseng in cancer prevention.

One possible mechanism for the anticancer effects of ginseng is its ability to improve immune function, as indicated by animal studies. In an interesting Italian study, 227 volunteers received either placebo or a standardized extract of ginseng (100 mg) for twelve weeks. All participants received an influenza vaccination four weeks into the study. After the flu shot, forty-two people in the placebo group had a cold or flu, compared to fifteen in the group taking ginseng. Influenza antibody levels and natural killer cell activities were higher in the ginseng group. Nine cases of minor side effects were reported by the 227 volunteers, eight (insomnia, nausea, stomach pain) in the ginseng group and one in the placebo group (insomnia).

Finnish researchers studied the effects of ginseng in thirty-six newly diagnosed non-insulin-dependent diabetics. Patients were treated for eight weeks with placebo or ginseng (100 mg or 200 mg per day). Ginseng treatment, especially at the higher dose, caused a significant improvement in measures of psychophysical performance, mood, sense of well-being, vigor, and physical activity. Importantly, chemical measures of diabetes status (hemoglobin A1C and fasting blood glucose) improved. The authors of this small (only twelve patients per experimental group) but well-designed study concluded that ginseng may be useful in the management of diabetes.

Several studies have evaluated the effects of ginseng on mood and well-being. The results suggest an effect, but more work is needed. A twelve-week Mexican study compared the effects of a multivitamin preparation to the same preparation with added ginseng extract on 625 urban-dwelling volunteers. Quality of life, as measured by an eleven-item questionnaire, improved almost twofold in the vitamin plus ginseng group compared to the vitamin alone.

There is very little objective information about the effect of ginseng on impotence. A Korean study of ninety men with erectile dysfunction showed a significant improvement in men who took ginseng, compared to those who took placebo, but the study was published in an obscure journal. Studies are badly needed to be able to better evaluate ginseng's effect on this condition.

Another popular use of ginseng that is not well supported is for the improvement of athletic performance. Animal studies of ginseng are generally positive, but the results of the very few controlled human studies do not suggest any benefit. In general, studies of ginseng in athletic performance do not follow established scientific methods and cannot be considered valid.

DANGERS

Ginseng, like many other herbal products, is remarkably safe. No serious side effects have been reported in the people participating in recent controlled clinical trials, although not all studies kept track of side effects. There have been a few reports of problems, but unreasonably high doses (6–10 times the usual doses) were being used in some cases or there was a question about the ginseng being tested. Sleeplessness, agitation, nervousness, diarrhea, swollen and tender breasts, postmenopausal vaginal bleeding, rashes, and blood pressure changes have been reported rarely. If your blood pressure is poorly controlled, avoid ginseng. Do not take it during pregnancy.

RECOMMENDATIONS

Ginseng has been used in China since antiquity. Later its popularity spread to other Asian countries, and now it is growing in North America. This fascinating plant contains a mixture of chemicals in its roots that certainly has some physiological effects when taken continuously for at least several months, but nothing has been proven conclusively. What evidence there is points to a subtle tonic effect that is poorly appreciated in Western medicine. Ginseng may increase your feeling of well-being and stimulate the immune system. The extent to which these effects can actually help you is unknown, as is the value of ginseng in male impotence and in improving athletic performance. A myriad of other proposed uses for ginseng are also unproven.

If you wish to take ginseng, we suggest using a standardized extract of Asian ginseng root. Most positive studies have been done using extracts standardized to 4 percent ginsenosides. Take 100 to 200 mg per day for at least two months to notice benefits.

SAW PALMETTO

Saw palmetto, *Serenoa repens,* is the dwarf palm or fan palm found in the southeastern United States; it is now cultivated for its medicinal value. The berry from this small tree has long been of interest for urinary tract problems.

European investigators studying the berry found that an extract of lipids from the dried berry contained a number of interesting steroidlike compounds called sitosterols. Several compounds in the berry act as antiandrogens, and later investigations in Europe revealed that the extract has useful activity for benign prostatic hypertropy (BPH). BPH is a noncancerous enlargement of the prostate gland that causes annoying urinary difficulties, low bladder retention volume (necessitating frequent urination), frequent waking to urinate at night, "dribbling" after urination, and decreased size and force of the urine stream. The problem stems from the prostate tissue pinching the urethra as it traverses the gland. BPH is a problem very commonly experienced by men over fifty; almost 90 percent of males over eighty have significant BPH. With BPH it is important to rule out prostate cancer before making the diagnosis. Conventional treatment for BPH involves either surgery or use of a drug such as finasteride (Proscar), which blocks the conversion of testosterone to 5-α-dihydrotestosterone, a hormone that has the ability to increase the growth of prostate tissue. Finasteride affects only the converting enzyme, so testosterone levels do not decline; though impotence has been reported as an adverse effect, it is not that common. Saw palmetto apparently works in a similar manner.

EFFECTS

Like finasteride, lipid extracts of dried saw palmetto berries inhibit the enzyme that converts testosterone to 5-α-dihydrotestosterone. Studies using prostate tissue indicate that saw palmetto also blocks the binding of dihydrotestosterone to the tissue and has anti-inflammatory activity that could decrease symptoms of BPH. There is no change in testosterone levels in men taking saw palmetto, so impotence is not a problem.

EVIDENCE OF EFFICACY

Extracts of saw palmetto have been used for some time in Europe and are now receiving attention in the United States. Recent clinical trials conducted in Europe support the use of this plant for BPH. For example, a randomized, double-blind clinical trial conducted at eighty-seven different health centers in nine European countries involving over a thousand patients who received either extract of saw palmetto (Permixon, 320 mg per day) or finasteride (5 mg per day) showed a 38 percent reduction in symptoms in both groups six months into the study, as well as changes in a number of other measurements that indicate substantial improvement in BPH. This comparison of saw palmetto and finasteride showed them to be equally effective. With respect to adverse effects, both were also well tolerated, but a sexual function score was higher with saw palmetto compared to finasteride. Thus the saw palmetto extract worked as well as finasteride in treating BPH but was not perceived by the patients to adversely affect sexual function. This study agrees with most previously reported, smaller studies and supports the use of the extract of this plant as a first-line treatment for early BPH.

DANGERS

The lipid extract of saw palmetto is very well tolerated. Headache and stomach and intestinal upset are possible but infrequent side effects.

RECOMMENDATIONS

Most well-designed and controlled studies of saw palmetto in BPH have used a product called Permixon. The results show therapeutic benefit. Other preparations of saw palmetto are available. If you wish to treat BPH with saw palmetto, choose a standardized extract that contains greater than 85 percent fatty acids and sterols and that contains 160 mg of dried extract per capsule; take 320 mg per day. Studies show it may take six months to experience the full benefit from saw palmetto treatment. Of course, a licensed health care provider should monitor your therapy and the progress of your condition.

ST. JOHN'S WORT

St. John's wort is *Hypericum perforatum,* a low perennial shrub that develops beautiful yellow flowers in the spring. In Europe it is also commonly called hypericum. The plant is abundant on the West Coast of the United States and in fact is used as an ornamental landscape plant.

St. John's wort has long been used for medicinal purposes. The plant juice has been applied directly to wounds to speed healing, and teas made with the leaves and tops of the plant have been used to treat urinary and lung diseases and mental depression. Today most attention is directed toward evaluating the effectiveness of St. John's wort and extracts of this plant in treating depression.

Depression, other than that which is self-limiting and initiated by a tragic event, is a common and debilitating disorder. There are many conventional antidepressants your doctor can prescribe, including TCAs (tricyclic antidepressants), SSRIs (selective serotonin reuptake inhibitors), and MAOIs (monoamine oxidase inhibitors). These drugs are effective, but many patients don't want to use them because of their side effects, which include weight gain, fatigue, headache, and low blood pressure. An effective herbal without frequent side effects would be a welcome addition for many doctors and patients. St. John's wort may be that herbal, and extracts of the flowering tops of the plant are now widely used in European countries for this purpose. Sixty-six million doses of St. John's wort extract were prescribed in Germany during 1994, and there St. John's wort is recognized as being useful for psychological disturbances, depression, anxiety, and nervous states.

EFFECTS

St. John's wort contains a red compound called hypericin that is a very mild MAO inhibitor. It also contains a phenolic compound called hyperforin, flavonoids, a volatile oil, and many other compounds. Hypericin has been considered the component with the antidepressant effect, but a recent German study of depressed patients indicates that hyperforin may be very important as well. So the actual identity of the plant component(s) with antidepressant activity is uncertain. Early studies demonstrated inhibition of MAO in laboratory tests but this is now thought to occur at doses unobtainable in the human brain. Other studies point to an alteration of receptors for chemical messengers in the brain as the mechanism or an effect on GABA. More work needs to be done to pinpoint the way St. John's wort works and what chemical or chemicals in the plant are important. As with most herbs, current thinking is that the benefit is due to a synergistic mixture of many chemicals that make up the plant or its extract.

EVIDENCE OF EFFICACY

More than twenty European clinical trials evaluating St. John's wort as a treatment for depression have been completed. The consensus is that St. John's wort is significantly better than placebo and equal to available conventional drugs for depression. A published meta-analysis (a statistical technique for combining and evaluating the evidence from multiple trials) examined the thirteen trials comparing St. John's wort against placebo and showed that 55 percent of people in the St. John's wort group improved on depression measures, compared to 22 percent taking placebo. An evaluation of three trials comparing St. John's wort to conventional antidepressants revealed a 63 percent improvement rate for St. John's wort and a 58 percent rate for the other drugs, an unimportant difference. Side effects were reported in 19.8 percent of the St. John's wort group and in 35.9

percent of the group taking other drugs. Thus while more studies are needed, one can conclude that St. John's wort extracts are more effective than placebo for the treatment of depression and may be equally effective as the conventional drugs to which it has been compared, with fewer side effects.

St. John's wort has also been evaluated for seasonal affective disorder, a depression common in the late fall and winter seasons when days are shorter in the Northern Hemisphere. A group of German patients with severe symptoms was treated with St. John's wort plus bright light or dim light. Both groups improved equally, indicating an application of this herb for severe "winter blues."

DANGERS

Information from various clinical trials indicate that St. John's wort has a low incidence of side effects. Stomach and intestinal upset, allergic reactions, fatigue, and emotional upset were reported. Additionally, St. John's wort has the potential of causing sun sensitivity, so a sunblock is recommended when people use this herb. Nevertheless, serious drug toxicity reactions have not been reported from these trials.

RECOMMENDATIONS

St. John's wort extracts offer an attractive alternative to conventional antidepressant drugs. The herb seems to be effective for mild to moderate depression, with few adverse effects when used in normal doses. More research is needed to directly compare the effectiveness of St. John's wort to our most effective synthetic drugs for depression. St. John's wort extracts may be useful, but if depression is serious enough to require drug treatment, a licensed health care provider should monitor your condition.

The recommended dose of St. John's wort is 300 mg of a standardized extract containing 0.3 percent hypericin taken three times a day. This is the dose used in the clinical trials that have shown antidepression effects. As is the case with many other herbal products, several months of treatment are needed to produce a noticeable improvement. There are many products available that are promoted as "mood elevators" that contain numerous herbs in addition to St. John's wort. These should be avoided because the contributions of the other herbs are unknown and because the amount of St. John's wort in the usual dose may be too low.

VALERIAN

Valerian, known as garden heliotrope and by several other common names, grows wild in damp places in Europe, Asia, and North America. It is also cultivated. The plant is a perennial growing to three to four feet with big white, pink, or lavender flower clusters comprised of many individual flowers. The root and rhizome of the plant have a very strong odor and have long attracted attention for their ability to combat anxiety. Powdered root products and tinctures and extracts have official status in drug compendia in many European countries and in Canada. In Germany, valerian is listed for treatment of restlessness and nervous disorders of sleep. Until recent years it had official status in the United States, but now it can be sold only as a dietary supplement.

EFFECTS

The root and rhizome of valerian contain 0.1 to 0.3 percent of a volatile oil that gives these plant parts their characteristic disagreeable odor. Remarkably, the compounds responsible for the antianxiety and sedative effect of valerian are still not known despite valerian's long history of medicinal use. The special combination of chemicals present in the root may be key to the physiological effects observed. Studies using brain nerve terminals have shown that an extract of valerian root stimulates the release of a neurotransmitter in the body called GABA. The resulting increase in brain GABA concentrations is likely to be how the plant improves sleep patterns and acts as a mild tranquilizer.

The roots, rhizomes, and extracts of valerian clearly have mild sedative and antianxiety effects in both laboratory animals and humans. But *mild* is the operative word. Valerian can be taken without a serious adverse effect and without the addiction potential so characteristic of sedative and tranquilizer drugs.

EVIDENCE OF EFFICACY

Several clinical studies have evaluated the effect of valerian on sleep, but these studies have limitations because they tested only a small number of patients or healthy volunteers and were of short duration. Nevertheless, the consensus from an evaluation of the better studies is that valerian is effective as a mild sedative.

For example, in 1982 investigators from Switzerland studied 128 volunteers who took either placebo, valerian extract (400 mg), or a proprietary sleep product containing both valerian and hops. Each product was taken in random order on nonconsecutive nights. Study subjects filled out questionnaires on their nightly sleep patterns. Valerian helped people fall asleep sooner, and people reported they slept better, especially those who had previous sleep problems. (One problem with the study is that the placebo was odor-free while valerian capsules had the plant's characteristic odor.) Other scientific studies are in general agreement with these findings. There is little evidence to support the use of valerian as a mild tranquilizer, but most sedatives have antianxiety effect when taken in low doses.

DANGERS

Animal studies have suggested that there is a possibility of liver damage with high doses of valerian, but close examination of the studies shows that other compounds in the products being tested (skullcap, for example) may be the culprit. Humans have been using valerian for many centuries, and there are no reports of serious adverse effects. Liver damage was not even evident in overdose situations. Because valerian is a mild sedative, it makes sense to avoid alcoholic beverages or other drugs causing drowsiness when taking a valerian product. In addition, be careful operating machinery or an automobile while taking valerian during the day because of the potential for drowsiness. Taking valerian at night did not cause sedation or "daytime hangover" the next day. A benzodiazepine drug taken for comparison purposes did have a morning-after effect. Other occasionally reported side effects include headache, restlessness, nausea, and blurred vision.

RECOMMENDATIONS

Valerian has been used for a long time as a mild sedative and tranquilizer. Clinical studies support this use and indicate that occasional use is safe. We suggest, as with any medication for sleep and anxiety, that valerian be used only as a temporary measure to get past the problem. It is most important to deal with the underlying reason for anxiety or trouble sleeping and not rely on a drug to solve the problem.

For sleep, 400 mg of the powdered root before bedtime is appropriate. For use of the liquid forms or of the extracts, follow the directions on the manufacturer's label. For anxiety, a lower dose taken two or three times a day could serve as a temporary measure, though we do not recommend self-medicating in this way. Because of the possibility that valerian may cause liver damage in high doses, you should not use it if you have liver disease. Because the effects of valerian on the fetus have not been tested, it should be avoided during pregnancy and breast-feeding, and it should not be used in children. Avoid alcohol and other sedative drugs while taking it. On balance, valerian is an old and underutilized medication that is a safe and effective mild sedative.

Part 5

DIETARY SUPPLEMENT
PROFILES

15

FIVE POPULAR DIETARY SUPPLEMENTS

The preparations discussed in this section are in reality a group of miscellaneous products that are neither vitamins nor minerals nor herbals. They are unified only by being classified as dietary supplements by the FDA. All can be found in nature and are considered natural products even though they may be prepared commercially by chemical synthesis. For example, melatonin is synthesized by the pineal gland in humans, yet almost all of the melatonin used in the commercially available products is prepared by chemical synthesis. Even though it has nothing to do with the diet, melatonin falls under the regulatory category of "dietary supplements" (see herbals chapter for a discussion of FDA regulation of dietary supplements). Below we discuss probiotics and four other popular nonherbal, nonvitamin, dietary supplements.

PROBIOTICS

Probiotics are living microorganisms taken by mouth to improve gastrointestinal or vaginal health. In the United States and Canada, all commercial probiotic products are made of anaerobic bacteria (they can't live in the presence of oxygen) normally found in the vaginal or intestinal tract. A product containing a special therapeutic yeast is also being introduced. They are sold in capsule form (containing freeze-dried bacteria) or in fermented dairy products such as special yogurts. These products are usually taken to prevent or treat diarrhea or vaginitis. Microorganisms

taken to treat a specific vaginal or intestinal infection are often
called biotherapeutic agents.

EFFECTS

In contrast to the rest of our body, where microorganisms are not
normally present, the vagina and intestinal tract are open to the
environment and are therefore nonsterile. Both places provide a
nice home for bacteria. They are warm, moist, and bathed in nutrients, but there is only a little oxygen in the vagina and almost
none in the lower intestinal tract. So bacteria (or yeasts) must be
able to live without oxygen.

Another function of bacteria in the vagina and GI tract is that
they help to protect us from invading external microbes. Collectively they resist the invasion of pathogenic bacteria to which
we are constantly exposed. The number of bacteria normally
found in these areas is astounding, especially the lower intestine. Usually we have 30 trillion bacteria in every ounce of colon
content; 20 to 40 percent of the weight of our feces is bacteria.
But this is a good thing, and problems develop only when these
bacteria are disturbed.

Antibiotics cure disease by killing bacteria that cause an infection, but there is a price to pay. Such drugs also kill some of
the normal bacteria in our intestinal tract and vagina, upsetting
the delicate balance of "friendly" bacteria that reside there.
When this happens, invading microorganisms usually found in
small numbers in the vagina and GI tract grow and can cause diarrhea and vaginitis, both common side effects of antibiotic
therapy. Some antibiotics carry a greater risk than others, but all
can cause intestinal and vaginal disturbances. A very serious
form of diarrhea called pseudomembranous colitis can also develop after antibiotic changes in intestinal bacteria. It is due to
the overgrowth of *Clostridium difficile,* an antibiotic-resistant
bacteria. Pseudomembranous colitis is an uncommon but life-
threatening infection in the colon that can recur again and again.

Probiotics play an important role in preventing and treating
antibiotic-induced diarrhea and vaginitis by introducing bacteria important to the protective ecology of both the GI tract and
the vagina. Replacing intestinal or vaginal bacteria destroyed by
antibiotic therapy helps to prevent or even treat overgrowths of
pathogenic bacteria that occur when the normal balance is upset

by antibiotics. This is the whole idea behind the use of probiotics. You take an oral dose of a bacteria or a mixture of bacteria or a yeast and their presence helps restore the normal microbial balance in the intestine or vagina. What doesn't make sense is using a second antibiotic to treat an antibiotic-induced infection (i.e., treating an antibiotic-associated diarrhea with another antibiotic). This should be avoided if possible.

Of course, antibiotics do not cause all diarrhea and vaginitis. Sometimes pathogens simply overwhelm the protective barrier created by normal bacteria and cause infections such as salmonella and shigella. Most traveler's diarrhea is caused by ingesting special pathogenic strains of *E. coli* that are new to people traveling to the areas in which they are found. They usually don't affect people who live in these areas because the people are accustomed to them. An antibiotic may be needed to treat these infections, but probiotics can be useful in preventing subsequent antibiotic-associated diarrhea. There is some evidence that probiotics may be useful in preventing some cases of traveler's diarrhea.

Bacteria of the *Lactobacillus* genus are most important for a healthy vaginal environment. They keep the vagina acidic, and many invading bacteria don't do well in an acidic environment. They can also make and release hydrogen peroxide and other substances that can inhibit pathogens. Also, they are present in such large numbers that they tend to crowd out invaders. Probiotic products taken to treat and prevent vaginitis are usually made of lactobacilli and, interestingly, are taken by mouth. These bacteria find their way into the vagina because of the close physical proximity of the anus and the opening of the vagina. Special strains of "tagged" lactobacilli have been isolated from the vaginal tract after oral ingestion. Vaginal probiotic suppositories can be used to directly introduce lactobacilli, but this is less common.

The intestinal tract is much more complex than the vagina. Bacteria normally found in the highest numbers there, including *Bacteriodes, Eubacterium,* and *Enterococcus,* can cause infections on their own, so they are not good probiotics. Also, these and other bacteria can harbor antibiotic resistance genes that may be donated to other bacteria. A probiotic bacterium must not cause an infection, must be able to survive stomach acid, must be able to survive in the intestines, must have the ability to act as a barrier to suppress the growth of an invading bacteria, and must disappear once the normal ecology is restored. Lacto-bacilli and other anaerobic bacteria called *bifidobacteria* meet these criteria and are used as intestinal probiotics, even though they are normally found in only small quantities in the intestine. *Saccharomyces boulardii,* a yeast, is also an effective probiotic.

EVIDENCE OF EFFICACY

There is ample evidence of the effectiveness of probiotics in preventing and even treating intestinal and vaginal infections. In Europe, it is routine to take a probiotic together with every anti-biotic prescription; probiotics are routinely used for diarrhea and to prevent traveler's diarrhea, and they are prescribed by doctors and are covered by government insurance plans. The situation is different in North America. Probiotics are consid-ered dietary supplements, not drugs. In the United States, this means that drug use claims made by the manufacturers of these products are limited and that the FDA does not closely scruti-nize them, as long as no serious adverse reactions occur. As we have previously discussed, there are huge variations in product quality and there is a lack of effective consumer information on the labels of "dietary supplement" products.

There is strong evidence from human clinical studies that certain probiotic bacteria can be very effective in intestinal and vaginal disease. In the following tables, we list infection types and the probiotic bacteria that have been successfully used (in controlled studies) to treat them. When choosing a commercial probiotic product to treat or prevent a specific infection, select one that contains the microbe demonstrated to be effective against the infection.

Probiotic Bacteria in Diarrhea

PROBIOTIC	DIARRHEA TYPE
Lactobacillus casei GG	Antibiotic, traveler's, infant, adult acute
Saccharomyces boulardii	Antibiotic, traveler's, pseudomembranous colitis, HIV-related, infant
Bifidobacterium longum	Antibiotic
Bifidobacterium longum plus *Lactobacillus acidophilus*	Antibiotic
Enterococcus faecium	Antibiotic, adult acute

PROBIOTIC   **DIARRHEA TYPE**

Bifidobacterium longum and
   Streptococcus thermophilus   Infant

Probiotic Bacteria in Other Infections

PROBIOTIC MICROORGANISM   **INFECTION**

Lactobacillus acidophilus   Recurrent Candida vaginitis
Lactobacilli   Recurrent urinary tract infection

Anyone who says probiotics are not helpful for significant infections is mistaken. One example of an infection where probiotics have been of help in treatment is recurrent Candida vaginitis. This yeast infection is common in women taking antibiotics and, for reasons that are not well understood, the infection often keeps recurring after treatment with antifungal drugs. Women often get into a cycle of repeated courses of antifungal medicine to treat this annoying problem. Yogurt has long been claimed to help against vaginitis, but no proof of this existed until 1995, when a study was done in which yogurt fermented with a hydrogen peroxide–producing strain of lactobacilli was given to thirty-three women with recurrent candidal vaginitis. The average number of infections was 2.54 without yogurt and only 0.38 during the yogurt phase, a significant difference. The special strain of lactobacilli that was in the yogurt was isolated from the vagina. Later, the same investigators reported on the successful use of vaginal suppositories containing *Lactobacillus casei* GG in a study of twenty-eight women with recurrent vaginitis.

Another example is the effective use of the therapeutic yeast *Saccharomyces boulardii* in the treatment of recurrent pseudomembranous colitis. Pseudomembranous colitis is a very serious inflammation of the colon that causes severe diarrhea and, if left untreated, can be life-threatening. It is due to overgrowth of *Clostridium difficile,* a bacterium resistant to most antibiotics. As in the vaginitis example above, effective treatments are available (in this case therapy with vancomycin or metronidazole), but the infection keeps returning after treatment is stopped. Like vaginitis, recurrent diarrhea severely affects quality of life. In a controlled study of 124 patients, two capsules of dried yeast taken twice a day reduced the recurrence rate to 26 percent, compared to 45 percent in the placebo-treated group. All patients received antibiotic treatment for ten days and took the yeast for thirty days.

DANGERS

The commercially available probiotics seem remarkably safe. There is always the worry of the probiotic itself causing an infection, but this should be a risk only to patients who have problems with their immune system. However, one study gave *Saccharomyces boulardii* in high doses (3 g per day) to AIDS patients without problems with yeast infections developing. One probiotic, *Enterococcus faecium,* carries the potential of transferring antibiotic resistance genes. The probiotic strain is apparently nonpathogenic, but other *Enterococcus* strains cause serious infections and are almost impossible to treat due to antibiotic resistance. Furthermore, they may transfer their resistance to other pathogens and cause them to be resistant as well. We do not recommend use of probiotic products containing *Enterococcus faecium.*

RECOMMENDATIONS

We believe that probiotics offer many benefits for people in the prevention and treatment of some infections.

- Probiotics should be routinely taken whenever an antibiotic drug is prescribed. Take the probiotic while the antibiotic is being taken and continue for at least three days after the antibiotic is finished. This will reduce the risk of antibiotic-associated diarrhea and, maybe pseudomembranous colitis (or *Clostridium difficile* diarrhea), though their use should be supervised by a licensed health care professional.
- Women with yeast infections should take a high-potency yogurt fermented with hydrogen peroxide–producing strains of lactobacilli every day or capsules of this bacterium. Continue until the recurrences stop.
- Daily probiotic use may be helpful against acute diarrhea in adults.

- Probiotics have been proven effective in infantile diarrhea (mostly caused by rotavirus), but their use should be undertaken under the care of a licensed health care professional. Infantile diarrhea can be serious, and professional medical attention is needed.
- Probiotics may be of some help in preventing traveler's diarrhea if taken daily during the trip. Be sure to take the usual precautions to avoid contaminated food and water.

What product should you purchase? This is a question that is most difficult to answer. In our opinion, the best-researched probiotic microorganisms are *Saccharomyces boulardii* and *Lactobacillus GG*. The Saccharomyces boulardii product that has shown therapeutic success in clinical trials for various types of diarrhea is made by a French pharmaceutical company. It is sold as capsules in many countries and now is available in the United States in pharmacies, health food stores, and related outlets. Lactobacillus GG is available in Finland and some European countries and has recently been introduced into the U.S. market in capsule form.

A variety of other Lactobacillus- and Bifidobacterium-containing products are also sold in the United States. Most of these probiotics have not been thoroughly tested in human clinical trials, so it is difficult to know which products are effective. If you choose to purchase one of these other Lactobacillus or Bifidobacterium probiotic products, make sure that the potency (live bacteria or yeast per dose) is stated on the label and the manufacturer should be one that you recognize as having a good reputation. Pick the most potent product and take it twice a day or according to the directions on the package. Your pharmacist can help select an appropriate product to use.

COENZYME Q₁₀ (UBIQUINONE)

The ubiquinones are a group of benzoquinone derivatives found in the mitochondia of living organisms. The most common ubiquinone is coenzyme Q_{10} or CoQ_{10}.

EFFECTS

In cell mitochondria, CoQ_{10} participates in the process of generating energy by passing along electrons. It accomplishes this by alternately being oxidized and reduced. Additionally, CoQ_{10} is a powerful free-radical scavenger (see Chapter 7). It is relatively lipid-soluble and, like vitamin E, can sit in our vital membranes and protect them from free radicals. Some claim that CoQ_{10} is an even more powerful free-radical scavenger than vitamin E. There is a great deal of interest in CoQ_{10} to treat and prevent diseases where free radicals are involved, especially heart disease.

EVIDENCE OF EFFICACY

The application of CoQ_{10} that has been most completely studied is the treatment of heart disease. Numerous studies in patients with angina and cardiac insufficiency show CoQ_{10} has some effect. However none of these studies included a placebo group for control purposes, so their results can be considered questionable.

A few small double-blind, controlled studies showed objective evidence of the effectiveness of CoQ_{10} compared to placebo. But other studies showed negative results using similar doses. In a large Italian study of over two thousand patients, 70 percent of those studied showed some improvement in a number of heart function measures. Side effects were seen in only 1.5 percent of people taking the drug. Improvement in at least three symptoms, such as shortness of breath, sweating, and palpitations, was noted in 54 percent. This study did not use a control group, however. CoQ_{10} before heart surgery has also been reported to be beneficial in decreasing signs of cardiac injury compared to placebo.

CoQ_{10} has been studied for other uses in a number of small clinical trials. The results of these showed some effect on breast cancer, some effect on high blood pressure, and no effect on athletic performance. Animal studies of CoQ_{10} to increase lifespan have shown no effect.

DANGERS

Adverse effects of CoQ_{10} treatment seem minimal. This compound is found in our diets and in our bodies. It seems nontoxic at the usual doses of 100 to 200 mg per day.

RECOMMENDATIONS

CoQ_{10} is an excellent antioxidant and free-radical scavenger that has many possible applications in the treatment and prevention of disease. Whether it is superior to vitamin E or other antioxidants remains to be determined. Certainly its role in the electron transport process of the mitochondria is an added dimension that may make it unique compared to other antioxidants. At present, evidence is strongest for a treatment benefit in heart disease. The idea is that CoQ_{10} may increase the heartbeat efficiency because of its role in the mitochondria in generating energy. Being a powerful antioxidant may make it helpful in preventing further oxidative damage to the heart and to the blood vessels feeding the heart.

Much larger studies using a control for comparison purposes need to be done before we know how valuable CoQ_{10} can be, however. Doses between 30 and 600 mg per day have been used, but most studies employ about 100 mg per day; daily intake should be sufficient to achieve blood levels of about 2 mcg per ml, but the amount necessary to achieve this goal may vary from patient to patient.

The usefulness of CoQ_{10} in other medical conditions should be considered unproven until more studies are completed. When CoQ_{10} therapy is being used for a serious illness such as heart disease, treatment should be supervised by a licensed health care professional.

GLUCOSAMINE AND CHONDROITIN

Glucosamine is an amino sugar and one of the building blocks for collagen, the main component of connective tissue. One type of connective tissue is cartilage, the dense white substance found in bone joints, the nose, ear, and tendons. Cartilage provides a smooth, slippery, tough coating that keeps our bones from rubbing against each other in movable joints such as knees and hips. Collagen makes cartilage strong, and mucopolysaccharide polymers such as chondroitin make up the ground substance that makes cartilage spongy and flexible.

EFFECTS

Using glucosamine and chondroitin as arthritis treatments has been popularized by the book *The Arthritis Cure,* by Dr. Jason Theodosakis. Dr. Theodosakis says that taking these two substances will stimulate cartilage repair. Glucosamine is supposed to stimulate the manufacture of cartilage and to make it easier for nutrients to penetrate cartilage by hydrating it (providing water). Chondroitin is supposed to hydrate cartilage also and to prevent it from breaking down. It has been suggested that together they provide relief for osteoarthritis sufferers by providing precursors for new cartilage.

EVIDENCE OF EFFICACY

The evidence to support the use of chondroitin and glucosamine comes mostly from studies conducted in Europe, where this approach is popular. Available published studies give the impression that glucosamine and chondroitin may help in arthritis, but they are hardly a "cure." The available studies are small or not well controlled but generally show that patients taking glucosamine obtained some relief of arthritis pain and stiffness. There are reasons to believe that glucosamine and chondroitin may help some people with osteoarthritis.

Glucosamine (in the form of glucosamine sulfate) is readily absorbed when taken by mouth, and it reaches the fluid in the joints. Surprisingly, chondroitin (as chondroitin sulfate) is not broken down completely in the gut by digestive enzymes, so some of it passes into the blood and can reach the joints. There are numerous uncontrolled clinical trials that suggest this combination works, but few of the more reliable and standard placebo-controlled trials used by experts to judge drug product effectiveness. One double-blind, placebo-controlled trial of 155 patients tested twice-weekly intramuscular injections of 400 mg of glucosamine sulfate for six weeks. Fifty-five percent of people given glucosamine responded with a significant reduction in disease severity, as compared to 33 percent of people given placebo. Another study tested oral glucosamine taken for 4 to 6 weeks versus placebo and versus NSAIDs such as ibuprofen. Both glucosamine and ibuprofen were better than placebo but were not different from each other in terms of beneficial results. The glucosamine group experienced fewer adverse effects.

The evidence for chondroitin is similarly suggestive but incomplete. A commercial chondroitin sulfate preparation was given by mouth or by injection for six months and compared to oral placebo and injected placebo. There were ten patients in each group. A statistically significantly improvement was observed for the chondroitin-treated groups, but this study was too small to draw conclusions on chondroitin for all people with osteoarthritis.

DANGERS

There is little published information on the adverse effects of these products.

RECOMMENDATIONS

Chondroitin and glucosamine may benefit some patients with osteoarthritis, but more controlled studies are needed to assess them. Both compounds appear to have few adverse effects, and we have spoken with many patients who claim to have obtained good results after taking both for a few months. The usual doses are 1 to 2 g a day of glucosamine and 800 to 1,600 mg a day of chondroitin.

As with all materials considered dietary supplements by the FDA, there are inferior products on the market, and we advise you to purchase a brand that is well established and recognized as being associated with a reputable company.

MELATONIN

Melatonin is a hormone synthesized by the pineal gland from tryptophan, a dietary amino acid. The pineal gland is a pea-sized gland attached to the brain on its back side. Melatonin is made and released into the blood at night. It is picked up from the blood circulation by the hypothalamus, the portion of the brain that controls body temperature, thirst, hunger, and sleep. Melatonin binds to specific receptors in the hypothalamus. We produce the most melatonin at puberty, and then melatonin production declines with age, with little produced after age seventy. Small amounts of melatonin are present in some foods (bananas, for example) but these amounts are thought to be insufficient to affect sleep.

EFFECTS

Melatonin works in the hypothalamus to help set our biological clocks, ensuring that we are awake and asleep at appropriate times in a twenty-four-hour day. Melatonin promotes sleep and reduces levels of cortisol, a stress hormone. Both light and melatonin strongly influence our sleeping patterns. It is difficult for most people to sleep during the day and stay up at night because daylight suppresses both sleep and melatonin release. Melatonin secretion reaches a peak at about 2 A.M. and then declines until you wake up in the morning. Very little melatonin is produced during the day.

Melatonin also functions as an antioxidant and free-radical scavenger (see Chapter 7). Of special importance is the ability of this small molecule to penetrate cells and even get into the cell nucleus, where it may help prevent damage to our DNA. There is considerable interest in the application of melatonin in diseases related to oxidative damage, such as arthritis, muscular dystrophy, and heart disease.

EVIDENCE OF EFFICACY

There is excellent evidence that melatonin can promote sleep. Since melatonin production declines as we age, this may be part of the reason why sleep habits often worsen with advancing age.

An unhealthy pattern of difficulty getting to sleep, nighttime awakening, and then napping during the day is set up. Good sleep is important for good health. Can melatonin help restore normal sleep patterns? Happily, it may.

Two recent, well-designed studies using a 2 mg controlled-release melatonin product showed that melatonin improved sleep for older subjects with insomnia. Subjects slept in their own bed but wore a device on the wrist that could sense motion. They took either placebo or melatonin two hours before bedtime for three weeks. Then they were switched to whatever medication (placebo or melatonin) they had not taken in the first part of the study. In one study, melatonin helped people fall asleep faster. Also, total wake time during the night was reduced from seventy-three minutes in the placebo phase to forty-nine minutes in the melatonin phase. In the second study, a standard-release 2 mg tablet was compared to 2 mg sustained-release tablet. Generally, the sustained-release tablet was slightly better than the standard-release tablet. Sleep improved even more during two months of treatment with melatonin and then deteriorated when the treatment was stopped. There were no significant side effects associated with melatonin treatment.

Can melatonin promote daytime sleep? One recent study indicates that it can. This study differed from most others in that subjects were young and did not have insomnia. The study took place in a controlled sleep-laboratory setting, and sleep was measured during the early afternoon after subjects had slept seven hours on the previous night. Several doses (1 mg, 10 mg, and 40 mg) of melatonin were tested. All doses helped people fall asleep faster, increased sleep time, and reduced time awake. Note that this study indicated that melatonin has the potential to put even well-rested people to sleep during the daytime, so melatonin use should be restricted to bedtime.

Can melatonin help us deal with jet lag experienced by travelers crossing several time zones? Studies of this question indicate that melatonin can be very valuable in resetting your biological clock to the destination time. Melatonin efficiently advanced bedtimes and maintained desirable sleep times in army personnel traveling from the United States to the Middle East, compared to a placebo. While the soldiers taking melatonin were awake, they did better on a vigilance test than those who took the placebo. Similar findings of the benefits of melatonin in treating jet lag have been reported in a study of long-haul flight crews.

Other uses of melatonin are considered experimental. It is clear that melatonin is a powerful antioxidant and has the ability to penetrate body cells. It has been shown to reduce heart disease and to prolong life in animal experiments. Doses of 20 mg per day have helped prevent weight loss in terminal cancer patients with solid tumors. Research is being conducted to determine the usefulness of melatonin in arthritis, in enhancing the immune system, in preventing osteoporosis, and as an adjunct in treating cancer.

DANGERS

The long-term use of melatonin has not been carefully studied for adverse effects, but less then 5 mg a day of melatonin is considered nontoxic. There are isolated reports of melatonin worsening depression. As noted, it can make you sleepy if taken during the day. In addition, high doses (75 mg) may have a contraceptive effect. To be on the safe side, women trying to get pregnant should avoid melatonin. Finally, the safety of melatonin in children and during pregnancy and lactation is not known.

RECOMMENDATIONS

People with sleep disorders should try to deal with the reason for their lack of sleep and not rely on a drug to solve the problem. Reducing stress and tension in one's life is a very important step toward good health and good sleep. Melatonin is not a tranquilizer and will not relieve stress and anxiety that may be causing the sleep problems. If you are under forty, it is unlikely that low melatonin levels are the cause of your insomnia.

If you are over forty, have trouble sleeping, and have tried the recommended nondrug techniques to get a good night's sleep with no success, melatonin is worth a try. Take 1 to 3 mg one hour before bedtime. Continue for two to three weeks to determine if this approach will help. Try a sustained-release product if the less expensive regular tablets do not seem to work. Avoid taking melatonin during the daytime because it may make you drowsy and affect your ability to drive. Don't take melatonin if you are also taking sedatives or tranquilizers, if you have a hormone imbalance or an autoimmune disease, or if you are trying to get pregnant or are pregnant. Don't give melatonin to children, because they already have high melatonin levels.

For jet lag prevention in adults, take 1 to 5 mg one hour before bedtime for five nights. Begin this treatment program as soon as you arrive at your destination. You should become adjusted to the new time zone after four or five nights, but note that most people can adjust to a new time zone in this same period *without* melatonin. Melatonin speeds the adjustment process for many people, however.

We do not recommend taking melatonin regularly unless recommended by a licensed health care provider. The many other suggested uses are unproven, and the effects of long-term use are unstudied.

Avoid the "all-natural" melatonin products. They may be made from animal pineal glands and carry the risk of impurities and pathogenic viruses and bacteria. Synthetic products are best. Synthetic melatonin is identical to the melatonin we produce in our pineal gland.

DHEA

Dihydroepiandrosterone, also called DHEA, has been known to exist in our bodies for some time. Interest in DHEA grew in the 1980s when several reports suggested it had antiaging properties. The United States Food and Drug Administration (FDA) briefly banned the sale of DHEA without a prescription, but sales resumed with the passage of DSHEA (see Part 6, "Herbal Medicines") in 1994. Under DSHEA, the FDA would have had to prove that DHEA was dangerous in order to remove it from the market. DHEA suppliers now can sell it as a dietary supplement without having to prove it has any effect on your body; at the same time, no therapeutic claims can be made for DHEA, so long as it is labeled as a dietary supplement. This is very different from traditional drug products, for which both effectiveness and safety must be conclusively proven before they can be sold.

EFFECTS

DHEA is a natural steroid made from cholesterol and secreted by the adrenal gland. It is not considered a hormone because it does not bind to special hormone receptors in the body. Rather, it floats around in the body and is eventually converted to androgens and estrogens. These classes of sex hormones have a variety of effects; all tissues may need small amounts of them. Enzymes present in tissues readily convert DHEA to androgens, and an enzyme called aromatase can convert androgens, in turn, to estrogens. DHEAS (DHEA combined with sulfate) blood levels are about four hundred times greater than DHEA levels and are used as a measure of DHEA status.

The connection between DHEA and aging comes from the observation that DHEA levels rise from birth, peak at about age thirty, and then gradually decline. By age eighty your DHEA level is only 10 to 20 percent of peak levels. To complicate matters, there are substantial differences in DHEA levels from one person to the next.

There are two important questions about DHEA:

- What does it mean to your health to have naturally high or low DHEA levels?
- Do DHEA supplements make you younger and healthier?

EVIDENCE OF EFFICACY

Most recent, well-done studies of DHEA point to considerable promise for this dietary supplement. There is tremendous scientific interest in DHEA, and we should have a clearer picture as time goes on. But we do not know how DHEA improves your health and what its possible side effects are.

One major area of DHEA research is improving quality of life in the elders. Researchers at the University of California, San Diego, gave DHEA, 50 mg a day, or an inactive placebo to thirteen men and seventeen women, ages forty to seventy. Each person took placebo or DHEA for three months, then switched to the other pill for another three months. Sixty-seven percent of the men and 84 percent of the women had an improved sense of well-being at the end of the DHEA phase. There was no improvement on placebo. Androgen levels increased in the men and women, but the increase in men was small. An increase in insulin-like growth factors was noted in both sexes. The volunteers had no change in sex drive. A few (eight men and eight women) were given 100 mg of DHEA daily and were followed by the researchers for one year. Blood levels of testosterone, androstenedione, and dihydrotestosterone (all anabolic steroids) were raised three- or four-fold in women, but not in men. Blood levels of DHEAS in these older women were *above* the upper limit expected of young adults.

Other measures of immune function, including muscle strength, weight loss (men only), and quality of life, improved while the volunteers were taking DHEA, compared to placebo. Overall, there were no adverse effects of DHEA, except for one woman who grew unwanted facial hair. While the results of this small study are promising, the unusually high androgen levels seen in women on DHEA are disquieting; other small studies of DHEA have also found increased androgen levels in women. DHEA doses below 50 mg per day would probably be more appropriate for future studies.

A French study of 622 subjects over age sixty-five revealed a correlation between low DHEA levels and poor health. Studies of the effects of DHEA supplements in this group are under way. Another study reported that six depressed patients showed improvement in their depressive symptoms and memory after four weeks of taking 30 to 90 mg per day of DHEA.

DHEA is also being studied to prevent heart disease. DHEA decreased hardening of the arteries, or atherosclerosis, in animals. In people, DHEA can increase levels of enzymes used by the body to keep blood from inappropriately clotting and platelets from sticking together. Low DHEA levels have been reported in people with high blood pressure and people with heart disease, but it is not known whether low DHEA levels cause the problem or are a result of it.

There is also some interest in DHEA's ability to stimulate the immune system and help the body fight infections and cancers. Animal studies show that high DHEA doses cause tumors to shrink and also decrease the numbers of chemically induced tumors.

DHEA has shown promise in improving systemic lupus

erythematosus (SLE). It has been thought that the ratio of androgens to estrogens could influence the progression of SLE, and
that DHEA would increase androgen levels. Twenty-eight female patients with mild to moderate SLE were given 200 mg per
day of DHEA or placebo for three months. SLE was improved
and disease flareups were reduced in people taking DHEA. Only
slight changes were seen in the placebo group.

The most common DHEA side effect was acne. Unwanted
facial hair was actually more common in people taking placebo.

DANGERS

There are safety concerns with DHEA, especially when it is
taken for a long time. In daily doses larger than 50 mg, DHEA
can increase androgen levels, causing masculinization in women.
DHEA-induced acne can also develop. The biggest worry, however, is cancer. If an organ is artificially stimulated to produce
well beyond its normal time, we worry about cancer developing
in that organ. Taking DHEA chronically gives artificially high
levels of testosterone and of insulin-like growth factor for an extended period of time. This could stimulate cancer development.
Indeed, a population study involving twenty thousand Maryland
residents showed that increased levels of DHEA (and androstenedione) in the body increased the risk of ovarian cancer. With
men, one might worry about the potential for DHEA to increase
prostate cancer and BPH (benign prostatic hypertropy). Studies
of DHEA supplements have mostly involved small numbers of
patients and been of short duration. Thus the true extent of DHEA
side effects is not known.

RECOMMENDATIONS

Many researchers are optimistic about DHEA's potential to improve health, especially in older adults, but we know very little
about the benefits of taking DHEA over a long period. Herbal dietary supplements have a long history of use, but DHEA is new.
Long-term studies are needed to evaluate DHEA's potential to
protect against heart disease, cancer, and infections.

DHEA is a steroid and has an impact on the amounts of other
steroid hormones in the body. It should be taken only under a

doctor's supervision. Doses of 25 to 50 mg per day give blood levels similar to those found in a young adult. Larger doses should be avoided, except possibly in treating SLE. We need to learn much more about DHEA before it can be recommended as a routine supplement.

Part 6

VITAMIN, MINERAL, AND HERBAL DRUG INTERACTIONS

The tables on the following pages will provide you with information that, although available to physicians and pharmacists, has not been made generally available to the consumer. These tables detail the possible effects that vitamins, minerals, and herbals can have on each other, on the drugs you take, and, in some cases, on the lab tests that your doctor orders to make a diagnosis or monitor your condition. For example:

- Colestipol and cholestyramine, used to help lower blood cholesterol, interfere with the absorption of many drugs and the fat-soluble vitamins A, D, E, and K.
- Women taking oral contraceptive pills may have more vitamin A in their blood than nonusers and can need more vitamin B_6 (pyridoxine).
- People taking digitalis drugs for heart failure should avoid taking excess calcium, unless prescribed by your doctor, because the combination can lead to abnormal heart rhythms.
- People who take lithium to control bipolar disorder, also known as manic-depression, should avoid iodine supplements because they will experience an abnormal depression of thyroid gland function.
- People who take iron supplements should consider taking vitamin C with their iron because the vitamin will increase the amount of iron absorbed into the bloodstream.
- If you take oral anticoagulant (blood-thinning) medicine, you should avoid taking megadoses of vitamin C because it can interfere with the anticoagulant's effect by preventing it from passing from your stomach into your bloodstream.

- People who take isoniazid for tuberculosis or hydralazine for high blood pressure need extra vitamin B_6 (pyridoxine).
- People taking an antidepressant must be cautious if they are also taking St. John's wort, an herbal product with antidepressant properties.

If you take vitamin, mineral, or herbal supplements, the following tables contain essential information for you. *Be sure your doctor also knows what vitamins and supplements you are taking.*

TABLE 12
Vitamin, Mineral, and Herbal Drug Interactions

	Can Interact With:	To:
Vitamin B$_1$ (thiamin)	Drugs used to relax muscles during surgery	Produce excessive muscle relaxation
Vitamin B$_2$ (riboflavin)	Certain urine tests	Produce false elevations in urine tests for chemicals known as catecholamines. These chemicals are essential to nervous system function.
		Cause discoloration of the urine. Riboflavin can interfere with any test in which color is important because it gives urine a yellowish color.
Vitamin B$_3$ (nicotinic acid, niacin)	Clonidine (Catapres) for high blood pressure	Eliminate flushing of the skin normally caused by nicotinic acid
	Lovastatin	Cause severe muscle aches and destruction (in one patient)
	Sulfinpyrazone for gout	Interfere with effects of sulfinpyrazone
	Certain blood tests	Elevate blood sugar. Very large doses of nicotinic acid are needed to produce this effect.
		Increase growth hormone levels in the blood
		Lower blood cholesterol by 15 to 30 percent. Large daily doses of about 3 g are needed to produce this effect.
		Increase blood levels of certain liver enzymes and chemicals. Nicotinic acid has been associated with jaundice in several patients.

	Can Interact With:	To:
Vitamin B₃	Certain urine tests	Produce false elevations in urine catecholamines, essential to nervous system function
		Increase the amount of sugar in the urine. Large doses of nicotinic acid must be taken to produce this effect.
Vitamin B₆ (pyridoxine)	Phenobarbital	Increase the rate at which phenobarbital is broken down in the body
	Levodopa (l-dopa) for Parkinsonism	Dramatically interfere with the effect of l-dopa. Doses as small as 10 mg may interfere with l-dopa. Avoid pyridoxine tablets, liquids, or multivitamins with the vitamin as an ingredient unless you are also taking Carbidopa, in which case the interaction does not occur.
	Phenytoin (Dilantin) for seizures	Increase the rate at which phenytoin is broken down; large doses of pyridoxine are needed to produce this effect.
	Isoniazid for tuberculosis	Produce B₆ deficiency. Extra vitamin B₆ is needed if you are taking Isoniazid.
	Cycloserine for tuberculosis	Produce B₆ deficiency. Vitamin B₆ may also prevent some of the side effects seen with cycloserine.
	Hydralazine (Apresoline) for high blood pressure	Produce B₆ deficiency. Extra B₆ is needed if you are taking hydralazine.
	Penicillamine for arthritis or Wilson's disease	Produce B₆ deficiency; take extra vitamin B₆.
	Oral contraceptives	Produce B₆ deficiency; take extra vitamin B₆.
Vitamin B₁₂ (cyanocobalamin)	Vitamin B₁₂	Increase the amount of vitamin B₁₂ absorbed
	Aminosalicylic acid (PAS)	Prevent B₁₂ from passing from the gut into the bloodstream

	Can Interact With:	To:
Vitamin B12	Alcohol	Excessive alcohol intake for more than two weeks can cause poor B12 absorption.
	Colchicine for gout	Cause less B12 to pass from the gut into the bloodstream
	Chloramphenicol, an antibiotic	Interfere with the effect of B12 on the body
	Neomycin, an antibiotic	Cause less B12 to pass from the gut into the bloodstream
	Vitamin B6	Assist in the absorption of B12
	Vitamin C	Assist in the absorption of B12, if vitamin C is taken in usual doses. Large doses of vitamin C may destroy natural vitamin B12 in food.
Folic acid	Chloramphenicol, an antibiotic	Cause folic acid deficiency
	Aminosalicylic acid	Reduce blood levels of folate
	Folic acid antagonists (e.g., methotrexate, trimethoprim)	May interfere with folic acid utilization in the body
	Pyrimethamine (Daraprim) for malaria	Interfere with the effect of pyrimethamine
	Oral contraceptives	May interfere with folic acid metabolism, leading to folate deficiency, though unlikely to cause anemia
	Phenytoin and similar antiseizure medicines	Decreased drug effect leading to increased seizures. Phenytoin can cause low folate levels and symptoms of folic acid deficiency. Avoid this combination.
	Sulfasalazine	May cause signs of folate deficiency
Vitamin C	Sulfa drugs, a category of anti-infectives	Increase the chance of drug crystals forming in the urine. Large amounts of vitamin C are needed to produce this effect.

	Can Interact With:	To:
Vitamin C	Aminosalicylic acid (PAS) for tuberculosis	Increase the chance of drug crystals forming in the urine. Large amounts of vitamin C are needed to produce this effect.
	Tricyclic antidepressants	Reduce antidepressant effect by increasing the rate at which it is eliminated from the body
	Alcohol	Slightly increase the rate at which alcohol breaks down in the body, possibly making you less sensitive to alcoholic beverages by removing the alcohol from your bloodstream more quickly. Large doses over a long period are needed for this effect.
	Estrogens	Increase estrogen levels, possibly leading to side effects
	Oral anticoagulants	Interfere with anticoagulant effect. Doses of 10 g a day or more are needed to interfere with the absorption of warfarin into the bloodstream.
	Oral contraceptives	Daily doses of vitamin C of 1 g or more lead to increased estrogen levels, possibly leading to side effects.
	Vitamin B_{12}	Assist in the absorption of B_{12}, if taken in normal doses. Large doses of vitamin C can destroy some natural B_{12} in food when mixed in the stomach.
	Iron	Increase iron absorbed from nonmeat foods
	Calcium	Assist in the absorption of calcium
	Copper	Reduce the amount of copper absorbed; large doses of vitamin C are needed to produce this effect

	Can Interact With:	To:
Vitamin C	Certain urine tests	Interfere with a test for the level of natural steroids in the urine
		Give a falsely high reading for sugar in the urine; large doses of vitamin C are needed for this effect
	Certain blood tests	Possible false bilirubin measurement (an indication of liver function)
		Possible low blood cholesterol readings in people under age twenty-five and higher readings in people with a history of cholesterol problems
		Give false high levels of uric acid
		Give possible false negative reading for blood in the stool
Vitamin A	Corticosteroid-type drugs for inflammation	Improve wound healing. People taking a corticosteroid normally experience some slowness in wound healing. Vitamin A cream may help reverse this effect, but vitamin A taken by mouth will not.
	Oral contraceptives	Interfere with vitamin A absorption into the bloodstream. The importance of this interaction is not known.
	Calcium	Assist in the absorption of calcium into the blood
	Isotretinoin (Accutane)	Isotretinoin is a vitamin A derivative. To avoid drug toxicity, do not take vitamin A if you are also taking isotretinoin.
	Mineral oil	May interfere with the absorption of vitamins A, D, E, and K
	Vitamin E	Increase the capacity of body tissues to store vitamin A, protecting against vitamin A toxicity

	Can Interact With:	To:
Vitamin A	Certain blood tests	Produce an unusually high sedimentation rate (test for normal body reaction to injury or disease)
		Produce a high prothrombin time (a test for blood clotting)
		Produce a low white and red blood cell count
		Produce high levels of certain enzymes and chemicals found in the liver (general tests for liver function). Large doses of vitamin A are needed for this effect.
	Zinc	Assist in the absorption of vitamin A
Vitamin D	Phenytoin for seizures	Interfere with the action of vitamin D on the body
	Antacids containing magnesium	Cause toxic blood levels of magnesium in people on dialysis
	Barbiturates	Decrease vitamin D activity. High doses of barbiturates must be taken over a long time to product this effect.
	Colestipol and cholestyramine resin for high cholesterol	Decrease absorption of vitamin D into the bloodsteam
	Digitalis drugs for heat failure	Cause high blood levels of calcium, thus perhaps causing abnormal heart rhythms
	Mineral oil	Interfere with the absorption of vitamin D. Do not take mineral oil within two hours of taking vitamin D.
	Thiazide diuretics	Cause high blood levels of calcium in people with poor parathyroid gland function

	Can Interact With:	To:
Vitamin D	Verapamil	Cause high blood levels of calcium, thus perhaps causing abnormal heart rhythms
	Certain blood tests	Interfere with the measurement of blood cholesterol
		Increase blood magnesium levels. This can be a severe problem in people with kidney disease, for whom magnesium can be toxic.
Vitamin E	Oral anticoagulant drugs	Cause bleeding. Large doses of vitamin E have been reported to interfere with blood clotting and may enhance the effect of anticoagulants.
	Mineral oil	May interfere with the absorption of vitamins A, D, E, and K
	Iron	Possibly interfere with iron's effect on anemic children
	Vitamin A	Increase the capacity of body tissues to store vitamin A, protecting against vitamin A toxicity
Vitamin K	Oral anticoagulants	Reduce anticoagulant action. This effect is well known, and vitamin K is used as an antidote for anticoagulant overdose.
	Mineral oil	May interfere with the absorption of vitamins A, D, E, and K
Calcium	Atenolol	Less atenolol in the blood, possibly leading to a reduced beta-blocker effect
	Digitalis drugs for heart failure	Produce abnormal heart rhythms, but large doses of calcium are needed to produce this effect. People taking digitalis should not take large amounts of calcium supplements.
	Tiludronate	Do not take calcium, magnesium, and aluminum inactivate tiludronate within two hours of taking the medicine.

	Can Interact With:	To:
Calcium	Iron supplements	Reduce absorption of iron into the blood. Take these two supplements at least two hours apart.
	Norfloxacin	Reduce amount of norfloxacin in the blood. Other drugs in the same chemical class, ciprofloxacin and ofloxacin, do not appear to be affected by taking calcium.
	Sodium polystyrene sulfonate	Lower its potassium-reducing effect
	Tetracycline antibiotics	Reduce the amount of tetracycline absorbed into the bloodstream. Separate calcium-containing foods, antacids, or supplements from the antibiotic by two hours.
	Thiazide diuretics	Cause high blood levels of calcium
	Vitamin C	Increase the amount of calcium absorbed
	Verapamil	Reduce the effectiveness of verapamil
	Phosphorous	Help maintain appropriate calcium/phosphorous balance in the body
	Certain blood tests	Indicate a high serum amylase level (used to evaluate the pancreas)
		Interfere with tests for blood magnesium
	Certain urine tests	Interfere with tests for natural steroids
Copper	Vitamin C	Reduce copper absorption. Large doses of vitamin C must be taken to produce this effect.
	Molybdenum	Maintain the appropriate ratio of copper to molybdenum in the body
	Iron	Decrease copper absorption

	Can Interact With:	To:
Copper	Zinc	Decrease copper absorption. Large doses of zinc must be taken to produce this effect.
Iodine	Lithium	Cause abnormally low thyroid activity. Lithium patients should avoid iodine, which suppresses the thyroid gland.
	Certain blood tests	Interfere with thyroid function tests
	Certain urine tests	Interfere with tests for natural steroids in the urine
	Allopurinol for gout	Increase iron storage in the liver. Do not take this combination.
Iron	Antacids	Reduce the amount of iron absorbed into the blood. These two should be taken at least two hours apart.
	Chloramphenicol, an antibiotic	Interfere with the effectiveness of iron in anemic people
	Cholestyramine resin for high cholesterol	Decrease the amount of iron absorbed into the blood. These two should be taken at least two hours apart.
	Pancreatic extract	Reduce the amount of iron absorbed into the blood
	Penicillamine for rheumatoid arthritis	Decrease the amount of penicillamine absorbed into the blood
	Tetracycline	Interfere with the amount of tetracycline absorbed into the blood. These two should be taken at least two hours apart.
	Vitamin C	Increase iron absorption into the bloodstream. Large doses of vitamin C are needed to produce this effect.
	Vitamin E	Interfere with the effect of iron in anemic children
	Calcium	Increase the absorption of calcium

	Can Interact With:	To:
Iron	Copper	Reduce the amount of copper absorbed
	Zinc	Reduce the absorption of iron. Large doses of zinc must be taken for this effect.
Magnesium	Aminoquinoline antimalarial drugs	Reduce drug absorption, possibly interfering with antimalarial effect
	Chlorpromazine, a tranquilizer	Reduce tranquilizer effect
	Digoxin	Interfere with the absorption of digoxin into the bloodstream
	Nitrofurantoin	Interfere with the absorption of nitrofurantoin into the bloodstream,
	Drugs to relax muscles during surgery	Produce excessive muscle relaxation, with possibly serious difficulties. This has been reported only with intravenous magnesium, but you should be sure to tell your surgeon if you are using a magnesium supplement.
	Oral anticoagulants	Reduce anticoagulant effect
	Penicillamine	Reduce penicillamine effect
	Tetracycline antibiotics	Reduce antibiotic effect
	Tiludronate	Reduce tiludronate absorption. Take these at least two hours apart.
Molybdenum	Copper	Maintain the appropriate ratio of copper to molybdenum in the body
Potassium	ACE inhibitors	Increase blood potassium levels
	Digitalis drugs	Low blood potassium levels can lead to digitalis toxicity. Be cautious about stopping your potassium if you are also taking a digitalis drug.
	Thiazide diuretics and loop diuretics	Lower potassium levels

	Can Interact With:	To:
Potassium	Potassium-sparing diuretics	Increase potassium levels, possibly to toxic levels
Phosphorous	Antacids	Bind phosphorous and prevent it from being absorbed
	Calcium and vitamin D	Reduce blood phosphate levels. May be a factor in the treatment of high blood calcium levels.
	Potassium supplements and potassium-sparing diuretics	Cause high blood potassium levels if taken together with a phosphate. People taking this combination should have their blood potassium levels checked periodically.
Zinc	Tetracycline antibiotics	Decrease the amount of tetracycline absorbed. Take these at least two hours apart.
	Vitamin A	Assist in vitamin A absorption
	Copper	Reduce copper absorption into the blood. Large doses of zinc are needed to produce this effect.
	Fluoroquinolone anti-infectives	Reduce absorption of fluoroquinolones, possibly reducing anti-infective effectiveness
	Iron	Reduce the absorption of iron. Large doses of zinc are needed to produce this effect.
Herbal medicines generally	Carbamazepine, digoxin, cyclosporine, phenytoin, warfarin, valproic acid	Produce drug side effects or toxicities. Mixing these medicines with an herbal product is discouraged.
Ginseng	Phenelzine	Cause hallucinations, headache, irritability, sleeplessness
	Warfarin	Reduce drug effect (based on a single clinical study)
St. John's Wort	Stimulants (amphetamines, ephedrine isometheptine (Midrin), phenylpropanolamine, pseudoephedrine	Produce excess stimulation, amphetamine-like effects

	Can Interact With:	To:
St. John's Wort	Dextromethorphan, fluoxetine, fluvoxamine, meperidine, nefazodone, paroxetine, sertraline, tramadol, venlafaxine	Produce excess drug effect
Danshen	Warfarin	May increase the blood-thinning effect of warfarin.
Ephedrine	Stimulants (amphetamines, ephedrine isometheptine (Midrin), phenylpropanolamine, pseudoephedrine	Increases the stimulant effect of these medicines.
	MAO Inhibitors	Sudden, very large increases in blood pressure, possibly requiring emergency treatment
Gingko Biloba	Warfarin	May increase the blood-thinning effect of warfarin.
Licorice	Blood pressure–lowering drugs	May counter the blood pressure–lowering effect of these medicines.
	Diuretics	May enhance the loss of body potassium that normally occurs with diuretics.
	Corticosteroid medicines	May alter the effects of corticosteroid drugs.
Kava	Tranquilizers, sleeping pills, and other nervous system depressants	May increase the level of nervous system depression.

Appendix

Vitamin and Mineral Content of Foods

HOW TO USE THESE TABLES

The following tables provide you with basic information about the amount of vitamins and minerals in our food. Many foods have more than one listing to reflect the amount of vitamins and minerals contained in different preparations of that food. There are also listings for foods that show the difference in nutrient content before and after cooking. Be sure to select the listing that most closely approximates the type of food you are measuring and its form.

The information contained in these tables was gleaned from a number of different sources, including the U.S. Department of Agriculture's publication 65, *Nutritive Value of American Foods*. The government has not published this data in booklet form for more than a decade, but it is available in detail on the internet at *http://www.nal.usda.gov/fnic/foodcomp*. What we've tried to do here is distill the massive amount of information to a usable form. Additional information on the composition of fast foods was obtained from the fast-food chains themselves.

To use these tables properly, you must keep an accurate record of the foods you eat every day. The food tables are divided into the following categories: dairy products, eggs, fish, and fowl; fast foods; fruits; grains and grain products; meats; sausage, cold cuts, and lunch meats; miscellaneous foods (including condiments, soups, and nuts); sugars, sweets, and desserts; and vegetables.

Most vitamins and minerals are available in a great variety of foods and are so widespread that most people do not have to think about obtaining sufficient quantities in their daily diets. Others are required in larger amounts than previously thought, so some supplementation for calcium, iron, and some of the B vitamins, for example, is relatively common. Still others are controversial in terms of their basic requirement for human nutrition. Detailed information on current requirements for each nutrient can be found in the chapter covering each one. Food sources for individual vitamins and minerals not included here can be found in the chart included in each individual vitamin and mineral profile.

You can also use your home computer and the internet to help track and analyze your diet's nutrient content. On pages 40–42, we include a partial list of software programs and internet sites that can help you; before buying any program you'll want to consider the extent of its nutrient content data base, ease of use, flexibility and, most important, does it do the job you need it to do? Nutrition software can cost a few dollars to hundreds or thousands of dollars, with pricing differences related to the program's sophistication, the depth of analysis offered, and their intended audience. Software packages intended for the general public cost less than those intended for nutrition and health care professionals.

Appendix: Vitamin and Mineral Content of Foods

Dairy Products

Item	Amount	Calories	Protein (g)	Calcium (mg)	Iron (mg)	Sodium (mg)	Potassium (mg)	Vitamin A (mcg)	Thiamin (mg)	Ribof (mg)	Niacin (mg)	Vitamin C (mg)	Vitamin B6 (mg)	Vitamin E (mg)	Folic Acid (mg)
Butter	1 tsp	36	0	1	0	49	1	165	0	0	0	0	0	0.1	0
Whipped	1 tsp	48	0	1	0	65	1	224	0	0	0	0	0	0.1	0
Buttermilk	1 cup	88	8.8	296	0.1	319	343	10	0.1	0.44	0.25	2.5	0.09	0.25	27
Natural cheeses															
Blue (Roquefort)	1 oz	103	6	88	0.14	186	22	347	0.01	0.17	0.3	0	0.05	0.2	3
Brick	1 oz	103	6	198	0.4	0	0	346	0	0.13	0.03	0	0.02	0	0
Camembert	1 oz	81	4.8	28	0.14	0	31	277	0.01	0.21	0.22	0	0.06	0	0
Cheddar	1 oz	111	72	100.3	196	23	367	0.01	0.13	0	0	0.02	0.4	0	2
Cottage cheese	½ cup	121	15.5	107	0.3	261	24	194	0.03	0.29	0.1	0	0.05	0.1	31
Cream cheese	1 oz	105	2.2	170	0.1	70	21	431	0.01	0.07	0	0	0.02	0.3	4
Cream cheese, whipped	1 oz	104	2.2	170	0.1	70	21	214	0.01	0.07	0	0	0.02	0.3	4
Limburger	1 oz	96	5.9	165	0.17	0	0	318	0.02	0.14	0.06	0	0.02	0	0
Parmesan	1 oz	118	11	340	0.11	219	45	318	0.01	0.22	0.06	0	0.03	0	0
Swiss	1 oz	103	7.7	258	0.25	198	29	318	0	0.11	0.03	0	0.02	0	0
Cheese, pasteurized process															
American	1 slice	70	4.4	132	0.2	216	15	342	0.01	0.08	0	0	0.02	0.3	3
American	1 oz	104	6.5	195	0.3	318	22	340	0.01	0.11	0	0	0.02	0.3	3

Item	Amount	Calories	Protein (g)	Calcium (mg)	Iron (mg)	Sodium (mg)	Potassium (mg)	Vitamin A (mcg)	Thiamin (mg)	Ribof (mg)	Niacin (mg)	Vitamin C (mg)	Vitamin B_6 (mg)	Vitamin E (mg)	Folic Acid (mg)
Swiss	1 slice	75	5.5	186	0.2	245	21	230	T	0.08	T	0	0.01	0.17	0
Swiss	1 oz	101	7.0	251	0.25	331	28	312	T	0.11	0.03	0	0.01	0.25	0
Cream															
Half and half	1 oz	41	0.96	33	0.01	14	39	145	0.01	0.05	0.01	0.3		0	0
Light cream	1 oz	63	0.9	31	0.01	13	37	259	0.01	0.05	0.01	0.3	0.01	0	0
Heavy cream	1 oz	105	0.65	22	0.01	10	27	459	T	0.03	0.01	0.3		0	0
Ice cream	½ cup	186	3.6	111	0	36	101	468	0.04	0.17	0.1	1	0.03	0.1	1
Ice milk	½ cup	144	3.5	116	0	35	107	220	0.05	0.18	0.1	1	0.03	0.1	1
Milk															
Whole	1 cup	159	8.5	288	0.1	122	351	350	0.07	0.41	0.2	2	0.1	0.24	1.5
Skim	1 cup	88	8.8	296	0.1	127	355	10	0.09	0.44	0.2	2	0.1	0.24	0.3
Low-fat	1 cup	145	10.3	352	0.1	150	431	200	0.1	0.52	0.2	2	0.1	0.24	0
Yogurt															
Made from whole milk	1 cup	152	7.4	72	0.1	115	323	340	0.07	0.39	0.2	2	0.1	0	0
Low-fat	1 cup	123	8.3	294	0.1	125	350	170	0.1	0.44	0.02	2	0.11	0	0

Eggs, Fish, and Fowl

Item	Amount	Calories	Protein (g)	Calcium (mg)	Iron	Sodium	Potassium	Vitamin A (mcg)	Thiamin	Ribof	Niacin	Vitamin C	Vitamin B_6 (mg)	Vitamin E (mg)	Folic Acid (mg)
Bass, sea, broiled	3 oz	216	135	0	0	0								0	0
Oven-fried and breaded	3 oz	165	18	0	0	0								0	0

Food	Portion														
Bluefish															
Baked or broiled	3 oz	132	22	24.3	0.6	87	42	6	0.09	0.09	1.5			0.21	2.5
Fried	3 oz	171	19	29.4	0.8	120			0.09	0.09	1.5			0.2	2.5
Caviar	1 oz	74	7.6	78	3.3	624	51						2.5	0.1	6.2
Chicken															
Light meat	3 oz	138	26.4	9.3	1	53	345	0.03	0.09	9.6	0	21			
Dark meat	3 oz	147	23.4	11	1.4	72	270	0.06	1.18	4.8	0	0.3			
Canned	3 oz	168	18.4	18	1.3	340	210	195	0.03	0.1	3.7	3			
A la king	3 oz	159	9	45	0.9	258	138	390	0.03	0.15	1.8	4			
Fricassee	3 oz	135	13	5.1	0.9	129	117	60	0.03	0.06	0.2				
Pot pie	3 oz	195	8.4	25.2	1.2	213	123	1,113	0.09	0.09	1.5	2			
Clams	5 small or ½ cup	98	15.8	55	4.1	1,010	184	110	0.01	0.11	1.1	11	80	0.3	3
Cod, cooked	3 oz	141	24	25.8	0.9	93	351	150	0.06	0.09	2.5				
Eggs															
Fried	1	86	5.5	24	1	135	56	570	0.04	0.12	T				
Hard-boiled	1	72	5.7	24	1	54	57	520	0.04	0.12	T				
Poached	1	72	5.7	24	1	119	57	520	0.04	0.12	T				
Scrambled	1	97	6.3	45	1	144	82	600	0.04	0.12	T				
Fish sticks	1	50	4.7	3	0.1				0.1	0.02	0.5				

Item	Amount	Calories	Protein (g)	Calcium (mg)	Iron (mg)	Sodium (mg)	Potassium (mg)	Vitamin A (mcg)	Thiamin (mg)	Ribof (mg)	Niacin (mg)	Vitamin C (mg)	Vitamin B6 (mg)	Vitamin E (mg)	Folic Acid (mg)
Flounder	3 oz	172	25.5	29	1.2	202	500		0.06	0.07	2.1	2	0.14		
Halibut, broiled	3 oz	145	21.4	14	0.7	114	211	578	0.04	0.06	7.1	3	289	0.5	14
Herring, smoked	1 fillet	84	8.9	26	0.6			10		0.11	1.3		0.06		36
Lobster meat	3 oz	78	15	54	0.6	177	150	0.09	0.06						
Lobster Newburgh	1 cup	485	26.5	218	2.3	573	428	0.18	0.28	0.2					
Mackerel, broiled	3 oz	197	18	5	1	0	0	144	0.12	0.2	6.4	0	0.5	1.3	0
Perch, fried	3 oz	189	16	28	1.1	129	237	0	0.09	0.09	1.5	0	0	0	0
Oysters	1 cup	158	20.2	226	13.2	175	290	7,400	.34	0.43	6	0.1	0	0	0
Rockfish, steamed	3 oz	90 *	15	0	0	57	372	0	0.03	0.09	0	0.9	0	0	0
Roe, herring	3 oz	99	18	12	1	0	0	0	0	0	0	1.8	0.12	0	0
Salmon															
Chinook	3 oz	177	15	129	8	0	306	192	0.03	0.12	6	0	0.24	0	5.7
Coho	3 oz	129	17	207	0.75	294	285	66	0.03	0.15	6	0	0	0	0
Fillet, broiled or baked	3 oz	155	23	68	1	99	377	1,360	.14	0.05	8.3	4	255	1.2	6
Baked	3 oz	150	18.4	12	1.2	114	435	161	0.18	0.07	10.8	4	1.2	595	6

Food	Serving														
Sardines, canned	2 med. (1 oz)	57	6.7	122	0.8	230	165	62	0.01	0.06	1.5	0	50	0.2	9
Scallops, cooked	3 oz	93	19.5	96	2.5	222	399	0	0	0	0	0	0	0	0
Shad, baked	3 oz	173	20	20.7	0.5	68	325	27	0.11	0.22	7.4	0	0	0	0
Shrimp	3 oz	80	17.8	66	1.4	107	173	34	0.02	0.03	2.8	9	42	0.4	2
Fried	3 oz	192	10.6	32.7	0.9	183	169	26	0.03	0.03	1.7	6	51.6	0.5	1.7
Sturgeon Steamed	4 oz	7.5	11	0.56	30	660	0	0	0	0	0	0	0	0	0
Smoked	1 oz	42	8.7	0	0	0	0	0	0	0	0	0	0	0	0
Swordfish, broiled	3 oz	138	22	21	0.9	0	0	1,614	0.03	0.03	8.7	0	0	0	0
Tile fish	3 oz	114	20												
Tuna In oil	3 oz	165	24	66	1.6	0	0	96	0.03	0.09	10	0	0.3	0.51	0
In water	3 oz	109	24	14	1.4	35	241	0	0	0.09	11.5	0	0	0	0
Salad	1 cup	349	30	41	2.7	0	0	590	0.08	0.23	10.3	2	0	0	0
Turkey	3 oz	224	23	9	1.8	79	377	144	0.09	0.17	9.7	2	340	0.3	9
Pot pie	1 piece	550	24.1	63	3.2	633	459	3,090	0.26	0.3	5.8	5			
Whitefish Cooked	1 oz	61	4.3	0	0.1	55	82	570	0.03	0.03	0.7	T	0.3		
Smoked	3 oz	129	17	18											

Fast Food

Item	Amount	Calories	Protein (g)	Calcium (mg)	Iron (mg)	Sodium (mg)	Potassium (mg)	Vitamin A (mcg)	Thiamin (mg)	Ribof (mg)	Niacin (mg)	Vitamin C (mg)	Vitamin B6 (mg)	Vitamin E (mg)	Folic Acid (mg)
Arby's															
Arby Q	1	389	17.6	56	9	1,268	456	T	0.27	0.4	9	T	N/A	N/A	N/A
Bacon Platter	1	593	22	48	3.6	880	491	80	0.38	0.34	3	4	N/A	N/A	N/A
Baked Potato															
Plain	1	240	5.8	T	2.7	58	1,333	T	0.09	0.14	3	33	N/A	N/A	N/A
Butter and sour cream	1	463	8	520	2.7	203	1,420	40	0.09	0.14	3	33	N/A	N/A	N/A
Broccoli and cheese	1	417	10	80	2.7	361	1,455	40	0.09	0.17	3	45	N/A	N/A	N/A
Beef 'N' Cheddar	1	508	24	120	6	1,166	321	T	0.5	0.62	10	1	N/A	N/A	N/A
Biscuit															
Plain	1	280	6	80	2.7	730	130	T	0.23	0.14	3	T	N/A	N/A	N/A
Bacon	1	318	7	80	2.7	904	157	T	0.23	0.14	3	T	N/A	N/A	N/A
Sausage	1	460	12	80	3.6	1,000	225	T	0.3	0.17	4	T	N/A	N/A	N/A
Ham	1	323	13	80	2.7	1,169	254	T	0.45	0.26	4	T	N/A	N/A	N/A
Chef Salad	14.5 oz	205	18	136	6	796	819	1,000	0.38	0.37	7	53	N/A	N/A	N/A
Chicken Breast															
Fillet	1	445	22	48	2.9	958	403	T	0.23	0.6	9	5	N/A	N/A	N/A
Chicken Cordon Bleu	1	518	30.5	48	3	1,463	464	T	0.38	0.65	10	5	N/A	N/A	N/A
Croissant															
Plain	1	260	6	32	2.7	300	95	T	0.15	0.14	2	T	N/A	N/A	N/A
Bacon/egg	1	430	17.4	16	3.8	720	266	80	0.3	0.39	3	T	N/A	N/A	N/A

Item	Serving												N/A	N/A	N/A	N/A
Ham/cheese	1	345	16	120	2.7	939	225	T	0.38	0.25	4	T	N/A	N/A	N/A	N/A
Sausage/egg	1	519	17.5	48	3.6	632	242	40	0.3	0.34	3	T	N/A	N/A	N/A	N/A
Curly Fries	3.5 oz	337	4	16	1.4	167	724	T	0.06	0.07	2	T	N/A	N/A	N/A	N/A
Egg Platter	1	460	15	48	3.6	591	412	80	0.38	0.34	4	4	N/A	N/A	N/A	N/A
Ham Platter	1	518	24	48	3.6	1,177	578	80	0.7	0.43	4	4	N/A	N/A	N/A	N/A
Junior Roast Beef	1	233	11.5	32	1.5	519	201	T	0.18	0.26	6	T	N/A	N/A	N/A	N/A
Regular Roast Beef	1	383	22	48	2.7	936	422	T	0.3	0.47	11	T	N/A	N/A	N/A	N/A
Garden Salad	11.6 oz	117	7	128	1.6	134	600	980	0.16	0.37	1	51	N/A	N/A	N/A	N/A
Giant Roast Beef	1	228	33	72	8	1,433	599	T	0.4	0.75	17	1	N/A	N/A	N/A	N/A
Fish Filet	1	526	23	136	4	872	450	T	0.35	0.3	5.6	3	N/A	N/A	N/A	N/A
French Dip Sandwich	1	368	22	40	4	1,018	367	T	0.2	0.46	8.4	T	N/A	N/A	N/A	N/A
French Dip 'N' Swiss	1	429	28	216	4.8	1,438	390	T	0.2	0.54	8.4	T	N/A	N/A	N/A	N/A
French fries	2.5 oz	246	2	T	1	114	240	T	0.06	T	2	4	N/A	N/A	N/A	N/A
Grilled Chicken Barbecue	1	386	23.4	56	4	1,002	596	50	0.3	0.29	13.6	3	N/A	N/A	N/A	N/A
Grilled Chicken Deluxe	1	430	23.6	56	2.5	901	659	80	0.3	0.29	13.6	8	N/A	N/A	N/A	N/A
Light Roast Beef Deluxe	1	294	18	104	4.5	826	392	40	0.2	0.45	8.4	7	N/A	N/A	N/A	N/A
Light Roast Turkey Deluxe	1	260	20	104	3.4	1,262	353	40	0.2	0.4	15.4	12	N/A	N/A	N/A	N/A
Light Roast Chicken Deluxe	1	276	24	104	2.8	777	432	40	0.5	0.75	9.4	7	N/A	N/A	N/A	N/A
Bac 'N' Cheddar Deluxe	1	512	21	88	4.4	1,094	491	40	0.5	0.62	10	11	N/A	N/A	N/A	N/A
Ham and Cheese	1	355	24.6	136	2.7	1,400	382	T	0.82	0.37	8	T	N/A	N/A	N/A	N/A
Muffin, Blueberry	1	240	4	16	0.7	200	84	T	0.09	.01	8	T	N/A	N/A	N/A	N/A
Philly Beef 'N' Swiss	1	197	24	240	6	1,144	409	T	0.3	0.62	9	20	N/A	N/A	N/A	N/A

Item	Amount	Calories	Protein (g)	Calcium (mg)	Iron (mg)	Sodium (mg)	Potassium (mg)	Vitamin A (mcg)	Thiamin (mg)	Ribof (mg)	Niacin (mg)	Vitamin C (mg)	Vitamin B6 (mg)	Vitamin E (mg)	Folic Acid (mg)
Roast Chicken Club	1	503	30.5	144	9	1,143	534	T	0.5	0.71	11	8	N/A	N/A	N/A
Sausage Platter	1	640	21	64	3.6	861	507	80	0.45	0.34	3	4	N/A	N/A	N/A
Super Roast Beef	1	552	24	72	6.5	1,174	533	30	0.38	0.56	12	9	N/A	N/A	N/A
Burger King															
Big King Sandwich	1	660	40	N/A	N/A	920									
Biscuit															
Bacon, egg & cheese	1	510	19	N/A	N/A	1,530									
Sausage		590	16	N/A	N/A	1,390									
BK Big Fish sandwich	1	700	26	N/A	N/A	980									
BK Broiler	1	550	30	N/A	N/A	480									
Cheeseburger	1	380	23	N/A	N/A	770									
Double	1	600	41	N/A	N/A	1,060									
Double, with bacon	1	640	44	N/A	N/A	1,240									
Chicken Sandwich	1	710	26	N/A	N/A	1,400									
Chicken Salad	1	200	21	N/A	N/A	110									
Chicken Tenders	8 pieces	310	21	N/A	N/A	710									
Croissanwich, with sausage egg, and cheese	1	600	22	N/A	N/A	1,140									
Dutch Apple Pie	1	300	3	N/A	N/A	230									
French Fries, medium, salted	1	400	3	N/A	N/A	820									
French Toast Sticks	1	500	4	N/A	N/A	490									

Item	Serving												
Hamburger	1	330	20	N/A	N/A	530							
Hash Browns	1	220	2	N/A	N/A	320							
Onion rings, regular	1	270	4	N/A	N/A	810							
Salad, garden, no dressing	1	100	6	N/A	N/A	115							
Salad, side, no dressing	1	60	3	N/A	N/A	55							
Shakes:													
Chocolate, medium	1	440	12	N/A	N/A	330							
Strawberry, medium	1	550	13	N/A	N/A	350							
Vanilla, medium	1	430	13	N/A	N/A	330							
Whopper	1	640	27	N/A	N/A	870							
With cheese	1	730	33	N/A	N/A	1,350							
Double	1	870	46	N/A	N/A	940							
Double, with cheese	1	960	52	N/A	N/A	1,420							
Whopper Jr.	1	420	21	N/A	N/A	530							
With cheese	1	460	23	N/A	N/A	770							
Dairy Queen													
DQ Homestyle Hamburger	1	290	17	48	2.7	630	40	N/A	N/A	N/A	4	N/A	N/A
DQ Homestyle Cheeseburger	1	340	20	120	3.6	850	100	N/A	N/A	N/A	4	N/A	N/A
DQ Homestyle Double Cheeseburger	1	540	35	200	4.5	1,130	150	N/A	N/A	N/A	4	N/A	N/A

Item	Amount	Calories	Protein (g)	Calcium (mg)	Iron (mg)	Sodium (mg)	Potassium (mg)	Vitamin A (mcg)	Thiamin (mg)	Ribof (mg)	Niacin (mg)	Vitamin C (mg)	Vitamin B6 (mg)	Vitamin E (mg)	Folic Acid (mg)
DQ Homestyle Bacon Double Cheeseburger	1	610	41	200	4.5	1,380	N/A	150	N/A	N/A	N/A	6	N/A	N/A	N/A
DQ Ultimate Burger	1	670	40	200	4.5	1,210	N/A	150	N/A	N/A	N/A	9	N/A	N/A	N/A
Hot Dog	1	240	9	48	1.8	730	N/A	20	N/A	N/A	N/A	4	N/A	N/A	N/A
Chili 'n' Cheese Dog	1	330	14	120	1.8	1,090	N/A	150	N/A	N/A	N/A	4	N/A	N/A	N/A
Chicken Strip Basket	1	1,000	35	48	4.5	2,260	N/A	40	N/A	N/A	N/A	9	N/A	N/A	N/A
Grilled Chicken Sandwich	1	310	24	16	2.7	1,040	N/A	0	N/A	N/A	N/A	4	N/A	N/A	N/A
French fries Medium	1	350	4	16	0.7	630	N/A	0	N/A	N/A	N/A	4	N/A	N/A	N/A
Large	1	440	5	32	1	790	N/A	0	N/A	N/A	N/A	5	N/A	N/A	N/A
Onion rings	1	320	5	16	1.4	180	N/A	0	N/A	N/A	N/A	0	N/A	N/A	N/A
Cookie Dough Blizzard Small chocolate chip	1	660	12	280	1.8	440	N/A	250	N/A	N/A	N/A	1	N/A	N/A	N/A
Medium chocolate chip	1	950	17	360	2.7	660	N/A	350	N/A	N/A	N/A	1	N/A	N/A	N/A
Dilly Bar, chocolate	1	210	3	80	0.4	75	N/A	60	N/A	N/A	N/A	0	N/A	N/A	N/A
Banana split	1	510	8	200	1.8	180	N/A	200	N/A	N/A	N/A	15	N/A	N/A	N/A
Dipped cone, small	1	340	6	160	1.8	130	N/A	100	N/A	N/A	N/A	1	N/A	N/A	N/A
Medium	1	490	8	200	1.8	190	N/A	150	N/A	N/A[	N/A	2	N/A	N/A	N/A
DQ Cone Small, chocolate	1	240	6	120	1	115	N/A	150	N/A	N/A	N/A	0	N/A	N/A	N/A
Medium, chocolate	1	340	8	200	1.8	160	N/A	150	N/A	N/A	N/A	1	N/A	N/A	N/A

Large, vanilla	1	410	10	280	1.8	N/A	200	200	N/A	N/A	N/A	2	N/A	N/A	N/A
DQ Sandwich	1	150	3	48	0.7	N/A	115	40	N/A	N/A	N/A	0	N/A	N/A	N/A
Frozen yogurt, nonfat	½ cup	100	3	80	0.7	N/A	70	0	N/A	N/A	N/A	0	N/A	N/A	N/A
Cone, medium	1	260	9	200	1.8	N/A	160	0	N/A	N/A	N/A	2	N/A	N/A	N/A
Cup, medium	1	230	8	200	1.4	N/A	150	0	N/A	N/A	N/A	1	N/A	N/A	N/A
Health Breeze, small	1	470	11	280	1.8	N/A	200	0	N/A	N/A	N/A	2	N/A	N/A	N/A
Health Breeze, medium	1	710	15	360	2.7	N/A	380	20	N/A	N/A	N/A	4	N/A	N/A	N/A
Sundae, medium, strawberry	1	280	8	240	1.4	N/A	580	0	N/A	N/A	N/A	6	N/A	N/A	N/A
Strawberry Breeze, small	1	320	10	280	1.8	N/A	160	0	N/A	N/A	N/A	6	N/A	N/A	N/A
Strawberry Breeze, medium	1	460	13	360	2.7	N/A	190	0	N/A	N/A	N/A	9	N/A	N/A	N/A
Fudge Bar, no sugar added	1	50	4	80	0	N/A	270	0	N/A	N/A	N/A	0	N/A	N/A	N/A
Fudge Cake Supreme	1	890	11	160	1.8	N/A	70	60	N/A	N/A	N/A	0	N/A	N/A	N/A
Lemon DQ Freez'r	½ cup	80	0	0	0	N/A	960	200	N/A	N/A	N/A	0	N/A	N/A	N/A
Malt								0							
Chocolate, small	1	650	15	360	1.8	N/A	370	300	N/A	N/A	N/A	2	N/A	N/A	N/A
Chocolate, medium	1	880	19	480	2.7	N/A	500	400	N/A	N/A	N/A	2	N/A	N/A	N/A
Misty Slush															
Small	1	220	0	0	0	N/A	20	0	N/A	N/A	N/A	0	N/A	N/A	N/A
Medium	1	290	0	0	0	N/A	30	0	N/A	N/A	N/A	0	N/A	N/A	N/A
Peanut Buster Parfait	1	730	16	240	1.8	N/A	400	150	N/A	N/A	N/A	1	N/A	N/A	N/A
Round Cake, frozen	⅛ cake	340	7	160	1.4	N/A	250	150	N/A	N/A	N/A	0	N/A	N/A	N/A

Item	Amount	Calories	Protein (g)	Calcium (mg)	Iron (mg)	Sodium (mg)	Potassium (mg)	Vitamin A (mcg)	Thiamin (mg)	Ribof (mg)	Niacin (mg)	Vitamin C (mg)	Vitamin B6 (mg)	Vitamin E (mg)	Folic Acid (mg)
Sandwich Cookie															
Blizzard															
Small, chocolate	1	520	10	280	1.8	380	N/A	200	N/A	N/A	N/A	1	N/A	N/A	N/A
Medium, chocolate	1	640	12	320	2.7	500	N/A	200	N/A	N/A	N/A	1	N/A	N/A	N/A
Shake															
Chocolate, small	1	560	13	360	1.8	310	N/A	300	N/A	N/A	N/A	2	N/A	N/A	N/A
Chocolate, medium	1	770	17	480	2.7	420	N/A	400	N/A	N/A	N/A	2	N/A	N/A	N/A
Starkiss	1	80	0	0	0	10	N/A	0	N/A	N/A	N/A	0	N/A	N/A	N/A
Strawberry Shortcake	1	430	7	200	1.8	360	N/A	100	N/A	N/A	N/A	6	N/A	N/A	N/A
Sundae															
Chocolate, small	1	280	5	160	1	140	N/A	100	N/A	N/A	N/A	0	N/A	N/A	N/A
Chocolate, medium	1	400	8	200	1.4	210	N/A	150	N/A	N/A	N/A	0	N/A	N/A	N/A
Treatzza Pizza															
Heath	1/8 pizza	180	3	48	0.7	160	N/A	40	N/A	N/A	N/A	0	N/A	N/A	N/A
M&M's	1/8 pizza	190	3	48	0.7	160	N/A	40	N/A	N/A	N/A	0	N/A	N/A	N/A
Vanilla Orange Bar, no sugar added	1	60	2	48	0	40	N/A	20	N/A	N/A	N/A	0	N/A	N/A	N/A
Domino's Pizza															
Cheese Pizza															
Hand Tossed 12"	2 slices	344	14	278	4	980	N/A	94	N/A	N/A	N/A	3	N/A	N/A	N/A
Thin Crust 12"—															
1/8 pizza	1	364	16	422	1.5	1,012	N/A	172	N/A	N/A	N/A	4	N/A	N/A	N/A
Deep Dish 12"	2 slices	560	24	451	5	1,184	N/A	232	N/A	N/A	N/A	3	N/A	N/A	N/A

	Serving															
Ham Pizza																
Hand Tossed 12"—																
2 slices	362	17	279	4	1,143	N/A	139	N/A	N/A	N/A	3		N/A	N/A	N/A	N/A
Thin Crust 12"—																
⅓ pizza	388	19	424	1.7	1,229	N/A	172	N/A	N/A	N/A	4		N/A	N/A	N/A	N/A
Deep Dish 12" 2 slices	577	26	453	5	1,347	N/A	232	N/A	N/A	N/A	3		N/A	N/A	N/A	N/A
Italian Sausage and Mushroom Pizza																
Hand Tossed 12" 2 slices	402	18	287	5	1,151	N/A	146	N/A	N/A	N/A	3		N/A	N/A	N/A	N/A
Thin Crust 12"—																
⅓ pizza	442	20	434	2	1,240	N/A	183	N/A	N/A	N/A	4		N/A	N/A	N/A	N/A
Deep Dish 12" 2 slices	618	26	460	5	1,356	N/A	240	N/A	N/A	N/A	4		N/A	N/A	N/A	N/A
Pepperoni Pizza																
Hand Tossed 12" 2 slices	406	18	282	4	1,179	N/A	142	N/A	N/A	N/A	3		N/A	N/A	N/A	N/A
Thin Crust 12"—																
⅓ pizza	447	20	428	1.8	1,277	N/A	177	N/A	N/A	N/A	4		N/A	N/A	N/A	N/A
Deep Dish 12" 2 slices	622	26	456	5	1,383	N/A	235	N/A	N/A	N/A	3		N/A	N/A	N/A	N/A
Veggie																
Hand Tossed 12" 2 slices	360	15	286	4	1,028	N/A	150	N/A	N/A	N/A	13		N/A	N/A	N/A	N/A
Thin Crust 12"—																
⅓ pizza	386	17	433	2	1,076	N/A	187	N/A	N/A	N/A	17		N/A	N/A	N/A	N/A
Deep Dish 12" 2 slices	576	24	460	5	1,233	N/A	243	N/A	N/A	N/A	13		N/A	N/A	N/A	N/A
X'tra Cheese and Pepperoni Pizza																
Hand Tossed 12" 2 slices	455	21	412	5	1,304	N/A	175	N/A	N/A	N/A	3		N/A	N/A	N/A	N/A
Thin Crust 12"—																
⅓ pizza	512	24	601	2	1,443	N/A	222	N/A	N/A	N/A	4		N/A	N/A	N/A	N/A
Deep Dish 12" 2 slices	671	30	586	5	1,508	N/A	269	N/A	N/A	N/A	3		N/A	N/A	N/A	N/A
Jack in the Box																
Apple Turnover 1	340	4	0	1.8	510	85	20	N/A	N/A	N/A	12		N/A	N/A	N/A	N/A

Item	Amount	Calories	Protein (g)	Calcium (mg)	Iron (mg)	Sodium (mg)	Potassium (mg)	Vitamin A (mcg)	Thiamin (mg)	Ribof (mg)	Niacin (mg)	Vitamin C (mg)	Vitamin B6 (mg)	Vitamin E (mg)	Folic Acid (mg)
Breakfast Jack	1	300	18	0	2.7	890	220	80	N/A	N/A	N/A	8	N/A	N/A	N/A
Carrot Cake	1	370	3	16	1.4	340	150	1,100	N/A	N/A	N/A	0	N/A	N/A	N/A
Cheeseburger	1	330	15	120	4.5	760	110	80	N/A	N/A	N/A	T	N/A	N/A	N/A
Cheesecake	1	310	8	80	0.4	210	15	0	N/A	N/A	N/A	0	N/A	N/A	N/A
Double Cheeseburger	1	450	24	200	3.6	970	320	100	N/A	N/A	N/A	0	N/A	N/A	N/A
Double Fudge Cake	1	300	3	32	1.8	320	250	60	N/A	N/A	N/A	0	N/A	N/A	N/A
Egg Rolls	3 pieces	440	15	64	4.5	1,020	500	150	N/A	N/A	N/A	12	N/A	N/A	N/A
	5 pieces	730	25	120	7.2	1,700	830	250	N/A	N/A	N/A	1	N/A	N/A	N/A
Garden Chicken Salad	1	200	23	160	0.7	420	560	700	N/A	N/A	N/A	12	N/A	N/A	N/A
Hamburger	1	280	13	64	4.5	560	220	40	N/A	N/A	N/A	T	N/A	N/A	N/A
¼ Pounder	1	510	26	120	3.6	1,080	320	60	N/A	N/A	N/A	9	N/A	N/A	N/A
Ice Cream Shake															
Vanilla, regular	1	610	12	320	0	320	730	150	N/A	N/A	N/A	0	N/A	N/A	N/A
Cappucino classic, regular	1	630	11	280	0	320	710	150	N/A	N/A	N/A	0	N/A	N/A	N/A
Chocolate regular	1	640	10	280	0.4	330	720	150	N/A	N/A	N/A	0	N/A	N/A	N/A
Oreo cookie classic, regular	1	740	13	320	0.4	490	730	150	N/A	N/A	N/A	0	N/A	N/A	N/A
Strawberry, regular	1	640	10	280	0	85	300	150	N/A	N/A	N/A	0	N/A	N/A	N/A
Jumbo Jack															
Hamburger	1	560	28	80	4.5	680	350	T	N/A	N/A	N/A	9	N/A	N/A	N/A
With cheese	1	650	32	200	5.4	1,090	380	100	N/A	N/A	N/A	9	N/A	N/A	N/A
Chicken Breast Pieces	5	360	27	16	1.8	970	430	40	N/A	N/A	N/A	1	N/A	N/A	N/A
Chicken and Fries	1	730	26	80	2.7	1,690	1,100	40	N/A	N/A	N/A	9	N/A	N/A	N/A

Item	Serving													
Chicken Caesar Sandwich	1	520	27	200	2.7	1,050	490	80	N/A	N/A	N/A	2	N/A	N/A
Chicken Fajita Pita	1	280	24	120	2.7	840	410	100	N/A	N/A	N/A	0	N/A	N/A
Chicken Filet (grilled)	1	520	27	160	4.5	1,240	510	100	N/A	N/A	N/A	0	N/A	N/A
Chicken Sandwich	1	450	16	64	1.8	1,030	265	40	N/A	N/A	N/A	1	N/A	N/A
Chicken Supreme	1	680	23	200	2.7	1,500	400	150	N/A	N/A	N/A	9	N/A	N/A
Chicken Teriyaki Bowl	1	670	29	120	0	1,620	620	600	N/A	N/A	N/A	0	N/A	N/A
Curly Fries														
Seasoned	1	420	6	32	2.7	1,030	630	80	N/A	N/A	N/A	0	N/A	N/A
Chili and cheese	1	650	12	80	2.7	1,640	810	250	N/A	N/A	N/A	T	N/A	N/A
Fish and Chips	1	720	19	16	2.7	1,580	1,060	20	N/A	N/A	N/A	12	N/A	N/A
French Fries														
Regular	1	360	4	0	0	740	610	0	N/A	N/A	N/A	24	N/A	N/A
Jumbo	1	430	4	0	1.4	890	740	0	N/A	N/A	N/A	27	N/A	N/A
Super scoop	1	610	6	16	1.8	1,250	1,040	0	N/A	N/A	N/A	42	N/A	N/A
Hash Brown	1	160	1	0	0.4	310	190	40	N/A	N/A	N/A	6	N/A	N/A
Jalapeños, stuffed	7 pieces	470	14	240	1	1,560	190	200	N/A	N/A	N/A	18	N/A	N/A
	10 pieces	680	20	400	1.8	2,220	270	300	N/A	N/A	N/A	30	N/A	N/A
Onion Rings	1	460	7	32	2.7	780	150	40	N/A	N/A	N/A	18	N/A	N/A
Philly Cheesesteak Sandwich	1	520	33	240	5.4	1,980	420	150	N/A	N/A	N/A	0	N/A	N/A
Pancakes with Bacon	1 order	400	13	64	1.8	980	280	0	N/A	N/A	N/A	0	N/A	N/A
Potato Wedges, Bacon/Cheddar	1	800	20	280	1.8	1,470	960	100	N/A	N/A	N/A	12	N/A	N/A
Sausage Croissant	1	670	21	120	3.6	940	180	200	N/A	N/A	N/A	1	N/A	N/A
Side Salad	1	50	2	160	0.7	75	160	150	N/A	N/A	N/A	0	N/A	N/A

Item	Amount	Calories	Protein (g)	Calcium (mg)	Iron (mg)	Sodium (mg)	Potassium (mg)	Vitamin A (mcg)	Thiamin (mg)	Ribof (mg)	Niacin (mg)	Vitamin C (mg)	Vitamin B6 (mg)	Vitamin E (mg)	Folic Acid (mg)
Sourdough Breakfast Sandwich	1	380	21	200	3.6	1,120	260	150	N/A	N/A	N/A	9	N/A	N/A	N/A
Sourdough Jack Hamburger	1	670	32	160	4.5	1,180	510	150	N/A	N/A	N/A	6	N/A	N/A	N/A
Spicy Crispy Chicken Sandwich	1	560	24	80	2.7	1,020	470	40	N/A	N/A	N/A	5	N/A	N/A	N/A
Supreme Croissant	1	570	21	80	3.6	1,240	340	150	N/A	N/A	N/A	12	N/A	N/A	N/A
Taco Regular	1	190	7	80	1	410	240	80	N/A	N/A	N/A	0	N/A	N/A	N/A
Monster	1	290	11	160	1.4	550	290	80	N/A	N/A	N/A	5	N/A	N/A	N/A
Ultimate Breakfast Sandwich	1	620	36	200	4.5	1,800	450	150	N/A	N/A	N/A	9	N/A	N/A	N/A
Ultimate Cheeseburger	1	1,030	50	240	6.3	1,200	520	100	N/A	N/A	N/A	1	N/A	N/A	N/A
Ultimate Cheeseburger with Bacon	1	1,150	57	240	7.2	1,770	610	100	N/A	N/A	N/A	1	N/A	N/A	N/A
Kentucky Fried Chicken															
BBQ Baked Beans	1 order	45	1	64	1.8	760	N/A	80	N/A	N/A	N/A	T	N/A	N/A	N/A
Biscuit		180	4	16	1	560	N/A	T	N/A	N/A	N/A	T	N/A	N/A	N/A
Chicken Sandwich Original Recipe	1	497	29	80	2.7	1,213	N/A	T	N/A	N/A	N/A	T	N/A	N/A	N/A
BBQ Flavored	1	256	17	48	4.1	782	N/A	T	N/A	N/A	N/A	4	N/A	N/A	N/A

Item	Serving													
Chunky Chicken														
Pot Pie	1	770	29	80	1.8	2,160	N/A	800	N/A	N/A	1	N/A	N/A	N/A
Coleslaw	5 oz	180	2	32	0.7	280	N/A	T	N/A	N/A	36	N/A	N/A	N/A
Colonel's Crispy														
Strips	1 order	261	20	T	0.5	658	N/A	T	N/A	N/A	T	N/A	N/A	N/A
Corn on the Cob	1 order	150	5	T	0.5	20	N/A	20	N/A	N/A	4	N/A	N/A	N/A
Green Beans	1 order	45	1	32	0.7	730	N/A	40	N/A	N/A	2	N/A	N/A	N/A
Cornbread	1	228	3	48	0.7	194	N/A	T	N/A	N/A	T	N/A	N/A	N/A
Spicy Buffalo														
Crispy Strips	1 order	350	22	16	1	1,110	N/A	T	N/A	N/A	T	N/A	N/A	N/A
Original Recipe														
Breast	1 order	400	29	32	1	1,116	N/A	T	N/A	N/A	T	N/A	N/A	N/A
Drumstick	1 order	140	13	T	0.7	422	N/A	T	N/A	N/A	T	N/A	N/A	N/A
Thigh	1 order	250	16	32	0.7	747	N/A	T	N/A	N/A	T	N/A	N/A	N/A
Wing	1 order	140	9	T	0.4	414	N/A	T	N/A	N/A	T	N/A	N/A	N/A
Extra Crispy														
Breast	1 order	470	31	32	1	930	N/A	T	N/A	N/A	T	N/A	N/A	N/A
Drumstick	1 order	190	13	T	0.7	260	N/A	T	N/A	N/A	T	N/A	N/A	N/A
Thigh	1 order	370	19	16	0.7	540	N/A	T	N/A	N/A	T	N/A	N/A	N/A
Hot and Spicy Chicken														
Breast	1 order	530	32	32	1	1,110	N/A	T	N/A	N/A	T	N/A	N/A	N/A
Drumstick	1 order	190	13	T	0.7	300	N/A	T	N/A	N/A	T	N/A	N/A	N/A
Thigh	1 order	370	18	T	0.7	570	N/A	T	N/A	N/A	T	N/A	N/A	N/A
Wing	1 order	210	10	32	0.4	340	N/A	T	N/A	N/A	T	N/A	N/A	N/A
Macaroni and Cheese	5 oz	180	7	120	T	860	N/A	200	N/A	N/A	T	N/A	N/A	N/A
Mashed Potatoes														
with Gravy	1 order	120	1	T	0.4	440	N/A	T	N/A	N/A	T	N/A	N/A	N/A

Item	Amount	Calories	Protein (g)	Calcium (mg)	Iron (mg)	Sodium (mg)	Potassium (mg)	Vitamin A (mcg)	Vitamin C (mg)	Niacin (mg)	Ribof (mg)	Thiamin (mg)	Vitamin B6 (mg)	Vitamin E (mg)	Folic Acid (mg)
Mean Greens	1 order	70	1	160	1.8	650	N/A	600	6	N/A	N/A	N/A	N/A	N/A	N/A
Potato Salad	1 order	230	4	16	2.7	540	N/A	100	T	N/A	N/A	N/A	N/A	N/A	N/A
Potato Wedges	1 order	180	5	16	1.8	750	N/A	T	1	N/A	N/A	N/A	N/A	N/A	N/A
Tender Roast Chicken (with skin)															
Breast	1 order	251	37	T	T	830	N/A	T	T	N/A	N/A	N/A	N/A	N/A	N/A
Drumstick	1 order	97	15	T	T	271	N/A	T	T	N/A	N/A	N/A	N/A	N/A	N/A
Thigh	1 order	207	18	T	T	504	N/A	T	T	N/A	N/A	N/A	N/A	N/A	N/A
Wing	1 order	121	12	T	T	331	N/A	T	T	N/A	N/A	N/A	N/A	N/A	N/A
Tender Roast Chicken (no skin)															
Breast	1 order	169	31	T	T	797	N/A	T	T	N/A	N/A	N/A	N/A	N/A	N/A
Drumstick	1 order	67	11	T	T	259	N/A	T	T	N/A	N/A	N/A	N/A	N/A	N/A
Thigh	1 order	106	13	T	T	312	N/A	T	T	N/A	N/A	N/A	N/A	N/A	N/A
McDonald's															
Apple Bran Muffin (lowfat)	1	300	6	80	1.4	380	N/A	T	T	N/A	N/A	N/A	N/A	N/A	N/A
Arch Deluxe	1	550	28	48	4.5	1,010	N/A	100	6	N/A	N/A	N/A	N/A	N/A	N/A
With bacon	1	590	32	48	4.5	1,150	N/A	100	6	N/A	N/A	N/A	N/A	N/A	N/A
Bacon, Egg and Cheese Biscuit	1	440	17	80	2.7	1,310	N/A	100	T	N/A	N/A	N/A	N/A	N/A	N/A
Big Mac	1	560	26	160	4.5	1,070	N/A	60	4	N/A	N/A	N/A	N/A	N/A	N/A
Biscuit	1	260	4	48	1.8	840	N/A	T	T	N/A	N/A	N/A	N/A	N/A	N/A
Apple Pie, baked	1	260	3	16	1	200	N/A	T	24	N/A	N/A	N/A	N/A	N/A	N/A

Item	Serving														
Breakfast Burrito	1	320	13	64	1.8	600	N/A	100	N/A	N/A	N/A	9	N/A	N/A	N/A
Cheeseburger	1	320	15	120	2.7	820	N/A	60	N/A	N/A	N/A	2	N/A	N/A	N/A
Chicken McNuggets	4 pieces	190	12	T	0.7	340	N/A	T	N/A	N/A	N/A	T	N/A	N/A	N/A
	6 pieces	290	18	16	1	510	N/A	T	N/A	N/A	N/A	T	N/A	N/A	N/A
	9 pieces	430	27	16	1.2	770	N/A	T	N/A	N/A	N/A	T	N/A	N/A	N/A
Chicken Salad Deluxe (grilled)	1 order	120	21	32	1.2	240	N/A	1,200	N/A	N/A	N/A	24	N/A	N/A	N/A
Cinnamon Roll	1	400	7	64	1.2	340	N/A	100	N/A	N/A	N/A	T	N/A	N/A	N/A
Crispy Chicken Deluxe Sandwich	1	500	26	48	2.7	1,100	N/A	60	N/A	N/A	N/A	5	N/A	N/A	N/A
Danish Apple	1	360	5	64	1	290	N/A	100	N/A	N/A	N/A	T	N/A	N/A	N/A
Cheese	1	410	7	64	1	340	N/A	150	N/A	N/A	N/A	T	N/A	N/A	N/A
Egg McMuffin	1	290	17	120	2.7	710	N/A	100	N/A	N/A	N/A	1	N/A	N/A	N/A
English Muffin	1	140	4	80	1.4	210	N/A	100	N/A	N/A	N/A	T	N/A	N/A	N/A
Fish Filet Deluxe Sandwich	1	560	23	48	2.7	1,060	N/A	60	N/A	N/A	N/A	2	N/A	N/A	N/A
French Fries Small	1 order	210	3	T	0.4	135	N/A	T	N/A	N/A	N/A	9	N/A	N/A	N/A
Large	1 order	450	6	16	1	290	N/A	T	N/A	N/A	N/A	18	N/A	N/A	N/A
Super	1 order	540	8	16	1.2	350	N/A	T	N/A	N/A	N/A	21	N/A	N/A	N/A
Garden Salad	1 order	35	2	32	1	20	N/A	1,200	N/A	N/A	N/A	24	N/A	N/A	N/A
Grilled Chicken Deluxe Sandwich	1	440	27	64	2.7	1,040	N/A	60	N/A	N/A	N/A	5	N/A	N/A	N/A
Hamburger	1	260	13	120	2.7	580	N/A	T	N/A	N/A	N/A	2	N/A	N/A	N/A
Hash Browns	1	130	1	T	0.4	330	N/A	T	N/A	N/A	N/A	2	N/A	N/A	N/A
Hotcakes Plain	1	310	9	80	2.7	610	N/A	T	N/A	N/A	N/A	T	N/A	N/A	N/A

Item	Amount	Calories	Protein (g)	Calcium (mg)	Iron (mg)	Sodium (mg)	Potassium (mg)	Vitamin A (mcg)	Thiamin (mg)	Ribof (mg)	Niacin (mg)	Vitamin C (mg)	Vitamin B6 (mg)	Vitamin E (mg)	Folic Acid (mg)
With syrup and margarine	1	580	9	80	2.7	760	N/A	80	N/A	N/A	N/A	T	N/A	N/A	N/A
Ice Cream Cone, vanilla, reduced-fat	1	150	4	80	0.4	75	N/A	60	N/A	N/A	N/A	1	N/A	N/A	N/A
Milk, low-fat	1 carton	100	8	240	T	115	N/A	100	N/A	N/A	N/A	2	N/A	N/A	N/A
McDonald Land Cookies	1 box	180	2	16	1.8	190	N/A	T	N/A	N/A	N/A	T	N/A	N/A	N/A
Orange Juice	6 oz	80	1	16	0.4	20	N/A	20	N/A	N/A	N/A	54	N/A	N/A	N/A
Quarter Pounder	1	420	23	120	4.5	820	N/A	20	N/A	N/A	N/A	2	N/A	N/A	N/A
Quarter Pounder with Cheese	1	530	28	120	4.5	1,290	N/A	80	N/A	N/A	N/A	2	N/A	N/A	N/A
Sausage	1 patty	170	6	T	0.4	290	N/A	T	N/A	N/A	N/A	T	N/A	N/A	N/A
Sausage Biscuit	1	430	10	48	2.7	1,130	N/A	T	N/A	N/A	N/A	T	N/A	N/A	N/A
With egg	1	510	16	80	2.7	1,210	N/A	60	N/A	N/A	N/A	T	N/A	N/A	N/A
Sausage McMuffin	1	360	13	120	1.8	740	N/A	40	N/A	N/A	N/A	T	N/A	N/A	N/A
With egg	1	440	19	120	2.7	810	N/A	100	N/A	N/A	N/A	T	N/A	N/A	N/A
Shake Small chocolate	1	360	11	280	0.7	250	N/A	60	N/A	N/A	N/A	1	N/A	N/A	N/A
Small strawberry	1	360	11	280	0.7	180	N/A	60	N/A	N/A	N/A	6	N/A	N/A	N/A
Small vanilla	1	360	11	280	0.4	250	N/A	60	N/A	N/A	N/A	1	N/A	N/A	N/A
Sundae Hot caramel	1	360	7	200	T	180	N/A	100	N/A	N/A	N/A	1	N/A	N/A	N/A
Hot fudge	1	340	8	200	0.7	170	N/A	100	N/A	N/A	N/A	1	N/A	N/A	N/A

Popeye's Chicken & Biscuits															
Apple pie	1 piece	290	3	32	1.8	820	N/A	0	N/A	N/A	N/A	0	N/A	N/A	N/A
Biscuits	1 order	250	4	32	2.7	430	N/A	80	N/A	N/A	N/A	0	N/A	N/A	N/A
Cajun rice	1 order	150	10	80	1.8	1,260	N/A	0	N/A	N/A	N/A	0	N/A	N/A	N/A
Coleslaw	1 order	149	1	16	2.7	271	N/A	0	N/A	N/A	N/A	2	N/A	N/A	N/A
Corn on the cob	1 order	127	4	0	1.8	20	N/A	0	N/A	N/A	N/A	4	N/A	N/A	N/A
French fries	3 oz	240	4	0	2.7	610	N/A	0	N/A	N/A	N/A	0	N/A	N/A	N/A
Mild															
Breast	1 order	270	23	32	2.7	660	N/A	60	N/A	N/A	N/A	0	N/A	N/A	N/A
Leg	1 order	120	10	0	1	240	N/A	40	N/A	N/A	N/A	0	N/A	N/A	N/A
Tender	1 order	110	6	0	0.7	160	N/A	0	N/A	N/A	N/A	0	N/A	N/A	N/A
Thigh	1 order	300	15	16	2.7	620	N/A	60	N/A	N/A	N/A	0	N/A	N/A	N/A
Wing	1 order	160	9	0	1	290	N/A	60	N/A	N/A	N/A	0	N/A	N/A	N/A
Nuggets	1 order	410	17	16	2.7	660	N/A	0	N/A	N/A	N/A	1	N/A	N/A	N/A
Onion rings	1 order	310	5	48	1.8	210	N/A	0	N/A	N/A	N/A	0	N/A	N/A	N/A
Potatoes and gravy	1 order	100	5	32	1.8	460	N/A	100	N/A	N/A	N/A	0	N/A	N/A	N/A
Red beans and rice	1 order	270	8	0	5.4	680	N/A	0	N/A	N/A	N/A	0	N/A	N/A	N/A
Shrimp	1 order	250	16	48	1.8	650	N/A	0	N/A	N/A	N/A	0	N/A	N/A	N/A
Spicy															
Breast	1 order	270	23	32	2.7	590	N/A	60	N/A	N/A	N/A	0	N/A	N/A	N/A
Leg	1 order	120	10	0	1	240	N/A	40	N/A	N/A	N/A	0	N/A	N/A	N/A
Tender	1 order	110	6	0	0.7	215	N/A	0	N/A	N/A	N/A	0	N/A	N/A	N/A
Thigh	1 order	300	15	16	2.7	450	N/A	60	N/A	N/A	N/A	0	N/A	N/A	N/A
Wing	1 order	160	9	0	1	290	N/A	60	N/A	N/A	N/A	0	N/A	N/A	N/A
Taco Bell															
Big Beef Mexi-Melt	1	290	16	400	1.2	850	N/A	250	N/A	N/A	N/A	4	N/A	N/A	N/A

Item	Amount	Calories	Protein (g)	Calcium (mg)	Iron (mg)	Sodium (mg)	Potassium (mg)	Vitamin A (mcg)	Thiamin (mg)	Ribof (mg)	Niacin (mg)	Vitamin C (mg)	Vitamin B6 (mg)	Vitamin E (mg)	Folic Acid (mg)
Big Beef Nachos Supreme	1	450	14	120	2.7	810	N/A	100	N/A	N/A	N/A	4	N/A	N/A	N/A
Border Wraps															
Chicken Fajita Wrap	1	470	17	120	1.4	1,290	N/A	350	N/A	N/A	N/A	4	N/A	N/A	N/A
Chicken Fajita Wrap Supreme	1	520	18	120	1.4	1,300	N/A	400	N/A	N/A	N/A	6	N/A	N/A	N/A
Steak Fajita Wrap	1	470	20	120	1.8	1,190	N/A	300	N/A	N/A	N/A	4	N/A	N/A	N/A
Steak Fajita Wrap Supreme	1	510	21	120	1.8	1,200	N/A	300	N/A	N/A	N/A	6	N/A	N/A	N/A
Veggie Fajita Wrap	1	420	10	120	1.4	980	N/A	350	N/A	N/A	N/A	6	N/A	N/A	N/A
Veggie Fajita Wrap Supreme	1	470	11	120	1.4	990	N/A	300	N/A	N/A	N/A	6	N/A	N/A	N/A
Burritos															
Bean	1	380	13	120	2.7	1,100	N/A	450	N/A	N/A	N/A	0	N/A	N/A	N/A
Burrito Supreme	1	440	17	120	2.7	1,230	N/A	500	N/A	N/A	N/A	5	N/A	N/A	N/A
Big Beef Supreme	1	520	24	120	2.7	1,520	N/A	600	N/A	N/A	N/A	5	N/A	N/A	N/A
7-Layer Burrito	1	530	16	200	3.6	1,280	N/A	300	N/A	N/A	N/A	5	N/A	N/A	N/A
Grilled Chicken Burrito	1	410	17	120	1.2	1,380	N/A	800	N/A	N/A	N/A	1	N/A	N/A	N/A
Big Chicken Supreme	1	510	23	120	1.8	1,900	N/A	450	N/A	N/A	N/A	0	N/A	N/A	N/A
Chili-Cheese Burrito	1	330	14	400	1.2	870	N/A	600	N/A	N/A	N/A	0	N/A	N/A	N/A

Item	Serving													
Chicken Club Burrito	1	550	20	200	1.2	1,250	N/A	150	N/A	N/A	5	N/A	N/A	N/A
Bacon Cheeseburger	1	570	16	400	2.7	1,460	N/A	300	N/A	N/A	5	N/A	N/A	N/A
Cheese Quesadilla	1	350	16	340	1.8	860	N/A	80	N/A	N/A	0	N/A	N/A	N/A
Chicken Quesadilla	1	410	23	340	1.8	1,170	N/A	150	N/A	N/A	0	N/A	N/A	N/A
Cinnamon Twists	1	140	1	0	0.4	190	N/A	40	N/A	N/A	0	N/A	N/A	N/A
Chocolate Taco Ice Cream Dessert	1	310	3	48	0.7	100	N/A	40	N/A	N/A	0	N/A	N/A	N/A
Mexican Pizza	1	570	21	200	3.6	1,040	N/A	400	N/A	N/A	5	N/A	N/A	N/A
Mexican Rice	1	190	5	120	1.4	760	N/A	1,000	N/A	N/A	1	N/A	N/A	N/A
Nachos	1	320	5	80	0.7	570	N/A	60	N/A	N/A	0	N/A	N/A	N/A
Nachos Bel Grande	1	770	2	160	3.6	1,310	N/A	150	N/A	N/A	4	N/A	N/A	N/A
Pintos 'n' Cheese	1	190	9	120	1.8	650	N/A	500	N/A	N/A	0	N/A	N/A	N/A
Tacos														
Regular	1	180	9	64	1	330	N/A	100	N/A	N/A	0	N/A	N/A	N/A
Soft Taco	1	220	11	64	1	580	N/A	100	N/A	N/A	0	N/A	N/A	N/A
Taco Supreme	1	220	10	80	1	350	N/A	150	N/A	N/A	0	N/A	N/A	N/A
Soft Taco Supreme	1	260	12	80	1.8	590	N/A	150	N/A	N/A	4	N/A	N/A	N/A
Double Decker	1	340	14	80	1.8	750	N/A	100	N/A	N/A	0	N/A	N/A	N/A
Double Decker Supreme	1	390	15	120	1.8	760	N/A	150	N/A	N/A	4	N/A	N/A	N/A
Grilled Steak Soft Taco	1	230	15	64	1.2	1,020	N/A	40	N/A	N/A	0	N/A	N/A	N/A
Grilled Steak Taco Supreme	1	290	16	80	1.2	1,040	N/A	80	N/A	N/A	12	N/A	N/A	N/A
Grilled Chicken Soft Taco	1	240	12	64	0.7	1,110	N/A	150	N/A	N/A	0	N/A	N/A	N/A

Item	Amount	Calories	Protein (g)	Calcium (mg)	Iron (mg)	Sodium (mg)	Potassium (mg)	Vitamin A (mcg)	Vitamin C (mg)	Niacin (mg)	Ribof (mg)	Thiamin (mg)	Vitamin B6 (mg)	Vitamin E (mg)	Folic Acid (mg)
BLT Soft Taco	1	340	11	80	0.7	610	N/A	40	4	N/A	N/A	N/A	N/A	N/A	N/A
Taco Salad with Salsa	1	850	30	600	6.3	1,780	N/A	1,600	24	N/A	N/A	N/A	N/A	N/A	N/A
No shell	1	420	24	200	4.5	1,520	N/A	1,600	21	N/A	N/A	N/A	N/A	N/A	N/A
Tostada	1	380	10	120	2.7	650	N/A	500	1	N/A	N/A	N/A	N/A	N/A	N/A.
Pizza Hut															
Apple Dessert Pizza	1	250	3	N/A	1	230	N/A	N/A	N/A	N/A	N/A	N/A	N/A	N/A	N/A
Breadstick	1	130	3	N/A	1	240	N/A	100	N/A	N/A	N/A	N/A	N/A	N/A	N/A
Buffalo Wings, hot	4 pieces	210	22	16	0.7	900	N/A	200	N/A	N/A	N/A	N/A	N/A	N/A	N/A
Buffalo Wings, medium	5 pieces	200	23	16	0.7	510	N/A	60	N/A	N/A	N/A	N/A	N/A	N/A	N/A
Cavatini Pasta	1 serving	480	21	120	3.6	1,170	N/A	250	N/A	N/A	N/A	N/A	N/A	N/A	N/A
Cavatini Supreme Pasta	1 serving	560	24	120	4.5	1,400	N/A	300	N/A	N/A	N/A	N/A	N/A	N/A	N/A
Cherry Dessert Pizza	1 slice	250	3	N/A	1.4	220	N/A	N/A	N/A	N/A	N/A	N/A	N/A	N/A	N/A
Garlic Bread	1 slice	150	3	32	1.2	240	N/A	100	N/A	N/A	N/A	N/A	N/A	N/A	N/A
Ham and Cheese Sandwich	1	550	33	240	4.5	2,150	N/A	150	N/A	N/A	N/A	N/A	N/A	N/A	N/A
Pizza, Beef, medium															
Thin 'n' Crispy	1 slice	240	13	80	1.8	790	N/A	200	N/A	N/A	N/A	N/A	N/A	N/A	N/A
Hand Tossed	1 slice	280	15	120	1.4	860	N/A	200	N/A	N/A	N/A	N/A	N/A	N/A	N/A
Pan	1 slice	310	14	120	2.7	720	N/A	200	N/A	N/A	N/A	N/A	N/A	N/A	N/A
Stuffed Crust	1 slice	340	20	200	3.6	1,270	N/A	250	N/A	N/A	N/A	N/A	N/A	N/A	N/A

Pizza, Cheese, medium

	Serving												
Thin 'n' Crispy	1 slice	210	12	160	1	530	N/A	200	N/A	N/A	N/A	N/A	N/A
Hand Tossed	1 slice	280	16	200	1.8	770	N/A	250	N/A	N/A	N/A	N/A	N/A
Pan	1 slice	300	15	200	1.8	610	N/A	200	N/A	N/A	N/A	N/A	N/A
Stuffed Crust	1 slice	380	21	280	2.7	1,160	N/A	250	N/A	N/A	N/A	N/A	N/A

Pizza, Chicken Supreme, medium

	Serving												
Thin 'n' Crispy	1 slice	220	14	80	1.4	550	N/A	250	N/A	N/A	N/A	N/A	N/A
Hand Tossed	1 slice	240	14	120	1.8	660	N/A	150	N/A	N/A	N/A	N/A	N/A
Pan	1 slice	280	14	80	1.8	570	N/A	150	N/A	N/A	N/A	N/A	N/A
Stuffed Crust	1 slice	390	21	240	3.6	1,130	N/A	250	N/A	N/A	N/A	N/A	N/A

Pizza, Ham, medium

	Serving												
Thin 'n' Crispy	1 slice	190	10	80	1.4	560	N/A	150	N/A	N/A	N/A	N/A	N/A
Hand tossed	1 slice	230	13	120	1.8	710	N/A	200	N/A	N/A	N/A	N/A	N/A
Pan	1 slice	250	12	80	1.8	590	N/A	150	N/A	N/A	N/A	N/A	N/A
Stuffed Crust	1 slice	380	22	200	3.6	1,250	N/A	300	N/A	N/A	N/A	N/A	N/A

Pizza, Italian Sausage, medium

	Serving												
Thin 'n' Crispy	1 slice	300	15	120	1.8	740	N/A	300	N/A	N/A	N/A	N/A	N/A
Hand Tossed	1 slice	300	15	120	2.7	780	N/A	150	N/A	N/A	N/A	N/A	N/A
Pan	1 slice	350	16	120	1.8	740	N/A	200	N/A	N/A	N/A	N/A	N/A
Stuffed Crust	1 slice	430	22	240	2.7	1,200	N/A	350	N/A	N/A	N/A	N/A	N/A

Pizza, Meat Lover's, medium

	Serving												
Thin 'n' Crispy	1 slice	310	16	120	1.8	900	N/A	300	N/A	N/A	N/A	N/A	N/A
Hand Tossed	1 slice	290	15	120	2.7	820	N/A	150	N/A	N/A	N/A	N/A	N/A
Pan	1 slice	360	17	120	1.8	870	N/A	200	N/A	N/A	N/A	N/A	N/A
Stuffed Crust	1 slice	500	25	240	3.6	1,510	N/A	300	N/A	N/A	N/A	N/A	N/A

Pizza, Personal Pan

	Serving												
Cheese	1 slice	630	28	280	5.4	1,160	N/A	500	N/A	N/A	N/A	N/A	N/A
Pepperoni	1 slice	670	29	200	7.2	1,250	N/A	500	N/A	N/A	N/A	N/A	N/A

Item	Amount	Calories	Protein (g)	Calcium (mg)	Iron (mg)	Sodium (mg)	Potassium (mg)	Vitamin A (mcg)	Thiamin (mg)	Ribof (mg)	Niacin (mg)	Vitamin C (mg)	Vitamin B$_6$ (mg)	Vitamin E (mg)	Folic Acid (mg)
Supreme	1 slice	710	32	200	2.7	1,380	N/A	500	N/A	N/A	N/A	N/A	N/A	N/A	N/A
Pizza, Pepperoni, medium															
Thin 'n' Crispy	1 slice	220	10	80	1.8	610	N/A	200	N/A	N/A	N/A	N/A	N/A	N/A	N/A
Hand Tossed	1 slice	260	12	120	1.8	750	N/A	250	N/A	N/A	N/A	N/A	N/A	N/A	N/A
Pan	1 slice	280	12	120	2.7	640	N/A	200	N/A	N/A	N/A	N/A	N/A	N/A	N/A
Stuffed Crust	1 slice	410	22	200	2.7	1,250	N/A	350	N/A	N/A	N/A	N/A	N/A	N/A	N/A
Pizza, Pepperoni Lover's, medium															
Thin 'n' Crispy	1 slice	270	15	120	1.8	780	N/A	200	N/A	N/A	N/A	N/A	N/A	N/A	N/A
Hand Tossed	1 slice	320	17	160	2.7	910	N/A	300	N/A	N/A	N/A	N/A	N/A	N/A	N/A
Pan	1 slice	350	17	160	2.7	800	N/A	250	N/A	N/A	N/A	N/A	N/A	N/A	N/A
Stuffed Crust	1 slice	480	24	240	3.6	1,440	N/A	400	N/A	N/A	N/A	N/A	N/A	N/A	N/A
Pizza, Pork, medium															
Thin 'n' Crispy	1 slice	270	14	20	1.8	780	N/A	200	N/A	N/A	N/A	N/A	N/A	N/A	N/A
Hand Tossed	1 slice	290	14	120	1.4	850	N/A	200	N/A	N/A	N/A	N/A	N/A	N/A	N/A
Pan	1 slice	300	14	120	2.7	720	N/A	200	N/A	N/A	N/A	N/A	N/A	N/A	N/A
Stuffed Crust	1 slice	420	22	240	3.6	1,290	N/A	250	N/A	N/A	N/A	N/A	N/A	N/A	N/A
Pizza, Supreme, medium															
Thin 'n' Crispy	1 slice	250	13	120	1.8	710	N/A	200	N/A	N/A	N/A	N/A	N/A	N/A	N/A
Hand Tossed	1 slice	270	13	120	1.4	760	N/A	200	N/A	N/A	N/A	N/A	N/A	N/A	N/A
Pan	1 slice	300	13	120	2.7	670	N/A	200	N/A	N/A	N/A	N/A	N/A	N/A	N/A
Stuffed Crust	1 slice	440	23	240	3.6	1,380	N/A	300	N/A	N/A	N/A	N/A	N/A	N/A	N/A
Pizza, Super Supreme, medium															
Thin 'n' Crispy	1 slice	280	15	120	1.8	810	N/A	300	N/A	N/A	N/A	N/A	N/A	N/A	N/A
Hand Tossed	1 slice	290	15	120	2.7	830	N/A	150	N/A	N/A	N/A	N/A	N/A	N/A	N/A
Pan	1 slice	340	15	120	2.7	790	N/A	250	N/A	N/A	N/A	N/A	N/A	N/A	N/A

Item	Serving													
Stuffed Crust	1 slice	470	24	240	3.6	1,440	N/A	300	N/A	N/A	N/A	N/A	N/A	N/A
Pizza, Veggie Lover's, medium														
Thin 'n' Crispy	1 slice	170	7	64	1.8	460	N/A	250	N/A	N/A	N/A	N/A	N/A	N/A
Hand Tossed	1 slice	240	11	120	1.8	650	N/A	200	N/A	N/A	N/A	N/A	N/A	N/A
Pan	1 slice	240	10	120	2.7	480	N/A	150	N/A	N/A	N/A	N/A	N/A	N/A
Stuffed Crust	1 slice	390	18	200	3.6	1,140	N/A	250	N/A	N/A	N/A	N/A	N/A	N/A
Spaghetti with Marinara Sauce	1	490	18	120	3.6	730	N/A	200	N/A	N/A	N/A	N/A	N/A	N/A
Spaghetti with Meat Sauce	1	600	23	80	3.6	910	N/A	350	N/A	N/A	N/A	N/A	N/A	N/A
Spaghetti with Meatballs	1	850	37	120	5.4	1,120	N/A	400	N/A	N/A	N/A	N/A	N/A	N/A
Supreme Sandwich	1	640	34	240	6	2,150	N/A	150	N/A	N/A	N/A	N/A	N/A	N/A
Wendy's														
Baked Potato														
Plain	10 oz	284	7	24	3.8	25	N/A	0	N/A	N/A	36	N/A	N/A	N/A
Bacon and cheese	1	380	17	144	4.3	1,390	N/A	100	N/A	N/A	36	N/A	N/A	N/A
Broccoli and cheese	1	411	9	168	4.5	470	N/A	350	N/A	N/A	72	N/A	N/A	N/A
Cheese	1	383	14	304	4.1	640	N/A	200	N/A	N/A	36	N/A	N/A	N/A
Chili and cheese	1	630	20	264	5	770	N/A	200	N/A	N/A	36	N/A	N/A	N/A
Sour cream and chives	1	380	8	64	4.3	40	N/A	300	N/A	N/A	48	N/A	N/A	N/A
Sour cream	1	60	1	24	0	15	N/A	400	N/A	N/A	0	N/A	N/A	N/A
Whipped margarine	1	60	0	0	0	115	N/A	100	N/A	N/A	0	N/A	N/A	N/A

Item	Amount	Calories	Protein (g)	Calcium (mg)	Iron (mg)	Sodium (mg)	Potassium (mg)	Vitamin A (mcg)	Thiamin (mg)	Ribof (mg)	Niacin (mg)	Vitamin C (mg)	Vitamin B6 (mg)	Vitamin E (mg)	Folic Acid (mg)
Big Bacon Classic	1	580	34	200	5.4	1,460	N/A	150	N/A	N/A	N/A	15	N/A	N/A	N/A
Breaded Chicken Sandwich	1	440	28	80	2.9	840	N/A	40	N/A	N/A	N/A	6	N/A	N/A	N/A
Chicken Nuggets	5 pieces	210	14	16	0.4	460	N/A	0	N/A	N/A	N/A	1	N/A	N/A	N/A
	4 pieces	170	11	8	0.4	370	N/A	0	N/A	N/A	N/A	1	N/A	N/A	N/A
Chicken Club Sandwich	1	470	31	88	3	970	N/A	40	N/A	N/A	N/A	6	N/A	N/A	N/A
Chili															
Small	8 oz	210	15	64	2.8	800	N/A	80	N/A	N/A	N/A	4	N/A	N/A	N/A
Large	12 oz	310	23	96	4.3	1,190	N/A	100	N/A	N/A	N/A	6	N/A	N/A	N/A
Cheddar cheese, shredded	2 Tbs	70	4	96	0	110	N/A	40	N/A	N/A	N/A	0	N/A	N/A	N/A
Saltines	2	25	1	8	0.4	80	N/A	0	N/A	N/A	N/A	0	N/A	N/A	N/A
Cheeseburger Kids Meal	1	320	17	136	3.2	830	N/A	60	N/A	N/A	N/A	0	N/A	N/A	N/A
Chocolate Chip Cookie	1	270	3	8	1.8	120	N/A	0	N/A	N/A	N/A	0	N/A	N/A	N/A
French fries															
Small	1	270	4	8	0.7	85	N/A	0	N/A	N/A	N/A	5	N/A	N/A	N/A
Medium	1	390	5	16	1	120	N/A	0	N/A	N/A	N/A	6	N/A	N/A	N/A
Biggie	1	470	7	24	1.2	150	N/A	0	N/A	N/A	N/A	9	N/A	N/A	N/A
Frosty Dairy Dessert															
Small	1	330	8	248	1	200	N/A	150	N/A	N/A	N/A	0	N/A	N/A	N/A
Medium	1	440	11	328	1.4	260	N/A	200	N/A	N/A	N/A	0	N/A	N/A	N/A

Item	Serving													
Large	1	540	14	400	1.8	320	N/A	250	N/A	N/A	N/A	0	N/A	N/A
Grilled Chicken Sandwich	1	310	27	80	2.7	790	N/A	40	N/A	N/A	N/A	6	N/A	N/A
Hamburger Kids Meal	1	270	15	88	3	610	N/A	20	N/A	N/A	N/A	0	N/A	N/A
Jr. Bacon Cheeseburger	1	380	20	136	3.4	850	N/A	80	N/A	N/A	N/A	6	N/A	N/A
Jr. Cheeseburger	1	320	17	136	3.2	830	N/A	60	N/A	N/A	N/A	1	N/A	N/A
Jr. Cheeseburger Deluxe	1	360	18	144	3.4	890	N/A	100	N/A	N/A	N/A	6	N/A	N/A
Jr. Hamburger	1	270	15	88	3	610	N/A	20	N/A	N/A	N/A	1	N/A	N/A
Plain Single	1	360	24	88	4.1	580	N/A	0	N/A	N/A	N/A	0	N/A	N/A
Single with Everything	1	420	25	104	4.7	920	N/A	60	N/A	N/A	N/A	6	N/A	N/A
Salads														
Caesar Side Salad	1	100	8	24	1.2	620	N/A	350	N/A	N/A	N/A	15	N/A	N/A
Deluxe Garden Salad	1	110	7	144	1.4	350	N/A	1,200	N/A	N/A	N/A	15	N/A	N/A
Grilled Chicken Salad	1	200	25	152	1.9	720	N/A	1,200	N/A	N/A	N/A	15	N/A	N/A
Grilled Chicken Caesar Salad	1	260	26	56	3.1	1,170	N/A	800	N/A	N/A	N/A	15	N/A	N/A
Side Salad	1	60	4	80	0.9	180	N/A	600	N/A	N/A	N/A	18	N/A	N/A
Taco Salad	1	380	26	296	4.1	1,040	N/A	450	N/A	N/A	N/A	27	N/A	N/A
Soft Breadstick	1	130	4	32	1.6	250	N/A	0	N/A	N/A	N/A	0	N/A	N/A
Spicy Chicken Sandwich	1	410	28	88	2.7	1,280	N/A	40	N/A	N/A	N/A	6	N/A	N/A

Item	Amount	Calories	Protein (g)	Calcium (mg)	Iron (mg)	Sodium (mg)	Potassium (mg)	Vitamin A (mcg)	Thiamin (mg)	Ribof (mg)	Niacin (mg)	Vitamin C (mg)	Vitamin B6 (mg)	Vitamin E (mg)	Folic Acid (mg)
Stuffed Pitas															
Chicken Caesar	1	490	34	267	3.2	1,320	N/A	50	N/A	N/A	N/A	15	N/A	N/A	N/A
Classic Greek	1	440	15	256	3.2	1,050	N/A	50	N/A	N/A	N/A	18	N/A	N/A	N/A
Garden Ranch															
Chicken	1	480	30	128	3.4	1,180	N/A	60	N/A	N/A	N/A	54	N/A	N/A	N/A
Garden Veggie	1	400	11	128	3.2	760	N/A	60	N/A	N/A	N/A	54	N/A	N/A	N/A
Taco Chips	1 order	210	3	32	0.4	180	N/A	0	N/A	N/A	N/A	0	N/A	N/A	N/A

Fruits

Item	Amount	Calories	Protein (g)	Calcium (mg)	Iron (mg)	Sodium (mg)	Potassium (mg)	Vitamin A (mcg)	Thiamin (mg)	Ribof (mg)	Niacin (mg)	Vitamin C (mg)	Vitamin B6 (mg)	Vitamin E (mg)	Folic Acid (mg)
Applesauce															
Sweetened	1 cup	232	0.5	10	1.3	5	166	100	0.05	0.03	0.1	3	0.06	0	0
Unsweetened	1 cup	100	0.5	10	1.2	5	190	100	0.05	0.02	0.1	2	0.06	0	0
Apricots															
Raw, whole	½ lb	109	2.2	36	1.1	2.5	599	5,755	0.07	0.09	1.3	22	0.15	1	5
Canned, in syrup	3 med. halves	86	0.6	11	0.3	1	234	1,740	0.02	0.02	0.4	4	0	0	0
Canned, In water	3 med. halves	38	0.7	12	0.3	1	246	1,830	0.02	0.02	0.4	4	0	0	0

Dehydrated, uncooked	17 large halves	260	5	67	5.5	26	979	10,900	0.01	0.16	3.3	12	0	0	0
Nectar	1 cup	143	0.8	23	0.5	T	379	2,380	0.03	0.03	0.5	8	0	0	0
Banana, raw	1 medium	101	1.3	10	0.8	1	440	190	0.05	0.06	0.7	10	0.5	0.7	11
Blackberries															
Raw	1 cup	84	1.7	46	1.3	1	245	200	0.03	0.03	0.4	21	0.1	4.5	37
Canned	1 cup	135	2	63	2.3	2.5	425	350	0.05	0.05	0.5	2	0	0	0
Blueberries															
Raw	1 cup	99	1.1	24	1.6	1.6	130	160	0.05	1	0.8	22	0.04	0	113
Frozen	1 cup	88	1.1	16	1.3	1.6	130	112	0.05	1	0.8	11	0.09	0	0
Cantaloupe	1/4 melon	30	0.7	14	0.4	12	251	3,400	0.04	0.03	6	33	0.08	0.1	T
Casaba melon	1/4 melon	92	4.1	48	1.4	41	854	178	0.14	0.1	2	44	0	0	0
Cherries, sweet, raw	15 large or 25 small	70	1.3	22	0.4	2	191	110	0.05	0.06	0.4	10	0.04	0	0
	1 cup	116	2.4	44	0.8	4	382	220	0.1	0.12	0.8	21	0.14	0	0

Item	Amount	Calories	Protein (g)	Calcium (mg)	Iron (mg)	Sodium (mg)	Potassium (mg)	Vitamin A (mcg)	Thiamin (mg)	Ribof (mg)	Niacin (mg)	Vitamin C (mg)	Vitamin B$_6$ (mg)	Vitamin E (mg)	Folic Acid (mg)
Coconut meat	1 cup	780	6	30	3.8	52	581	0	0.12	0.04	1.2	7	0.1	2	62
Cranberries	1 cup	46	0.4	14	0.5	2	82	40	0.03	0.02	0.1	11	0.03	0	2
Juice cocktail	1 cup	165	0.25	13	0.75	2.5	25	T	0.03	0.03	T	41	0	0	0
Sauce	5½ Tbs	146	0.1	6	0.2	1	30	4	T	T	T	2	0	0	0
Dates, whole without pits	10 medium	274	2.2	59	0.3	1	648	50	0.09	1	2.2	0	0.17	0	26
Figs, whole	2 large or 3 small	80	1.2	35	0.6	2	194	80	0.06	0.05	0.4	2	0.12	0	7
Fruit cocktail	1 cup	91	1	22	1	12	412	150	0.02	0.01	0.5	2	0.06	0	0
Grapefruit Fresh	½ medium	41	0.5	16	0.4	1	135	10	0.04	0.02	0.2	36	0.06	4	4
Sections	1 cup	87	1	61	0.8	2	257	20	0.08	0.04	0.4	76	0.06	0	0
Juice	1 cup	96	1.2	22	0.5	2	399	200	0.1	0.05	0.5	93	0.27	0	0
Grapefruit/Orange juice	1 cup	106	1.5	25	0.7	2	454	250	0.12	0.05	0.5	84	0.05	0	0

Food	Amount												
Grape													
Drink	1 cup	135	0.3	8	3	88	0	0.03	0.03	40	0	0	0
Juice	1 cup	167	0.5	28	5	293	0	0.1	0.05	T	0	0	0
Regular, fresh	10 grapes	45	0.4	8	2	115	70	0.03	0.02	3	0.06	0.5	4
Seedless, fresh	10 grapes	34	0.3	6	2	87	50	0.03	0.02	2	0.06	0.5	4
Honeydew melon	¼ melon	40	0.6	30	23	251	40	0.4	0.3	23	0.08	0.6	29
Lemon													
Raw	1 wedge	5	0.2	5	T	26	T	0.01	T	10	0.13	0	0
Juice	1 cup	61	0.7	22	2	344	50	0.07	0.02	112	0.11	0	0
Lime													
Raw	1 wedge	19	0.5	5	1	69	10	0.02	0.01	25	0	0	0
Juice	1 cup	64	0.7	22	2	256	20	0.05	0.02	79	0.1	0	0
Mango	1	152	1.6	23	16	437	11,090	0.12	2.5	81	0	0	0
Orange													
Juice, canned	1 cup	120	2	25	2	496	500	0.07	0.05	100	0.12	0	30
Juice, fresh	1 cup	112	1.7	27	2	496	500	0.22	0.07	124	0.08	0	10
Juice, frozen	1 cup	122	1.7	25	2	503	540	0.23	0.03	120	0.07	0	0
Whole, fresh	1	71	1.8	56	1	271	280	0.14	0.06	85	0.12	0.4	10
Papaya	1	119	1.8	61	9	711	5,320	0.12	0.12	170	0	0	0

Item	Amount	Calories	Protein (g)	Calcium (mg)	Iron (mg)	Sodium (mg)	Potassium (mg)	Vitamin A (mcg)	Thiamin (mg)	Ribof (mg)	Niacin (mg)	Vitamin C (mg)	Vitamin B6 (mg)	Vitamin E (mg)	Folic Acid (mg)
Peaches															
Canned, in syrup	1 cup	200	1	10	0.8	5	333	1,100	0.03	0.05	1.5	8	0	0	0
Canned, in water	1 cup	76	1	10	0.7	5	334	1,100	0.02	0.07	1.5	7	0.45	0	4
Dried	1 cup	419	5	77	9.6	26	1,520	6,240	0.02	0.3	8.5	29	0	0	0
Raw	1 fruit	51	0.8	12	0.7	1	269	1,770	0.03	0.07	1.3	9	0.04	0	4
Nectar	1 cup	120	0.5	10	0.5	2	194	1,070	0.02	0.05	1	T	0	0	0
Pears															
Canned, in syrup	1 cup	194	0.5	13	0.5	3	214	10	0.03	0.05	0.3	3	0	0	0
Canned, in water	1 cup	78	0.5	12	0.5	2	215	10	0.02	0.05	0.2	2	0.34	0	0
Dried	1 cup	482	5.6	63	2.3	13	1,031	130	0.02	0.32	1.1	13	0	0	0
Raw	1	100	1.1	13	0.5	3	213	30	0.03	0.07	0.2	7	0.003	0.9	4
Nectar	1 cup	130	0.8	8	0.3	3	98	T	T	0.05	T	T	0	0	0
Pineapple															
Canned, in water	1 slice	78	0.3	12	0.3	0.1	101	50	0.08	0.02	2	1	0	0	0
Juice, canned, unsweetened	1 cup	138	1	4	0.1	T	373	130	0.13	0.05	0.5	23	0	0	0
Juice, frozen	1 cup	130	1	28	0.8	3	340	30	0.13	0.05	0.5	30	0	0	0
Raw	1 cup	206	0.6	28	0.8	2	234	112	0.14	0.04	0.4	28	0.15	1	2
Plums															
Canned, in syrup	1 cup	214	1	23	2.3	3	367	3,130	0.05	0.05	1	5	0	0	0
Canned, in water	1 cup	114	1	22	2.5	5	368	3,110	0.05	0.05	1	5	0	0	0
Raw	1 fruit	32	0.3	8	0.3	1	112	160	0.02	0.02	0.3	4	0	0	0

Food	Amount														
Prunes															
Dried, with pits	½ lb	579	4.8	116	8.5	18	1,574	3,630	0.2	0.39	3.7	7	0	0	11
Juice	1 cup	197	1	4	10.6	5	602	0	0.03	0.03	1	5	0	0	0
Pumpkin, canned	1 cup	81	2.5	61	1	5	588	15,680	0.07	0.12	1.5	12	0.25	0	0
Raisins															
Raw, whole	1 cup	419	3.6	90	5.1	39	1,106	30	0.16	0.12	0.7	1	0.22	0	14
Cooked, with sugar	1 cup	628	3.5	86	4.7	38	1,047	30	0.12	0.09	0.6	T	0	0	0
Raspberries															
Black, raw	1 cup	98	2	40	1.2	1	267	T	0.04	0.12	1.2	24	0.27	20	0
Red, canned	1 cup	85	1.7	36	1.5	2	277	220	0.02	0.1	1.2	22	0	0	0
Red, frozen	1 cup	245	1.8	33	1.5	3	250	180	0.05	0.15	1.5	53	0	0	23
Red, raw	1 cup	70	1.5	27	1.1	1	207	160	0.04	0.11	1.1	31	0	20	0
Rhubarb, cooked, with sugar	1 cup	381	1.4	211	1.6	5	548	220	0.05	0.14	0.8	16	0	0	0
Strawberries															
Frozen, with sugar	1 cup	278	1.3	36	1.8	3	286	80	0.05	0.15	1.3	135	0.1	0	0
Raw	1 cup	56	1	32	1.5	2	246	90	0.04	0.1	0.9	88	0.08	0.3	7
Tangerine															
Juice, unsweetened	1 cup	106	1.2	44	0.5	2	440	1,040	0.15	0.05	0.2	54	0.007	0	0
Juice, sweetened	1 cup	125	1.2	44	0.5	2	440	1,040	0.15	0.05	0.2	54	0.007	0	0
Juice, frozen	1 cup	114	1.2	45	0.5	2	432	1,020	0.14	0.04	0.3	67	0	0	0
Raw	1	39	0.7	34	0.3	0.2	108	360	0.05	0.02	0.1	27	0	0	0

Item	Amount	Calories	Protein (g)	Calcium (mg)	Iron (mg)	Sodium (mg)	Potassium (mg)	Vitamin A (mcg)	Thiamin (mg)	Ribof (mg)	Niacin (mg)	Vitamin C (mg)	Vitamin B6 (mg)	Vitamin E (mg)	Folic Acid (mg)
Watermelon	1 cup	41	0.8	11	16	0.8	2	158	0.05	0.05	0.3	11	0.11	0	30

Grains and Grain Products

Item	Amount	Calories	Protein (g)	Calcium (mg)	Iron (mg)	Sodium (mg)	Potassium (mg)	Vitamin A (mcg)	Thiamin (mg)	Ribof (mg)	Niacin (mg)	Vitamin C (mg)	Vitamin B6 (mg)	Vitamin E (mg)	Folic Acid (mg)
Biscuit															
Homemade	1	103	2.1	3.4	0.4	175	33	T	0.06	0.06	0.5	T			0.06
From mix	1	91	2.0	19	0.6	272	82	T	0.08	0.07	0.6	T			0.2
Bran flakes	1 cup	106	3.6	19	12.4	207	137	1,650	0.41	0.49	0.41	12	0.39		0.2
Breads															
Cracked wheat	1 slice	66	2.2	22	0.3	132	34	T	0.03	0.02	0.3	T	0.23		
French	1 slice	58	1.8	9	0.4	116	1	0	0.06	0.09	0.5	0	0.10	0	
Italian	1 slice	54	1.8	16	0.4	117	15	0	0.06	0.04	0.05	0	0.09	0	
Raisin	1 slice	66	1.7	18	0.3	91	58	T	0.1	0.02	0.02	T			
Rye	1 slice	61	2.3	19	0.4	139	36	0	0.05	0.02	0.4	0	0.25	0.73	4.0
Pumpernickel	1 slice	79	2.8	27	0.8	182	145	0	0.07	0.04	0.4	0	0.04	0.98	
White	1 slice	76	2.4	24	0.7	142	29	T	0.07	0.06	0.7	T			
Whole wheat	1 slice	61	2.6	25	0.8	132	68	T	0.06	0.03	0.7	T	0.45		
Corn bread	1 piece	161	5.8	94	0.9	490	122	120	0.1	0.15	0.5	1			
Crackers															
Butter	10	151	2.3	49	0.2	360	37	70	T	0.01	0.3	0			
Cheese	10	44	1.0	31	0.1	95	10	30	T	0.01	0.1	0			

Graham	1 large	55	1.1	6	0.2	95	55	0	0.01	0.03	0.2	0	
Saltines	10	123	2.6	6	0.3	312	34	0	T	0.01	0.3	0	
Soda	10	33	0.7	2	0.1	83	9	0	T	T	0.1	0	
Macaroni, enriched	1 cup	192	6.5	14	1.4	1	103		0.23	0.13	0.18		
Macaroni and cheese, cooked	1 cup	430	16.8	362	1.8	1,086	240	860	0.2	0.4	0.18		
Muffins													
From mix	1	130	2.8	96	0.6	192	44	100	0.07	0.08	0.6	T	
Blueberry	1	112	2.9	34	0.6	253	46	90	0.06	0.08	0.5	T	
Bran	1	104	3.1	57	1.5	179	172	90	0.06	0.1	1.6	T	
Noodles, cooked	1 cup	200	6.6	16	1.4	3	70	110	0.22	0.13	1.9	T	
Oatmeal													
Instant, cooked	1 cup	166	6.2	24	1.4	257	0	0	0.14	0	0		
Regular, cooked	1 cup	132	4.8	22	1.4	523	146	0	0.19	0.5	0.2		
Pancakes, from mix	1	61	1.9	58	0.3	152	42	70	0.04	0.06	0.2	T	
Pastina, egg	1 cup	651	21.9	60	4.9	9		370	1.5	0.65	10.2	T	11.5
Popovers, homemade	1	90	3.5	38	0.6	88	60	130	0.06	0.1	0.4	T	

Item	Amount	Calories	Protein (g)	Calcium (mg)	Iron (mg)	Sodium (mg)	Potassium (mg)	Vitamin A (mcg)	Thiamin (mg)	Ribof (mg)	Niacin (mg)	Vitamin C (mg)	Vitamin B6 (mg)	Vitamin E (mg)	Folic Acid (mg)
Rice															
Long-grain brown, cooked	1 cup	232	4.9	23	1	550	137	0	0.18	0.04	2.7	T	1.1	4.8	41.8
Instant white, cooked	1 cup	180	3.6	21	1.8	767	57	0	0.23	0.02	2.1	T	0.34	1.2	
Pudding with raisins	1 cup	387	9.5	260	1.1	188	469	290	0.08	0.37	0.5	T			
Rolls															
Home-baked	1	119	2.9	16	0.7	98	41	30	0.09	0.09	0.8	T	0.12		
Hard	1	156	4.9	24	0.4	313	49	T	0.03	0.05	0.4	T			
Frankfurter or hamburger	1	119	3.3	30	0.8	202	38	T	0.11	0.07	0.9	T			
Rye wafers	10	224	8.5	34	2.5	573	390	T	0.21	0.16	0.8	T			
Salt sticks	1	106	3.3	16	0.3	548	33	T	0.02	0.03	0.3	T			
Spaghetti, cooked	1 cup	166	5	12	1	2	92	0	0.2	1.2	1.6	0	30	0	4
Waffle															
Homemade	1	209	7	85	1.3	356	109	250	0.13	0.19	1.0	T			
Frozen	1	86	2.4	41	0.6	219	54	40	0.06	0.05	0.4	T			
From mix	1	206	6.6	179	1	515	146	170	0.11	0.17	0.7	T			
Zwieback	1 piece	30	0.7	1	T	18	11	T	T	T	0.1				

Meats

Item	Amount	Calories	Protein (g)	Calcium (mg)	Iron (mg)	Sodium (mg)	Potassium (mg)	Vitamin A (mcg)	Thiamin (mg)	Ribof (mg)	Niacin (mg)	Vitamin C (mg)	Vitamin B6 (mg)	Vitamin E (mg)	Folic Acid (mg)
Bacon															
Cooked	2 slices	86	3.8	2	0.5	155	350	0.08	0.05	0.8		0			
Canadian	1 slice	58	5.7	3	0.9	537	91	0	0.19	0.04	1.1	0			
Beef															
Boneless for stew	¼ lb	371	29.5	13	3.8	52	236	50	0.06	0.22	4.5	0			
Chuck roast or steak	¼ lb	400	18.4	10	2.7	64	294	70	0.08	0.17	4.4	0			
Flank steak	¼ lb	222	34.6	16	4.3	61	277	13	0.06	0.26	5.2	0			
Porterhouse	¼ lb	527	22.4	10	2.9	55	250	85	0.07	0.18	4.8	0			
T-bone steak	¼ lb	537	22.1	9	3	54	248	85	0.06	0.18	4.7	0			
Rib roast	¼ lb	499	22.7	10	3	55	253	88	0.06	0.17	4.1	0			
Round steak	¼ lb	296	32.2	14	4	90	363	30	0.09	0.25	6.3	0	0.4	0.3	4
Hamburger	¼ lb	248	31.1	14	4	76	348	23	0.1	0.26	6.8	0	0.5	0.4	5
Hamburger, lean	¼ lb	324	27.5	14	3.6	67	308	43	0.1	0.24	6.1	0	0.5	0.4	5
Corned beef, cooked	¼ lb	422	26	10	3.3	1,069	68	T	0.02	0.21	1.7	0	0.1	0.1	4
Chile con carne with beans, canned	1 cup	298	16.8	72	3.8	1,189	522	134	0.07	0.16	2.9	4	0.2	0.4	20
Lamb															
Leg	¼ lb	317	29	13	1.9	70	322	T	0.17	0.31	6.2	3	0	0.31	4
Chops, loin	1 chop	18	2.6	1	0.2	6	30	T	0.01	0.03	0.6	0			
Chops, rib	1 chop	17	2.2	1	0.2	6	25	T	0.01	0.02	0.5	0			

Item	Amount	Calories	Protein (g)	Calcium (mg)	Iron (mg)	Sodium (mg)	Potassium (mg)	Vitamin A (mcg)	Thiamin (mg)	Ribof (mg)	Niacin (mg)	Vitamin C (mg)	Vitamin B6 (mg)	Vitamin E (mg)	Folic Acid (mg)
Liver															
Beef	¼ lb	260	30.0	12.5	10.0	209	431	60,555	0.30	4.75	18.7	31	0.95	2.0	326
Calf	¼ lb	296	33.5	14.8	16.1	134	14	37,083	0.27	4.73	18.7	42	0.75	1.5	329
Chicken	¼ lb	187	30.0	12.5	9.7	69	171	14,198	0.19	3.05	13.3	18	0.85	1.8	427
Pork															
Ham, cooked	¼ lb	424	26.0	11.3	3.4	64	292	T	0.58	0.26	5.2	0	0.36		8.8
Ham, cooked, lean	¼ lb	246	33.7	15	4.3	83	377	T	0.73	0.33	6.5	0	0.45		11
Loin and loin chops, lean, baked or roasted	¼ lb	288	33.4	15	4.3	82	374	T	1.23	0.35	7.4	0	0.45		11
Spareribs, cooked	¼ lb	499	23.6	10	3.0	42	189	T	0.49	0.24	3.9				

Sausage, Cold Cuts, and Lunch Meats

Item	Amount	Calories	Protein (g)	Calcium (mg)	Iron (mg)	Sodium (mg)	Potassium (mg)	Vitamin A (mcg)	Thiamin (mg)	Ribof (mg)	Niacin (mg)	Vitamin C (mg)	Vitamin B6 (mg)	Vitamin E (mg)	Folic Acid (mg)
Brockwurst	3 oz	228	9.7												
Boiled ham	3 oz	202	16	9.5	2.4				0.12	0.04	0.71				
Bologna	3 oz	262	10.4	6	1.5	1,120	198		0.04	0.06	0.71				
Braunschweiger (smoked liverwurst)	3 oz	275	12.7	8.5	5			1,777	0.05	0.4	2.2				

Food	Portion									
Brown 'n' serve sausage	3 oz	364	14.2				0.06	0.05	0.85	0.72
Capicola	3 oz	430,	17.4				0.04	0.03	0.44	0.08
Country-style sausage	3 oz	297	13	7.8	2					
Deviled ham	3 oz	302	12	6.8	1.8					
Frankfurter, Raw, 5" long	1	176	7.1	4	1.1	627	0.09	0.08	1.5	0.14
Frankfurter, Cooked, 5" long	1	170	6.9	3	0.8	125	0.08	0.11	0.08	
Knockwurst	1 link	189	9.6	1.4	0.37		0.12	0.01	0.11	
Knockwurst	3 oz	340	12.2	6.8	1.8		0.05	0.06	0.71	
Liverwurst, fresh	3 oz	265	14	7.8	4.6	1,728	0.05	0.35	1.55	0.05
Meat loaf	3 oz	172	13.7	7.8	1.6		0.04	0.09	0.68	
Mortadella	1 slice	79	5.1	3	0.8					
Mortadella	3 oz	272	17.6	10.3	2.7					
Polish sausage	3 oz	262	13.5	7.8	2	125	0.09	0.05	0.85	
Pork sausage, cooked	1 link	62	2.4	1	0.3	35	0.01	0	0.5	
Salami	3 oz	388	20.5	12.2	3.1		0.1	0.07	1.44	0.01
Scrapple	3 oz	185	7.6	4.4	1		0.24	0.1	2.3	0.03
Summer sausage	3 oz	265	16	9.5	2.4		0.03	0.07	1.15	
Vienna sausage, canned	1 link	38	2.2	1	0.3		0	0	0.02	0

Miscellaneous Foods

Item	Amount	Calories	Protein (g)	Calcium (mg)	Iron (mg)	Sodium (mg)	Potassium (mg)	Vitamin A (mcg)	Thiamin (mg)	Ribof (mg)	Niacin (mg)	Vitamin C (mg)	Vitamin B6 (mg)	Vitamin E (mg)	Folic Acid (mg)
Coffee	1 cup	2	T	4	0.2	2	65	0	0	T	0.5	0	T	0	0
Hot chocolate	1 cup	288	8.3	260	0.5	120	370	360	0.08	0.4	0.3	3	0	0	0
Jam and preserves	1 Tbs	54	0.1	4	0.2	2	18	T	T	0.1	T	T	0	0	0
Maple syrup	1 cup	794	0	328	3.8	32	554	0	0	0	0	0	0	0	0
Margarine															
Regular	1 Tbs	102	0.1	3	0	140	3	469	0	0	0	0	0	8	0
Whipped	1 Tbs	68	0.06	0.9	0	93	2	313	0	0	0	0	0	5	0
Marmalade	1 Tbs	51	0.1	7	0.1	3	7	0	T	T	T	1	0	0	0
Mustard															
Brown	1 Tbs	14	0.9	19	0.3	196	20	0	0	0	0	0	0	0	0
Yellow	1 Tbs	11	0.7	13	0.3	188	20	0	0	0	0	0	0	0	0
Nuts															
Almonds	2 Tbs	195	6	76	1.5	1	1	0	0.08	0.3	1.2	T	0.06	0	288
Brazil nuts, shelled	2 Tbs	239	3.9	50.6	0.9	30	195	0	0.3	0.03	0.44	0	0.04	4.71	T
Cashews	2 Tbs	152	4.7	10.3	1	4	126	27	0.12	0.07	0.5	0	0	1.6	0
Chestnuts, shelled	2 Tbs	53	0.8	7.3	0.5	1.6	124	0	0.06	0.06	0.16	0	0.09	0	0

English walnuts, shelled	2 Tbs	172	4	27	0.9	T	123	8	0.09	0.04	0.25	0.5	0.2	6	2
Filberts, shelled	2 Tbs	173	3.4	57	0.9	0.5	192	0	0.17	0	0.25	T	0.15	7.6	17
Peanuts															
Shelled, whole	2 Tbs	159	7.1	19.7	0.6	1.4	192	0	0.09	0.04	4.7	0	0	0	0
Roasted, salted	2 Tbs	159	7	20	0.6	114	183	0	0.09	0.04	4.7	0	0	0	0
Pecans, shelled	2 Tbs	187	2.5	19.8	0.7	T	164	35	0.23	0.04	0.25	T	0.05	5.4	5
Pine nuts, shelled	2 Tbs	173	3.5	2.8	1.4	0	0	10	0.35	0.07	1.26	T	0	0	0
Pistachio nuts															
Shelled	2 Tbs	162	5.3	35.6	2	275	0	62	0.18	0	0.38	0	0	1.4	0
In the shell	2 Tbs	81	2.6	17.8	1	132	0	31	0.09	0	0.19	0	0	0.7	
Walnuts shelled	2 Tbs	171	5.6	T	1.6	T	125	82	0.06	0.03	0.19	0	0	0	0
Water chestnuts	2 Tbs	17	0.3	9	0.1	4	105	0	0.03	0.04	0.21	0.8	0	0	0
Peanut butter	1 Tbs	94	4		0.3	97	100	0	0	0	0.14	0	0	0	0
Pizza															
Cheese	1 slice	153	7.8	144	0.7	456	85	410	0.4	0.13	0.7	5	0	0	0
Individual frozen															
Cheese	1 slice	179	6.9	114	0.7	472	83	320	0.04	0.12	0.7	4	0	0	0
Sausage	1 slice	157	5.2	11	0.8	488	113	380	0.06	0.08	1	6	0	0	0

Item	Amount	Calories	Protein (g)	Calcium (mg)	Iron (mg)	Sodium (mg)	Potassium (mg)	Vitamin A (mcg)	Thiamin (mg)	Ribof (mg)	Niacin (mg)	Vitamin C (mg)	Vitamin B6 (mg)	Vitamin E (mg)	Folic Acid (mg)
Popcorn															
Plain	1 cup	23	0.8		0.2	T	0	0	0	0.01	0.1	0	0.01	0	0
With oil and salt	1 cup	41	0.0	1	0.2	175	0	0	0	0.01	0.2	0	0.01	0	0
Potato sticks	1 cup	190	2.2	15	0.6	0	46	T	0.07	0.02	1.7	14	0	0	0
Pretzels	4 oz	442	11	25	1.7	1,905	148	0	0.09	0.14	3.2	0	0	0	0
Salad dressings															
Roquefort	1 Tbs	76	0.7	12T	164	6	30	T	0.02	T	T	0	0	0	
Low-cal	1 Tbs	3	0.25	T	170	4	10	T	0.01	T	T	0	0	0	
French	1 Tbs	66	0.1	20.1	219	13	0	0	0	0	0	0	0	0	
Low-cal	1 Tbs	15	0.1	20.1	126	13	0	0	0	0	0	0	0	0	
Italian	1 Tbs	83	T	2T	314	2	T	T	T	T	0	0	0	0	
Low-cal	1 Tbs	8	T	5	118	2	T	T	T	T	0	0	0	0	
Mayonnaise	1 Tbs	101	0.2	30.1	84	5	T	0.01	0.01	0	0	0	0	0	
Russian	1 Tbs	74	0.2	30.1	130	24	100	0.01	0	0.1	1	0	0	0	
Thousand island	1 Tbs	80	0.1	20.1	112	18	50	T	T	T	T	0	0	0	
Low-cal	1 Tbs	27	0.1	20.1	105	17	50	T	T	T	T	0	0	0	
Sesame seeds	1 cup	873	27.3	165	3.6	0	0	0	0.27	0.2	8.1	0	0	0	0
Soups															
Cream of asparagus	1 cup	65	2.4	26	0.7	984	120	310	0.05	0.1	0.7	0	0	0	0
Beef bouillon	1 cup	31	5	T	0.5	782	130	T	T	0.2	1.2	0	0	0	0

Food	Measure													
Beef noodle	1 cup	67	3.8	7	1	917	77	50	0.05	0.07	1	T	0	0
Chicken consomme	1 cup	22	3.4	121.2	0	0	0	0	0	0	0	0	0	0
Chicken gumbo	1 cup	55	3.1	190.5	950	108	220	0.02	0.05	1.2	5	0	0	
Chicken noodle	1 cup	62	3.4	10	0.5	979	56	50	0.02	0.02	5	0	0.12	0
Chicken with rice	1 cup	48	3.1	70.2	917	98	140	T	0.02	0.7	0.7	T	0	0
Chicken vegetable	1 cup	76	4.2	17	0.5	1,034	98	2,160	0.02	0.05	1	0	0	0
Clam chowder, Manhattan	1 cup	81	2.2	34	1	938	184	880	0.02	0.02	1	0	0	0
Cream of chicken	1 cup	94	2.9	240.5	970	79	410	0.02	0.05	0.5	T	0	0	
Cream of mushroom	1 cup	134	2.4	410.5	955	98	70	0.02	0.12	0.7	T	0	0	
Minestrone	1 cup	105	4.9	37	1.1	995	314	2,350	0.07	0.05	1	T	0	0
Onion	1 cup	65	5.3	29	0.5	1,051	103	T	T	0.02	1	0	0	
Pea, split	1 cup	145	8.6	29	1.5	941	0	440	0.25	0.15	1.5	1	0	0
Tomato	1 cup	88	2	15	0.7	970	230	1,000	0.05	0.05	1.2	12	0.1	0
Turkey noodle	1 cup	79	4.3	14	0.7	998	77	190	0.05	0.05	1.2	0	0	0
Vegetable beef	1 cup	78	5.1	23	0.7	1,046	162	2,700	0.05	0.05	1	0	0	0
Vegetarian vegetable	1 cup	78	2.2	20	1	838	172	2,940	0.05	0.05	1	0	0	0
Dehydrated soups														
Beef noodle	1 cup	67	2.4	10	0.5	420	41	20	0.1	0.05	0.7	T	0	0
Chicken noodle	1 cup	53	1.9	7	0.2	578	19	50	0.07	0.05	0.05	T	0	0
Chicken and rice	1 cup	48	1.2	7	T	622	10	T	T	T	T	0.2	0	0
Onion	1 cup	36	1.4	10	0.2	689	58	T	T	T	T	2	0	0
Pea	1 cup	123	7.6	20	2	796	294	50	0.15	0.15	1.5	T	0	0
Tomato vegetable with noodles	1 cup	65	1.4	7	0.2	1,025	29	480	0.05	0.02	0.5	5	0	0
Soy Sauce	1 cup	12	1	15	0.9	1,319	66	0	T	0.05	0.1	0	0	0

Item	Amount	Calories	Protein (g)	Calcium (mg)	Iron (mg)	Sodium (mg)	Potassium (mg)	Vitamin A (mcg)	Thiamin (mg)	Ribof (mg)	Niacin (mg)	Vitamin C (mg)	Vitamin B6 (mg)	Vitamin E (mg)	Folic Acid (mg)
Spaghetti in tomato sauce with cheese															
Homemade	1 cup	260	8.8	80	1.3	955	408	1,080	0.25	0.18	2.3	1.3	0	0	0
Canned	1 cup	345	10	73	5	1,733	549	1,680	0.64	0.5	8.2	18	0	0	0
Spaghetti with meatballs and tomato sauce															
Homemade	1 cup	332	18.6	124	3.7	1,009	665	1,590	0.25	0.3	4	22	0	0	0
Canned	1 cup	258	12.3	53	3.3	1,220	245	1,000	0.15	0.18	2.3	5	0	0	0
Sunflower seeds (hulled)	1 cup	812	34.8	174	10.3	44	1,334	70	2.84	0.33	7.8	1.8	0	19	0
Tartar sauce	1 Tbs	74	0.2	3	0.1	99	11	30	T	T	T	T	0	0	0
Yeast, baker's	1 oz	24	3.4	4	1.4	5	173	T	0.2	0.47	3.2	T	0	0	0

Sugars, Sweets, and Desserts

Item	Amount	Calories	Protein (g)	Calcium (mg)	Iron (mg)	Sodium (mg)	Potassium (mg)	Vitamin A (mcg)	Thiamin (mg)	Ribof (mg)	Niacin (mg)	Vitamin C (mg)	Vitamin B6 (mg)	Vitamin E (mg)	Folic Acid (mg)
Cakes, homemade															
Angel food	1 slice	241	6.3	8	0.2	253	79	0	T	0.13	0.18	0	N/A	N/A	N/A
Boston cream pie	1 slice	312	5.2	69	0.5	192	92	216	0.03	0.11	0.21	T	N/A	N/A	N/A
Caramel	1 slice	597	5.8	132	2.4	397	101	315	0.03	0.11	0.16	T	N/A	N/A	N/A
Chocolate, iced	1 slice	550	6.7	104	1.5	351	230	239	0.03	0.15	0.3	T	N/A	N/A	N/A
Chocolate cupcake	1	162	2	31	0.4	103	68	70	0.01	0.04	0.1	T	N/A	N/A	N/A
Fruitcake	1 slice	57	0.7	11	0.4	24	74	20	0.02	0.02	0.1	T	N/A	N/A	N/A

Food	Serving														
Gingerbread, iced	1 piece	362	3.9	51	0.3	269	66	134	0.02	0.07	0.02	T	N/A	N/A	N/A
Gingerbread, plain	1 piece	283	3.5	50	0.3	233	61	132	0.02	0.07	0.16	T	N/A	N/A	N/A
Pound	1 slice	142	1.7	6	0.2	33	18	80	0.01	0.03	0.1	0	N/A	N/A	N/A
White, iced	1 slice	587	5.2	75	0.2	366	91	173	0.02	0.09	0.16	T	N/A	N/A	N/A
Yellow, iced	1 slice	549	6.3	102	0.9	313	162	240	0.03	0.12	0.3	T	N/A	N/A	N/A
Cakes, made from mixes															
Angel food	1 slice	206	4.5	75	0.2	116	48	0	0.04	0.09	0.08	0	N/A	N/A	N/A
Coffee cake	1 piece	139	2.7	26	0.7	185	47	69	0.08	0.07	0.6	T	N/A	N/A	N/A
Cupcakes, iced	1	172	2.2	62	0.4	161	56	80	0.02	0.05	0.1	T	N/A	N/A	N/A
Devil's food	1 slice	469	6.1	82	1.1	363	180	208	0.04	0.11	0.41	T	N/A	N/A	N/A
Honey spice	1 slice	543	6.3	110	1.2	378	127	248	0.03	0.14	0.31	T	N/A	N/A	N/A
Marble	1 slice	432	5.7	102	1.1	338	159	118	0.02	0.11	0.26	T	N/A	N/A	N/A
White	1 slice	513	5.6	141	0.7	234	162	85	0.03	0.11	0.28	T	N/A	N/A	N/A
Yellow	1 slice	467	5.7	126	0.8	314	151	194	0.03	0.11	0.27	T	N/A	N/A	N/A
Candy															
Butterscotch	1 oz	113	T	5	0.4	19	1	40	0	T	T	0	N/A	N/A	N/A
Candy corn	1 oz	91	T	4	0.3	53	1	0	T	T	T	0	N/A	N/A	N/A
Caramels	1 oz	113	1.1	42	0.4	64	54	T	0.01	0.05	0.1	T	N/A	N/A	N/A
Chocolate															
Bittersweet	1 oz	135	2.2	16	1.4	1	174	10	0.01	0.05	0.3	0	N/A	N/A	N/A
Milk	1 oz	147	2.2	65	0.3	27	109	80	0.02	0.1	0.1	T	N/A	N/A	N/A
Semisweet	1 oz	144	1.2	9	0.7	1	92	10	T	0.02	0.1	T	N/A	N/A	N/A
Chocolate-coated															
Almonds	1 oz	161	3.5	58	0.8	17	155	T	0.03	0.15	0.5	T	N/A	N/A	N/A

Item	Amount	Calories	Protein (g)	Calcium (mg)	Iron (mg)	Sodium (mg)	Potassium (mg)	Vitamin A (mcg)	Thiamin (mg)	Ribof (mg)	Niacin (mg)	Vitamin C (mg)	Vitamin B$_6$ (mg)	Vitamin E (mg)	Folic Acid (mg)
Coconut	1 oz	124	0.8	14	0.3	56	47	0	0.01	0.02	0.1	0	N/A	N/A	N/A
Fudge, peanuts, and caramel	1 oz	123	2.2	51	0.4	58	85	T	0.05	0.06	0.5	T	N/A	N/A	N/A
Peanuts	1 oz	119	3.5	25	0.3	13	107	T	0.08	0.04	1.6	T	N/A	N/A	N/A
Raisins	1 oz	101	1.3	36	0.6	15	143	36	0.02	0.05	0.1	T	N/A	N/A	N/A
Fudge (chocolate)	1 oz	122	1.1	29	0.4	65	55	T	0.01	0.04	0.1	0	N/A	N/A	N/A
Gumdrops	1 oz	98	T	2	0.1	10	1	0	0	T	T	0	N/A	N/A	N/A
Jelly beans	1 oz	101	T	3	0.3	3	T	0	0	T	T	0	N/A	N/A	N/A
Peanut brittle	1 oz	119	1.6	10	0.7	9	43	0	0.05	0.01	1	0	N/A	N/A	N/A
Cookies															
Assorted															
sandwich-type	1	55	0.57	4	0.08	41	8	9	T	T	T	T			
Brownies with nuts	1	97	1.3	8	0.4	50	38	40	0.04	0.02	0.1	T			
Chocolate chip, homemade	1	52	0.5	5	0.2	35	12	10	0.01	0.01	0.1	T			
Chocolate chip, commercial	1	50	0.57	4	0.2	42	14	13	T	0.01	0.04	T			
Fig bars	1	50	0.5	11	0.15	35	28	15	T	0.1	0.05	T			
Macaroon	1	90	1	5	0.15	7	88	0	0.01	0.03	0.1	0			
Oatmeal-raisin	1	60	0.8	3	0.04	16	48	8	0.02	0.01	0.75	T			

Food	Portion												
Peanut butter sandwich	1	80	1.2	5	0.1	21	21	25	T	0.01	0.35	T	0.45
Sugar wafer	1	17	0.17	.1	0.01	7	2	5	T	T	0.02	0	
Vanilla wafer	1	14	0.16	1	0.01	8	2	4	T	T	0.01	0	
Danish pastry, plain	1	480	8.4	57	1	415	127	363	0.08	0.17	0.9	T	
Pies													
Apple	1 piece	302	2.6	9	0.4	365	94	40	0.02	0.02	0.5	1	
Banana	1 piece	252	7.5	1	0.2	231	290	T	0.15	0.3	1	N/A	
Blueberry	1 piece	286	2.8	13	0.7	316	77	40	0.02	0.02	0.4	4	
Cherry	1 piece	308	3.1	17	0.4	359	124	520	0.02	0.02	0.6	T	
Coconut custard	1 piece	268	6.8	107	0.8	282	186	260	0.07	0.22	0.3	0	
Lemon meringue	1 piece	268	3.9	15	0.5	296	53	180	0.3	0.08	0.2	3	
Mince	1 piece	320	3	33	1.2	529	210	T	0.08	0.05	0.5	1	
Peach	1 piece	300	3	12	0.6	316	176	860	0.02	0.05	8	4	
Pecan	1 piece	431	5.3	48	2.9	228	127	160	0.16	0.07	0.3	T	
Pumpkin	1 piece	241	4.6	58	0.6	244	182	2,810	0.03	0.11	0.6	T	
Puddings, made from commercial mix, with milk	1 cup	322	8.11	465	6.8	335	354	340	0.05	0.39	0.3	2	
Sherbet	1 cup	259	1.7	31	T	19	42	120	0.02	0.06	T	4	

Vegetables

Item	Amount	Calories	Protein (g)	Calcium (mg)	Iron (mg)	Sodium (mg)	Potassium (mg)	Vitamin A (mcg)	Thiamin (mg)	Ribof (mg)	Niacin (mg)	Vitamin C (mg)	Vitamin B6 (mg)	Vitamin E (mg)	Folic Acid (mg)
Artichoke	1 heart	20	4.3	78	1.7	46	458	230	0.11	0.03	1.1	12	0	0	0
Asparagus spears															
Canned, green	1 cup	51	5.8	46	4.6	571	402	1,940	0.15	0.24	0.2	36	0.13	0	23
Canned, white	1 cup	53	5.1	39	2.4	571	339	190	0.12	0.15	1.7	36	0.08	0	0
Cooked, boiled whole	1 cup	36	4	38	1.1	2	329	1,620	0.29	0.32	2.5	47	0	0	0
Frozen, cooked	1 cup	44	6.1	42	2.1	2	452	1,480	0.3	0.27	2.1	49	0.39	0	0
Beans, boiled and cut, French style	1 cup	31	2	62	0.8	5	189	675	0.09	0.11	0.6	14	0.11	0	0
Beans, canned, without pork	1 cup	300	16	170	5	844	670	150	0.18	0.1	1.6	4	0	0	0
Beans, kidney															
Canned	1 cup	225	14	73	4.5	8	660	T	0.13	0.10	1.5	0	0	0	0
Cooked	1 cup	300	20	95	6	7.5	850	T	0.28	0.15	1.8	0	1.1	0	0
Beans, lima															
Canned, drained	1 cup	220	12	64	3.6	540	510	436	0.06	0.12	1.2	14	0	0	0
Cooked	1 cup	178	12	75	4	1.6	675	448	0.29	0.16	2.0	29	0	0	0
Frozen	1 cup	188	12	56	4.2	160	681	368	0.12	0.08	1.6	27	0.27	0	0

Beans. white															
Raw	1 cup	680	44	288	15.6	38	2,392	0	1.3	0.44	4.8	0	0	0	0
Cooked	1 cup	224	15	95	5.1	13	790	0	0.27	0.13	1.3	0	2	0	0
Beans, yellow or wax															
Canned	1 cup	48	2.8	90	3	472	190	200	0.06	0.1	0.6	10	0.08	0	5
Cooked	1 cup	22	1.4	50	0.6	3	243	250	0.08	0.1	0.8	26	0.8	0	0
Frozen, cooked	1 cup	54	2.4	70	1.4	2	320	200	0.14	0.16	0.8	12	0.15	0	0
Bean sprouts, mung															
Cooked	1 cup	28	3.2	17	0.9	4	156	20	0.09	0.1	0.7	6	0	0	0
Raw	1 cup	21	2.2	42	0.8	3	134	12	0.08	0.08	0.5	12	0	0	0
Beets															
Canned	1 cup	62	1.6	32	1.2	392	276	34	0.02	0.04	0.2	6	0	0	0
Cooked	1 cup	54	1.8	24	0.8	72	244	34	0.06	0.06	0.6	10	0	0	0
Broccoli															
Cooked	1 cup	39	4.7	132	1.2	15	460	3,900	0.09	0.18	0.8	135	0	0	0
Raw	1-5½" stalk	32	3.6	103	1.1	15	328	2,500	0.01	0.23	9	113	0.2	1.9	2
Brussels sprouts,															
cooked	1 cup	54	6.3	48	1.5	15	409	780	0.12	0.21	1.2	130	04.3	0	0
Cabbage															
Cooked	1 cup	33	1.8	22	0.5	23	272	216	0.07	0.07	0.5	70	0	0	0
Red, raw	1 cup	31	2	42	0.8	26	268	40	0.09	0.06	0.4	61	0	0	0

Item	Amount	Calories	Protein (g)	Calcium (mg)	Iron (mg)	Sodium (mg)	Potassium (mg)	Vitamin A (mcg)	Thiamin (mg)	Ribof (mg)	Niacin (mg)	Vitamin C (mg)	Vitamin B6 (mg)	Vitamin E (mg)	Folic Acid (mg)
Carrots															
Cooked	1 cup	47	1.4	50	0.9	50	333	15,750	0.08	0.08	0.8	9	0	0	0
Raw	1 large	42	1.1	37	0.7	47	341	11,000	0.06	0.05	0.6	8	0.15	0.5	8
Cauliflower															
Cooked	1 cup	28	2.9	26	0.9	11	268	80	0.11	0.1	0.8	69	0	0	0
Raw	1 cup	27	2.7	25	1.1	13	295	60	0.11	0.1	0.7	78	0.32	0.15	31
Celery															
Cooked	1 cup	18	1	39	0.3	110	200	388	0.03	0.4	0.4	8	0	0	0
Raw	1 stalk	7	0.4	16	0.1	50	1,361	10	0.01	0.01	0.1	4	0.03	0.25	4
Chickpeas	1 cup	720	41	300	14	62	1,600	100	0.62	0.3	4	0	1.1	5.1	2
Coleslaw, with mayonnaise	1 cup	173	1.6	53	0.5	144	239	190	0.06	0.06	0.4	T	0	0	0
Collard greens, cooked	1 cup	150	3.2	853	3.6	0	1,188	35,380	0.5	0.9	5.4	345	0	0	0
Cucumber	1 medium	8	0.5	13	0.6	3	80	125	0.15	0.2	0.1	6	0.02	0	0
	½ cup	19	1	11	0.6	1	150	10	0.5	0.4	0.5	3	0	0	0
Eggplant, cooked	½ cup	19	2.1	90	0.8	29	148	4,956	T	T	0.7	62	0	0	0
Kale, cooked	½ cup	19													
Lentils	1 cup	212	15.6	50	4.2	0	498	40	0.14	0.12	1.2	0	1.2	5	0

Food	Serving														
Lettuce, iceberg, NY, and Great Lakes	1 cup	28	2.4	70	4	18	528	1,980	0.12	0.12	0.6	16	0.01	1	23
Mushrooms	4 large or 10 small	28	2.7	6	0.8	15	414	T	0.01	0.46	4.2	3	0.14	0.1	3
Okra, cooked	8–9 pods	29	2	92	0.5	2	174	490	0.13	0.18	0.9	20	0	0	0
Olives	10	45	0.5	24	0.6	926	21	120	0	0	0	0	0.006	0	0
Onion Cooked	1 cup	61	2.5	50	0.8	15	231	80	0.06	0.06	0.04	15	0	0	0
Onion Raw	1 cup	65	26	46	0.9	17	267	70	0.05	0.07	0.3	17	0.22	0.4	20
Parsley	1 cup	26	2.2	122	3.7	7	436	5,100	0.07	0.16	0.7	103	0.09	1.8	30
Peas Canned	1 cup	99	5	30	2.5	353	144	675	135	74	1.4	13		0	0
Peas Fresh, cooked	1 cup	107	8.1	35	2.7	2	294	210	420	165	3.5	30		0	0
Peas Frozen	1 cup	102	7.7	28	2.8	172	202	900	405	135	2.6	20		0	0
Peas Raw	1 cup	105	7.9	33	2.4	2	395	800	438	172	3.6	34		0	0
Peas and Carrots, frozen	4 oz	60	3.6	28	1.3	95	178	10,545	0.22	0.08	1.5	9	0	0	0
Peppers Green, raw	1	36	2	15	1.1	21	349	690	0.13	0.13	0.8	210	0.52	1.4	20
Peppers Hot chili	1 cup	51	2.2	22	1.2	0	0	23,500	0.02	0.22	1.5	21		0	0
Peppers Sweet green, cooked	1	29	1.6	15	0.8	14	238	690	0.1	0.11	0.7	T	0.41	0	0

Item	Amount	Calories	Protein (g)	Calcium (mg)	Iron (mg)	Sodium (mg)	Potassium (mg)	Vitamin A (mcg)	Thiamin (mg)	Ribof (mg)	Niacin (mg)	Vitamin C (mg)	Vitamin B6 (mg)	Vitamin E (mg)	Folic Acid (mg)
Pickles															
Oil	1	7	0.5	17	0.7	928	130	70	T	0.01	T	4	0.04	0	0
Sour	1	7	0.3	11	2.1	879	0	70	T	0.01	T	5	0.04	0	0
Sweet	1	22	0.1	2	0.2	0	0	10	T	T	T	1	0.02	0	0
Relish	1 cup	338	1.2	49	2	1,744	0	0	0	0	0	0		0	0
Potatoes															
Baked	1	145	4	14	1.1	6	782	T	0.15	0.07	2.7	31	0	0	0
Boiled	1	173	4.8	16	1.4	7	926	T	0.2	0.09	3.4	36	0	0.5	0
French fried	1/4 lb	311	6	17	1.5	7	967	T	0.15	0.09	3.5	24	0	0	0
Frozen, french fried	10	110	1.8	5	0.9	2	326	T	0.07	0.01	1.3	11	0	0	0
Mashed with milk	1 cup	137	4.4	50	0.8	632	548	40	0.17	0.11	2.1	21	0	0	0
Scalloped au gratin with cheese	1 cup	355	13	311	1.2	1,095	750	780	0.15	0.29	2.2	25	0	0	0
Potato chips	10 chips	113	1.1	8	0.4	226	0	T	0.04	0.01	1	3	T	0	1
Potato salad, homemade, without eggs	1/4 lb	112	3	36	0.7	599	362	160	0.09	0.08	1.3	13	0	0	0
Radish	1 small	2	0.1	3	0.1	2	32	1	0.003	0.003	0.03	3	T	0	T
Rutabaga, cooked	1 cup	60	1.5	100	0.5	7	284	940	0.1	0.1	1.4	44	0	0	0
Sauerkraut	1 cup	42	2.4	85	1.2	1,755	329	120	0.07	0.09	0.5	33	0.29	0	0

Food	Serving														
Soybeans, cooked	1 cup	177	15	90	4	0	0	990	0.47	0.2	1.8	26	0.3	0	892
Soybean curd (tofu)	3½ oz	72	7.8	128	1.9	7	42	0	0.06	0.03	0.1	0	0	0	363
Spinach															
Boiled	1 cup	42	5.4	166	490	582	14,300	0.12	0.26	1	50		0.34	0	3
Canned	1 cup	44	4.8	212	4.6	424	454	14,400	0.04	0.22	0.6	26	0.15	0	42
Frozen, cooked	1 cup	48	5.8	210	5	98	724	16,200	0.16	0.28	0.5	56	0.4	0	0
Squash															
Acorn, baked	1 cup	126	3.6	56	1.6	2		8,400	0.1	0.26	1.4	26	0	0	0
Acorn, boiled	1 cup	83	2.9	45	1.7	2	750	2,700	0.1	0.25	0	20	0	0	0
Summer, cooked	1 cup	28	1.8	50	0.8	2	282	780	0.1	0.16	0.16	20	0	0	0
Winter, cooked	1 cup	95	3	50	1.2	25	645	8,750	0.1	0.25	1	20	0	0	0
Winter, frozen, cooked	1 cup	72	2.4	50	52	2	414	7,800	0.06	1.42	1	16	0	0	0
Succotash, frozen, cooked	½ lb	211	9.6	30	2.3	86	558	680	0.2	0.12	3	14	0.4	0	0
Sweet potatoes															
Baked	1	161	2.4	46	1	14	342	9,230	0.1	0.08	0.8	26	0	0	0
Boiled	1	172	2.6	48	1.1	15	367	11,940	0.14	0.09	0.9	26	0	0	0
Candied	2 halves	168	1.3	37	0.9	42	190	6,300	0.06	0.04	0.4	10	0	0	0
Canned	1 small	108	2	25	0.8	48	200	7,800	0.05	0.04	0.6	14	0	0	0
Tomatoes															
Canned	1 cup	42	2	12	1	260	424	1,800	0.1	0.06	1.4	34	0	0	0

Item	Amount	Calories	Protein (g)	Calcium (mg)	Iron (mg)	Sodium (mg)	Potassium (mg)	Vitamin A (mcg)	Thiamin (mg)	Ribof (mg)	Niacin (mg)	Vitamin C (mg)	Vitamin B6 (mg)	Vitamin E (mg)	Folic Acid (mg)
Catsup	1 Tbs	16	0.3	3	0.1	156	54	210	0.01	0.01	0.2	2	0.16	0	0
Chili sauce	1 Tbs	16	0.4	3	0.1	201	56	210	0.01	0.01	0.2	2	0.16	0	0
Juice															
Canned or bottled	1 cup	46	2.2	17	2.2	486	552	1,940	0.12	0.07	1.9	39	0.5	0	0
Cocktail	1 cup	51	1.7	24	2.2	486	537	1,940	0.12	0.05	1.5	36	0.4	0	0
Low-sodium	1 cup	46	1.9	17	2.2	7	549	1,940	0.12	0.07	1.7	39	0.4	0	0
Paste	1 cup	215	8.9	71	9.2	100	2,237	8,650	0.52	0.31	8.1	128	0	0	0
Puree	1 cup	97	4.2	32	4.2	1,000	1,060	4,000	0.22	0.12	3.5	82	0	0	0
Ripe	1 medium	33	1.6	20	0.8	4	366	1,350	0.09	0.06	1	34	0.22	0.8	14
Turnips, cooked	1 cup	34	1.2	53	0.6	51	282	T	0.06	0.08	0.5	33	0	0	0
Turnip greens, cooked	1 cup	30	3.3	276	1.7	0	0	9,450	0.23	0.36	0.9	103	0	0	0
Vegetable juice cocktail	1 cup	41	2.2	29	1.2	484	535	1,690	0.12	0.07	1.9	22	0	0	0
Vegetables, mixed	1 cup	116	5.8	46	2.4	96	348	9,010	0.22	0.13	2	15	0	0	0
Yams, cooked	1 cup	210	4.8	8	1.2	0	0	T	0.18	0.08	1.2	18	0	0	0

Bibliography

Antioxidants

Ames, B. N., Shigenaga, M. K., and Hagen, T. M. Oxidants, antioxidants, and the degenerative diseases of aging. *Proceedings of the National Academy of Sciences of the United States of America* 90 (1993): 7915–7922.

Anonymous. The effect of vitamin E and beta carotene on the incidence of lung cancer and other cancers in male smokers: The Alpha-Tocopherol, Beta Carotene Cancer Prevention Study Group. *New England Journal of Medicine* 330 (1994): 1029–1035.

Buring, J. E., and Hennekens, C. H. Antioxidant vitamins and cardiovascular disease. *Nutrition Reviews* 55 (1997): S53–S58.

Diaz, M. N., Frei, B., Vita, J. A., and Keaney, J. F. Mechanisms of disease: Antioxidants and atherosclerotic heart disease. *New England Journal of Medicine* 337 (1997): 408–418.

Heinonen, O. P., Albanes, D., Virtamo, J., et al. Prostate cancer and supplementation with alpha-tocopherol and beta-carotene: Incidence and mortality in a controlled trial. *Journal of the National Cancer Institute* 90 (1998): 440–446.

Hennekens, C. H., Buring, J. E., Manson, J. E., et al. Lack of effect of long-term supplementation with beta carotene on the incidence of malignant neoplasms and cardiovascular disease. *New England Journal of Medicine* 334 (1996): 1145–1149.

Hodis, H. N., Mack, W. J., LaBree, L., et al. Serial coronary angiographic evidence that antioxidant vitamin intake reduces progression of coronary artery atheroslerosis. *Journal of the American Medical Association* 273 (1995): 1849–1854.

Kushi, L. H., Folsom, A. R., Prineas, R. J., Mink, P. J., Wu, Y., and Bostick, R. M. Dietary antioxidant vitamins and death from coronary heart disease in postmenopausal women. *New England Journal of Medicine* 334 (1996): 1156–1162.

Losonczy, K. G., Harris, T. B., and Havlik, R. J. Vitamin E and vitamin C supplement use and risk of all-cause and coronary heart disease mortality in older persons: The Established Populations for Epidemiologic Studies of the Elderly. *American Journal of Clinical Nutrition* 64 (1996): 190–196.

Meydani, M. Vitamin E. *Lancet* 345 (1995): 170–175.

Meydani, S. N., Meydani, M., Blumberg, J. B., et al. Vitamin E supplementation and in vivo immune response in healthy elderly subjects: A randomized controlled trial. *Journal of the American Medical Association* 277 (1997): 1380–1386.

Omenn, G. S., Goodman, G. E., Thornquist, M.D., et al. Effects of a combination of beta carotene and vitamin A on lung cancer and cardiovascular disease. *New England Journal of Medicine* 334 (1996): 1150–1155.

Rimm, E. B., Stampfer, M. J., Ascherio, A., Giovannucci, E., Colditz, G. A., and Willett, W. C. Vitamin E consumption and the risk of coronary heart disease in men. *New England Journal of Medicine* 328 (1993): 1450–1456.

Sano, M., Ernesto, C., Thomas, R. G., et al. A controlled trial of selegiline, alphatocopherol, or both as treatment for Alzheimer's disease: The Alzheimer's Disease Cooperative Study. *New England Journal of Medicine* 336 (1997): 1216–1222.

Stampfer, M. J., Hennekens, C. H., Manson, J. E., Colditz, G. A., Rosner, B., and Willett, W. C. Vitamin E consumption and the risk of coronary disease in women. *New England Journal of Medicine* 328 (1993): 1444–1449.

Biotin

Hill, M. J. Intestinal flora and endogenous vitamin synthesis. *European Journal of Cancer Prevention* 6 suppl. (1997): 1:S43–45.

Hymes, J., and Wolf, B. Biotinidase and its roles in biotin metabolism. *Clinica Chimica Acta* 255 (1996): 1–11.

Mock, D. M. Skin manifestations of biotin deficiency. *Seminars in Dermatology* 10 (1991): 296–302.

Mock, D. M. Determinations of biotin in biological fluids. *Methods in Enzymology* 279 (1997): 265–275.

Chamomile

Fidler, P., Loprinzi, C. L., O'Fallon, J. R., et al. Prospective evaluation of a chamomile mouthwash for prevention of 5-FU-induced oral mucositis. *Cancer* 77 (1996): 522–525.

Forster, H. B., Niklas, H., and Lutz, S. Antispasmodic effects of some medicinal plants. *Planta Medica* 40 (1980): 309–319.

Mucsi, I., Gyulai, Z., and Béládi, I. Combined effects of flavonoids and acyclovir against herpes viruses in cell cultures. *Acta Microbiologica Hungarica* 39 (1992): 137–147.

Pereira, F., Santos, R., and Pereira, A. Contact dermatitis from chamomile tea. *Contact Dermatitis* 36 (1997): 307.

Rekka, E. A., Kourounakis, P., and Kourounakis, P. N. Investigation of the effect of chamazulene on lipid peroxidation and free radical processes. *Research Communications in Molecular Pathology and Pharmacology* 92 (1996): 361–364.

Safayhi, H., Sabieraj, J., Sailer, E. R., and Ammon, H. P. Chamazulene: An antioxidant-type inhibitor of leukotriene B4 formation. *Planta Medica* 60 (1994): 410–413.

Subiza, J., Subiza, J. L., Alonso, M., et al. Allergic conjunctivitis to chamomile tea. *Annals of Allergy* 65 (1990): 127–132.

Subiza, J., Subiza, J. L., Hinojosa, M., et al. Anaphylactic reaction after the ingestion of chamomile tea: A study of cross-reactivity with other composite pollens. *Journal of Allergy and Clinical Immunology* 84 (1989): 353–358.

Coenzyme Q$_{10}$ (Ubiquinone)

Digiesi, V., Cantini, F., Oradei, A., et al. Coenzyme Q$_{10}$ in essential hypertension. *Molecular Aspects of Medicine* 15 suppl. (1994): 257–263.

Langsjoen, H., Langsjoen, P., Willis, R., and Folkers, K. Usefulness of coenzyme Q$_{10}$ in clinical cardiology: A long-term study. *Molecular Aspects of Medicine* 15 suppl. (1994): 165–175.

Langsjoen, P. H., Vadhanavikit, S., and Folkers, K. Effective treatment with coenzyme Q$_{10}$ of patients with chronic myocardial disease. *Drugs Under Experimental and Clinical Research* 11 (1985): 577–579.

Langsjoen, P., Willis, R., and Folkers, K. Treatment of essential hypertension with coenzyme Q$_{10}$. *Molecular Aspects of Medicine* 15 suppl. (1994): 265–272.

Lockwood, K., Moesgaard, S., Yamamoto, T., and Folkers, K. Progress on therapy of breast cancer with vitamin Q$_{10}$ and the regression of metastases. *Biochemical and Biophysical Research Communications* 212 (1995): 172–177.

Lonnrot, K., Metsa Ketela, T., and Alho, H. The role of coenzyme Q-10 in aging: A follow-up study on life-long oral supplementation of Q-10 in rats. *Gerontology* 41 suppl. (1995): 109–120.

Permanetter, B., Rossy, W., Weingartner, F., Bauer, R., Seidl, K. F., and Klein, G. Lack of effectiveness of coenzyme Q$_{10}$ (ubiquinone) in long-term treatment of dilated cardiomyopathy. *Zeitschrift für Kardiologie* 78 (1989): 360–365.

Porter, D. A., Costill, D. L., Zachwieja, J. J., et al. The effect of oral coenzyme Q$_{10}$ on the exercise tolerance of middle-aged, untrained men. *International Journal of Sports Medicine* 16 (1995): 421–427.

Taggart, D. P., Jenkins, M., Hooper, J., et al. Effects of short-term supplementation with coenzyme Q$_{10}$ on myocardial protection during cardiac operations. *Annals of Thoracic Surgery* 61 (1996): 829–833.

DHEA

Berr, C., Lafont, S., Debuire, B., Dartigues, J. F., and Baulieu, E. E. Relationships of dehydroepiandrosterone sulfate in the elderly with functional, psychological, and mental status, and short-term mortality: A French community-based study. *Proceedings of the National Academy of Sciences of the United States of America* 93 (1996): 13410–13415.

Casson, P. R., and Carson, S. A. Androgen replacement therapy in women: Myths and realities. *International Journal of Fertility and Menopausal Studies* 41 (1996): 412–422.

Casson, P. R., Faquin, L. C., Stentz, F. B., et al. Replacement of dehydroepiandrosterone enhances T-lymphocyte insulin binding in postmenopausal women. *Fertility and Sterility* 63 (1995): 1027–1031.

Flood, J. F., Morley, J. E., and Roberts, E. Memory-enhancing effects in male mice of pregnenolone and steroids metabolically derived from it. *Proceedings of the National Academy of Sciences of the United States of America* 89 (1992): 1567–1571.

Helzlsouer, K. J., Alberg, A. J., Gordon, G. B., et al. Serum gonadotropins and steroid hormones and the development of ovarian cancer. *Journal of the American Medical Association* 274 (1995): 1926–1930.

Jesse, R. L., Loesser, K., Eich, D. M., Qian, Y. Z., Hess, M. L., and Nestler, J. E. Dehydroepiandrosterone inhibits human platelet aggregation in vitro and in vivo. *Annals of the New York Academy of Sciences* 774 (1995): 281–290.

van Vollenhoven, R. F., Engleman, E. G., and McGuire, J. L. Dehydroepiandrosterone in systemic lupus erythematosus: Results of a double-blind, placebo-controlled, randomized clinical trail. *Arthritis and Rheumatism* 38 (1995): 1826–1831.

Wolkowitz, O. M., Reus, V. I., Roberts, E., et al. Dehydroepiandrosterone (DHEA) treatment of depression. *Biological Psychiatry* 41 (1997): 311–318.

Yen, S. S., Morales, A. J., and Khorram, O. Replacement of DHEA in aging men and women: Potential remedial effects. *Annals of the New York Academy of Sciences* 774 (1995): 128–142.

Echinacea

Bauer, R. Echinacea drugs—effects and active ingredients. *Zeitschrift für Arztliche Fortbildung* 90 (1996): 111–115.

Braunig, B., Dorn, M., et al. Echinacea purpurea root for strengthening the immune response in flu-like infections. *Zeitschrift für Phytotherapie* 13 (1992): 7–13.

Coeugniet, E., and Kuhnast, R. Adjuvant immunotherapy with different formulations of Echinacin®. *Therapiewoche* 36 (1986): 3352–3358.

Dorsch, W. Clinical application of extracts of Echinacea purpurea or Echinacea pallida: Critical evaluation of controlled clinical studies. *Zeitschrift für Arztliche Fortbildung* 90 (1996): 117–122.

Gaisbauer, M., Schleich, T., Stickl, H. A., and Wilczek, I. The effect of Echinacea purpurea Moench on phagocytosis in granulocytes measured by chemiluminescence. *Arzneimittel-forschung* 40 (1990): 594–598.

Melchart, D., Walther, E., Linde, K., Brandmaier, R., Lersch, C. Echinacea root extracts for the prevention of upper respiratory tract infections. A double-blind, placebo controlled randomized trial. *Archiv Fam Med* 7 (1998): 541–545.

Parnham, M. J. Benefit-risk assessment of the squeezed sap of the purple coneflower (Echinacea purpurea) for long-term oral immunostimulation. *Phytomedicine* 3 (1996): 95–102.

Roesler, J., Emmendorffer, A., Steinmuller, C., Luettig, B., Wagner, H., and Lohmann Matthes, M. L. Application of purified polysaccharides from cell cultures of the plant Echinacea purpurea to test subjects mediates activation of the phagocyte system. *International Journal of Immunopharmacology* 13 (1991): 931–941.

Scaglione, F., and Lund, B. Efficacy in the treatment of the common cold of a preparation containing an Echinacea extract. *International Journal of Immunotherapy* 11 (1995): 163–166.

Schoneberger, D. The influence of the pressed juice from Echinacea purpurea on the course and severity of colds. *Forum Immunologie* 8 (1992): 2–12.

See, D. M., Broumand, N., Sahl, L., and Tilles, J. G. In vitro effects of echinacea and ginseng on natural killer and antibody-dependent cell cytotoxicity in healthy subjects and chronic fatigue syndrome or acquired immunodeficiency syndrome patients. *Immunopharmacology* 35 (1997): 229–235.

Feverfew

Groenewegen, W. A., and Heptinstall, S. A comparison of the effects of an extract of feverfew and parthenolide, a component of feverfew, on human platelet activity in-vitro. *Journal of Pharmacy and Pharmacology* 42 (1990): 553–557.

Groenewegen, W. A., Knight, D. W., and Heptinstall, S. Progress in the medicinal chemistry of the herb feverfew. *Progress in Medicinal Chemistry* 29 (1992): 217–238.

Heptinstall, S. Feverfew—an ancient remedy for modern times? *Journal of the Royal Society of Medicine* 81 (1988): 373–374.

Heptinstall, S., Awang, D. V., Dawson, B. A., Kindack, D., Knight, D. W., and May, J. Parthenolide content and bioactivity of feverfew (Tanacetum parthenium (L.) Schultz-Bip.): Estimation of commercial and authenticated feverfew products. *Journal of Pharmacy and Pharmacology* 44 (1992): 391–395.

Johnson, E. S., Kadam, N. P., Hylands, D. M., and Hylands, P. J. Efficacy of feverfew as prophylactic treatment of migraine. *British Medical Journal (Clinical Research Ed.)* 291 (1985): 569–573.

Knight, D. W. Feverfew: Chemistry and biological activity. *Natural Product Reports* 12 (1995): 271–276.

Murphy, J. J., Heptinstall, S., and Mitchell, J. R. Randomised double-blind placebo-controlled trial of feverfew in migraine prevention. *Lancet* 2 (1988): 189–192.

Pattrick, M., Heptinstall, S., and Doherty, M. Feverfew in rheumatoid arthritis: A double blind, placebo controlled study. *Annals of the Rheumatic Diseases* 48 (1989): 547–549.

Folic Acid

Butterworth, C. E., Jr., Hatch, K. D., Soong, S. J., et al. Oral folic acid supplementation for cervical dysplasia: A clinical intervention trial. *American Journal of Obstetrics and Gynecology* 166 (1992): 803–809.

Czeizel, A. E., and Dudás, I. Prevention of the first occurrence of neural-tube defects by periconceptional vitamin supplementation. *New England Journal of Medicine* 327 (1992): 1832–1835.

den Heijer, M., Koster, T., Blom, H. J., et al. Hyperhomocysteinemia as a risk factor for deep-vein thrombosis. *New England Journal of Medicine* 334 (1996): 759–762.

Graham, I. M., Daly, L. E., Refsum, H. M., et al. Plasma homocysteine as a risk factor for vascular disease: The European Concerted Action Project. *Journal of the American Medical Association* 277 (1997): 1775–1781.

Kim, Y., and Mason, J. B. Folate, epithelial dysplasia and colon cancer. *Proceedings of the Association of American Physicians* 107 (1995): 218–227.

Requejo, A. M., Ortega, R. M., Navia, B., Gaspar, M. J., Quintas, E., and López Sobaler, A. Folate and vitamin B_{12} status in a group of preschool children. *International Journal for Vitamin and Nutrition Research* 67 (1997): 171–175.

Rimm, E. B., Willett, W. C., Hu, F. B., et al. Folate and vitamin B_6 from diet and supplements in relation to risk of coronary heart disease among women. *Journal of the American Medical Association* 279 (1998): 359–364.

Shimakawa, T., Nieto, F. J., Malinow, M. R., Chambless, L. E., Schreiner, P. J., and Szklo, M. Vitamin intake: A possible determinant of plasma homocyst(e)ine among middle-aged adults. *Annals of Epidemiology* 7 (1997): 285–293.

Stampfer, M. J., Malinow, M. R., Willett, W. C., et al. A prospective study of plasma homocyst(e)ine and risk of myocardial infarction in US physicians. *Journal of the American Medical Association* 268 (1992): 877–881.

Tucker, K. L., Mahnken, B., Wilson, P. W., Jacques, P., and Selhub, J. Folic acid fortification of the food supply: Potential benefits and risks for the elderly population. *Journal of the American Medical Association* 276 (1996): 1879–1885.

Ubbink, J. B., Vermaak, W. J., van der Merwe, A., and Becker, P. J. Vitamin B-12, vitamin B-6, and folate nutritional status in men with hyperhomocysteinemia. *American Journal of Clinical Nutrition* 57 (1993): 47–53.

Wald, N. Folic acid and the prevention of neural tube defects. *Annals of the New York Academy of Sciences* 29 (1993): 112–129.

Garlic

Adler, A. J., and Holub, B. J. Effect of garlic and fish-oil supplementation on serum lipid and lipoprotein concentrations in hypercholesterolemic men. *American Journal of Clinical Nutrition* 65 (1997): 445–450.

Auer, W., Eiber, A., Hertkorn, E., et al. Hypertension and hyperlipidaemia: Garlic helps in mild cases. *Br J Clin Pract Symp Suppl* 69 (1990): 3–6.

Isaacsohn, J. L., Moser, M., Stein, E. A., et al. Garlic powder and plasma lipids and lipoproteins: A multicenter, randomized, placebo-controlled trial. *Archiv Intern Med* 158 (1998): 1189–1194.

Jain, A. K., Vargas, R., Gotzkowsky, S., and McMahon, F. G. Can garlic reduce levels of serum lipids? A controlled clinical study. *American Journal of Medicine* 94 (1993): 632–635.

Lea, M. A. Organosulfur compounds and cancer. *Advances in Experimental Medicine and Biology* 54 (1996): 147–154.

Ledezma, E., DeSousa, L., Jorquera, A., et al. Efficacy of ajoene, an organosulphur derived from garlic, in the short-term therapy of tinea pedis. *Mycoses* 39 (1996): 393–395.

Mader, F. H. Treatment of hyperlipidaemia with garlic-powder tablets: Evidence from the German Association of General Practitioners' multicentric placebo-controlled double-blind study. *Arzneimittel-orschung* 40 (1990): 1111–1116.

Silagy, C., and Neil, A. Garlic as a lipid lowering agent—a meta-analysis. *Journal of the Royal College of Physicians of London* 28 (1994): 39–45.

Steiner, M., Khan, A. H., Holbert, D., and Lin, R. I. A double-blind crossover study in moderately hypercholesterolemic men that compared the effect of aged garlic extract and placebo administration on blood lipids. *American Journal of Clinical Nutrition* 64 (1996): 866–870.

Vorberg, G., and Schneider, B. Therapy with garlic: Results of a placebo-controlled, double-blind study. *Br J Clin Pract Symp Suppl* 69 (1990): 7–11.

Warshafsky, S., Kramer, R. S., and Sivak, S. L. Effect of garlic on total serum cholesterol: A meta-analysis. *Annals of Internal Medicine* 119 (1993): 599–605.

Weber, N. D., Andersen, D. O., North, J. A., Murray, B. K., Lawson, L. D., and Hughes, B. G. In vitro virucidal effects of Allium sativum (garlic) extract and compounds. *Planta Medica* 58 (1992): 417–423.

Ginger

Arfeen, Z., Owen, H., Plummer, J. L., Ilsley, A. H., Sorby Adams, R. A., and Doecke, C. J. A double-blind randomized controlled trial of ginger for the prevention of postoperative nausea and vomiting. *Anaesthesia and Intensive Care* 23 (1995): 449–452.

Backon, J. Ginger in preventing nausea and vomiting of pregnancy; a caveat due to its thromboxane synthetase activity and effect on testosterone binding. *European Journal of Obstetrics, Gynecology, and Reproductive Biology* 42 (1991): 163.

Bone, M. E., Wilkinson, D. J., Young, J. R., McNeil, J., and Charlton, S. Ginger root—a new antiemetic: The effect of ginger root on postoperative nausea and vomiting after major gynaecological surgery. *Anaesthesia* 45 (1990): 669–671.

Grontved, A., Brask, T., Kambskard, J., and Hentzer, E. Ginger root against seasickness: A controlled trial on the open sea. *Acta Oto-Laryngologica* 105 (1988): 45–49.

Grontved, A., and Hentzer, E. Vertigo-reducing effect of ginger root: A controlled clinical study. *ORL: Journal of Oto-rhino-laryngology and Its Related Specialties* 48 (1986): 282–286.

Mowrey, D. B., Clayson, D. E. Motion sickness, ginger, and psychophysics. *Lancet* 1 (1982): 655–657.

Phillips, S., Ruggier, R., and Hutchinson, S. E. Zingiber officinale (ginger)—an antiemetic for day case surgery. *Anaesthesia* 48 (1993): 715–717.

Stewort, J. J., Wood, M. J., Wood, C. D., and Mims, M. E. Effects of ginger on motion sickness susceptibility and gastric function. *Pharmacology* 42 (1991): 111–120.

Ginkgo Biloba

Blume, J., Kieser, M., and Holscher, U. Placebo-controlled double-blind study of the effectiveness of ginkgo biloba special extract EGb 761 in trained patients with intermittent claudication. *Vasa* 25 (1996): 265–274.

Ernst, E. Ginkgo biloba in treatment of intermittent claudication: A systematic research based on controlled studies in the literature. *Fortschritte der Medizin* 11 (1996): 85–87.

Haase, J., Halama, P., and Horr, R. Effectiveness of brief infusions with ginkgo biloba special extract EGb 761 in dementia of the vascular and Alzheimer type. *Zeitschrift für Gerontologie und Geriatrie* 29 (1996): 302–309.

Hopfenmuller, W. Evidence for a therapeutic effect of ginkgo biloba special extract: Meta-analysis of 11 clinical studies in patients with cerebrovascular insufficiency in old age. *Arzneimittelorschung* 44 (1994): 1005–1013.

Kanowski, S., Herrmann, W. M., Stephan, K., Wierich, W., and Horr, R. Proof of efficacy of the ginkgo biloba special extract EGb 761 in outpatients suffering from mild to moderate primary degenerative dementia of the Alzheimer type or multi-infarct dementia. *Pharmacopsychiatry* 29 (1996): 47–56.

LeBar, P. L., Katz, M. M., Berman, N., et al. A placebo-controlled, double-blind, randomized trial of an extract of ginkgo biloba for dementia. *Journal of the American Medical Association* 278 (1997): 1327–1332.

Mouren, X., Caillard, P., and Schwartz, F. Study of the anti-ischemic action of EGb 761 in the treatment of peripheral arterial occlusive disease by TcPo2 determination. *Angiology* 45 (1994): 413–417.

Pietri, S., Séguin, J. R., d'Arbigny, P., Drieu, K., and Culcasi, M. Ginkgo biloba extract (EGb 761) pretreatment limits free radical-induced oxidative stress in patients undergoing coronary bypass surgery. *Cardiovascular Drugs and Therapy* 11 (1997): 121–131.

Rai, G. S., Shovlin, C., and Wesnes, K. A. A double-blind, placebo controlled study of ginkgo biloba extract ("tanakan") in elderly outpatients with mild to moderate memory impairment. *Current Medical Research and Opinion* 12 (1991): 350–355.

Rowin, J., and Lewis, S. L. Spontaneous bilateral subdural hematomas associated with chronic ginkgo biloba ingestion. *Neurology* 46 (1996): 1775–1776.

Sticher, O. Quality of ginkgo preparations. *Planta Medica* 59 (1993): 2–11.

Ginseng

Bahrke, M. S., and Morgan, W. P. Evaluation of the ergogenic properties of ginseng. *Sports Medicine* 18 (1994): 229–248.

Caso Marasco, A., Vargas Ruiz, R., Salas Villagomez, A., and Begona Infante, C. Double-blind study of a multivitamin complex supplemented with ginseng extract. *Drugs Under Experimental and Clinical Research* 22 (1996): 323–329.

Chen, X. Cardiovascular protection by ginsenosides and their nitric oxide releasing action. *Clinical and Experimental Pharmacology and Physiology* 23 (1996): 728–732.

Choi, H. K., Seong, D. H., and Rha, K. H. Clinical efficacy of Korean red ginseng for erectile dysfunction. *International Journal of Impotence Research* 7 (1995): 181–186.

D'Angelo, L., Grimaldi, R., Caravaggi, M., et al. A double-blind, placebo-controlled clinical study on the effect of a standardized ginseng extract on psychomotor performance in healthy volunteers. *Journal of Ethnopharmacology* 16 (1986): 15–22.

Morris, A. C., Jacobs, I., McLellan, T. M., Klugerman, A., Wang, L. C., and Zamecnik, J. No ergogenic effect of ginseng ingestion. *International Journal of Sport Nutrition* 6 (1996): 263–271.

Salvati, G., Genovesi, G., Marcellini, L., et al. Effects of Panax Ginseng C.A. Meyer saponins on male fertility. *Panminerva Medica* 38 (1996): 249–254.

Scaglione, F., Cattaneo, G. Alessandria, M., and Cogo, R. Efficacy and safety of the standardised ginseng extract G115 for potentiating vaccination against the influenza syndrome and protection against the common cold. *Drugs Under Experimental and Clinical Research* 22 (1996): 65–72.

See, D. M., Broumand, N., Sahl, L., and Tilles, J. G. In vitro effects of echinacea and ginseng on natural killer and antibody-dependent cell cytotoxicity in healthy subjects and chronic fatigue syndrome or acquired immunodeficiency syndrome patients. *Immunopharmacology* 35 (1997): 229–235.

Sotaniemi, E. A., Haapakoski, E., and Rautio, A. Ginseng therapy in non-insulin-dependent diabetic patients. *Diabetes Care* 18 (1995): 1373–1375.

Thommessen, B., and Laake, K. No identifiable effect of ginseng (Gericomplex) as an adjuvant in the treatment of geriatric patients. *Aging (Milano)* 8 (1996): 417–420.

Tode, T., Kikuchi, Y., Kita, T., Hirata, J., Imaizumi, E., and Nagata, I. Inhibitory effects by oral administration of ginsenoside Rh2 on the growth of human ovarian cancer cells in nude mice. *Journal of Cancer Research and Clinical Oncology* 120 (1993): 24–26.

Yun, T. K. Experimental and epidemiological evidence of the cancer-preventive effects of Panax ginseng C.A. Meyer. *Nutrition Reviews* 54 (1996): S71–S81.

Yun, T. K., and Choi, S. Y. Preventive effect of ginseng intake against various human cancers: A case-control study on 1987 pairs. *Cancer Epidemiology, Biomarkers and Prevention* 4 (1995): 401–408.

Glucosamine and Chonodroitin

Conte, A., Volpi, N., Palmieri, L., Bahous, I., and Ronca, G. Biochemical and pharamacokinetic aspects of oral treatment with chondroitin sulfate. *Arzneimittel-orschung* 45 (1995): 918–925.

Pavelka, K., Jr., Sedlácková, M., Gatterová, J., Becvár, R., and Pavelka, K. S. Glycosaminoglycan polysulfuric acid (GAGPS) in osteoarthritis of the knee. *Osteoarthritis and Cartilage* 3 (1995): 15–23.

Pipitone, V. R. Chondroprotection with chondroitin sulfate. *Drugs Under Experimental and Clinical Research* 17 (1991): 3–7.

Rovati, L. C. Clinical research in osteoarthritis: Design and results of short-term and long-term trials with disease-modifying drugs. *International Journal of Tissue Reactions* 14 (1992): 243–251.

Rovetta, G. Galactosaminoglycuronoglycan sulfate (matrix) in therapy of tibiofibular osteoarthritis of the knee. *Drugs Under Experimental and Clinical Research* 17 (1991): 53–57.

Setnikar, I., Pacini, M. A., and Revel, L. Antiarthritic effects of glucosamine sulfate studied in animal models. *Arzneimittel-orschung* 41 (1991): 542–545.

Herbal Remedies (General)

Bisset, N. G. *Herbal Drugs and Phytopharmaceuticals.* Boca Raton, FL: Medpharm Scientific Publishers/CRC Press, 1994.

The Review of Natural Products. St. Louis: Facts and Comparisons Publishing Group, 1996.

Robbers, J. E., Speedie, M. K., and Tyler, V. E. *Pharmacognosy and Pharmacobiotechnology.* Baltimore, MD: Williams and Wilkins, 1996.

Tyler, V. E. *Herbs of Choice.* Binghamton, NY: Pharmaceutical Products Press, 1994.

Tyler, V. E. *The Honest Herbal,* third edition. Binghamton, NY: Pharmaceutical Products Press, 1993.

Melatonin

Brzezinski, A. Melatonin in humans. *New England Journal of Medicine* 336 (1997): 186–195.

Cagnacci, A., Arangino, S., Angiolucci, M., Maschio, E., Longu, G., and Melis, G. B. Potentially beneficial cardiovascular effects of melatonin administration in women. *Journal of Pineal Research* 22 (1997): 16–19.

Garfinkel, D., Laudon, M., Nof, D., and Zisapel, N. Improvement of sleep quality in elderly people by controlled-release melatonin. *Lancet* 346 (1995): 541–544.

Hagan, R. M., and Oakley, N. R. Melatonin comes of age? *Trends in Pharmacological Sciences* 16 (1995): 81–83.

Haimov, I., Lavie, P., Laudon, M., Herer, P., Vigder, C., and Zisapel, N. Melatonin replacement therapy of elderly insomniacs. *Sleep* 18 (1995): 598–603.

Hughes, R. J., and Badia, P. Sleep-promoting and hypothermic effects of daytime melatonin administration in humans. *Sleep* 20 (1997): 124–131.

Lamberg, L. Melatonin potentially useful but safety, efficacy remain uncertain. *Journal of the American Medical Association* 276 (1996): 1011–1014.

Lissoni, P., Tancini, G., Barni, S., et al. Treatment of cancer chemotherapy-induced toxicity with the pineal hormone melatonin. *Supportive Care in Cancer* 5 (1997): 126–129.

Reiter, R., Tang, L., Garcia, J. J., and Munoz Hoyos, A. Pharmacological actions of melatonin in oxygen radical pathophysiology. *Life Sciences* 60 (1997): 2255–2271.

Probiotics

Chapoy, P. Treatment of acute infantile diarrhea: Controlled trial of *Saccharomyces boulardii*. *Annales de Pediatrie* 32 (1985): 561–563.

Colombel, J. F., Cortot, A., Neut, C., and Romond, C. Yoghurt with *Bifidobacterium longum* reduces erythromycin-induced gastrointestinal effects. *Lancet* 2 (1987): 43.

Elmer, G. W., Moyer, K. A., Vega, R., et al. Evaluation of *Saccharomyces boulardii* for patients with HIV-related diarrhea and healthy volunteers receiving antifungals. *Microecology and Therapy* 25 (1995): 23–31.

Elmer, G. W., Surawicz, C. M., and McFarland, L. V. Biotherapeutic agents: A neglected modality for the treatment and prevention of selected intestinal and vaginal infections. *Journal of the American Medical Association* 275 (1996): 870–876.

Hilton, E., Isenberg, H. D., Alperstein, P., France, K., and Borenstein, M. T. Ingestion of yogurt containing *Lactobacillus acidophilus* as prophylaxis for candidal vaginitis. *Annals of Internal Medicine* 116 (1992): 353–357.

Hilton, E., Rindos, P., and Isenberg, H. D. *Lactobacillus* GG vaginal suppositories and vaginitis. *Journal of Clinical Microbiology* 33 (1995): 1433.

Isolauri, E., Juntunen, M., Rautanen, T., Sillanaukee, P., and Koivula, T. A human *Lactobacillus* strain (*Lactobacillus casei* sp Strain GG) promotes recovery from acute diarrhea in children. *Pediatrics* 88 (1991): 90–97.

Kollaritsch, V. H., Holst, H., Grobara, P., and Wiedermann, G. Prophylaxe der Reisediarrhöe mit *Saccharomyces boulardii*. *Fortschritte der Medizin* 111 (1993): 153–156.

McFarland, L. V., Surawicz, C. M., Greenberg, R. N., et al. A randomized placebo-controlled trial of *Saccharomyces boulardii* in combination with standard antibiotics for *Clostridium difficile* disease. *Journal of the American Medical Association* 271 (1994): 1913–1918.

McFarland, L. V., Surawicz, C. M., Greenberg, R. N., et al. Prevention of ß-lactam-associated diarrhea by *Saccharomyces boulardii* compared to placebo. *American Journal of Gastroenterology* 90 (1995): 439–448.

Oksanen, P. J., Salminen, S., Saxelin, M., et al. Prevention of travelers' diarrhoea by *Lactobacillus* GG. *Annals of Medicine* 22 (1990): 53–56.

Orrhage, K., Brismar, B., and Nord, C. E. Effects of supplements of *Bifidobacterium longum* and *Lactobacillus acidophilus* on the intestinal microbiota during administration of clindamycin. *Microbial Ecology in Health and Disease* 7 (1994): 17–25.

Reid, G., Bruce, A. W., and Taylor, M. Influence of three-day antimicrobial therapy and *Lactobacillus* vaginal suppositories on recurrence of urinary trace infections. *Clinical Therapeutics* 14 (1992): 11–16.

Saavedra, J. M., Bauman, N. A., Oung, I., Perman, J. A., and Yolken, R. H. Feeding of *Bifidobacterium bifidum* and *Streptococcus thermophilus* to infants in hospital for prevention of diarrhea and shedding of rotavirus. *Lancet* 344 (1994): 1046–1049.

Siitonen, S., Vapaatalo, H., Salminen, S., et al. Effect of *Lactobacillus* GG yoghurt in prevention of antibiotic associated diarrhoea. *Annals of Medicine* 22 (1990): 57–59.

Surawicz, C. M., Elmer, G. W., Speelman, P., McFarland, L. V., Chinn, J., and van Belle, G. Prevention of antibiotic-associated diarrhea by *Saccharomyces boulardii:* A prospective study. *Gastroenterology* 96 (1989): 981–988.

Wunderlich, P. F., Braun, L., Fumagalli, I., et al. Double-blind report on the efficacy of lactic acid-producing *Enterococcus* SF68 in the prevention of antibiotic-associated diarrhoea and in the treatment of acute diarrhoea. *Journal of International Medical Research* 17 (1989): 333–338.

Saw Palmetto

Carraro, J. C., Raynaud, J. P., Koch, G., et al. Comparison of phytotherapy (Permixon) with finasteride in the treatment of benign prostate hyperplasia: A randomized international study of 1,098 patients. *Prostate* 29 (1996): 231–240.

Champault, G., Patel, J. C., and Bonnard, A. M. A double-blind trial of an extract of the plant Serenoa repens in benign prostatic hyperplasia. *British Journal of Clinical Pharmacology* 18 (1984): 461–462.

Délos, S., Carsol, J. L., Ghazarossian, E., Raynaud, J. P., and Martin, P. M. Testosterone metabolism in primary cultures of human prostate epithelial cells and fibroblasts. *Journal of*

Steroid Biochemistry and Molecular Biology 55 (1995): 375–383.

Paubert Braquet, M., Richardson, F. O., Servent Saez N., et al. Effect of Serenoa repens extract (Permixon) on estradiol/testosterone-induced experimental prostate enlargement in the rat. *Pharmacological Research* 34 (1996): 171–179.

Plosker, G. L., and Brogden, R. N. Serenoa repens (Permixon): A review of its pharmacology and therapeutic efficacy in benign prostatic hyperplasia. *Drugs and Aging* 9 (1996): 379–395.

Ravenna, L., Di Silverio, F., Russo, M. A., et al. Effects of the lipidosterolic extract of Serenoa repens (Permixon) on human prostatic cell lines. *Prostate* 29 (1996): 219–230.

Shimada, H., Tyler, V. E., and McLaughlin, J. L. Biologically active acylglycerides from the berries of saw-palmetto (Serenoa repens). *Journal of Natural Products* 60 (1997): 417–418.

Strauch, G., Perles, P., Vergult, G., et al. Comparison of finasteride (Proscar) and Serenoa repens (Permixon) in the inhibition of 5-alpha reductase in healthy male volunteers. *European Urology* 26 (1994): 247–252.

St. John's Wort

Golsch, S., Vocks, E., Rakoski, J., Brockow, K., and Ring, J. Reversible increase in photosensitivity to UV-B caused by St. John's wort extract. *Hautarzt* 48 (1997): 249–252.

Hansgen, K. D., Vesper, J., and Ploch, M. Multicenter double-blind study examining the antidepressant effectiveness of the hypericum extract LI 160. *Journal of Geriatric Psychiatry and Neurology* 7 suppl. (1994): S15–S18.

Harrer, G., Hubner, W. D., and Podzuweit, H. Effectiveness and tolerance of the hypericum extract LI 160 compared to maprotiline: A multicenter double-blind study. *Journal of Geriatric Psychiatry and Neurology* 7 suppl. (1994): S24–S28.

Hubner, W. D., Lande, S., and Podzuweit, H. Hypericum treatment of mild depressions with somatic symptoms. *Journal of Geriatric Psychiatry and Neurology* 7 suppl. (1994): S12–S14.

Linde, K., Ramirez, G., Mulrow, C. D., Pauls, A., Weidenhammer, W., and Melchart, D. St. John's wort for depression—an overview and meta-analysis of randomised clinical trials. *BMJ (Clinical Research Ed.)* 31 (1996): 253–258.

Martinez, B., Kasper, S., Ruhrmann, S., and Moller, H. J. Hypericum in the treatment of seasonal affective disorders. *Journal of Geriatric Psychiatry and Neurology* 7 suppl. (1994): S29–S33.

Sommer, H., and Harrer, G. Placebo-controlled double-blind study examining the effectiveness of an hypericum preparation in 105 mildly depressed patients. *Journal of Geriatric Psychiatry and Neurology* 7 suppl. (1994): S9–S11.

Vorbach, E. U., Hubner, W. D., and Arnoldt, K. H. Effectiveness and tolerance of the hypericum extract LI 160 in comparison with imipramine: Randomized double-blind study with 135 outpatients. *Journal of Geriatric Psychiatry and Neurology* 7 suppl. (1994): S19–S23.

Woelk, H., Burkard, G., and Grunwald, J. Benefits and risks of the hypericum extract LI 160: Drug monitoring study with 3250 patients. *Journal of Geriatric Psychiatry and Neurology* 7 suppl. (1994): S34–S38.

Valerian

Balderer, G., and Borbély, A. A. Effect of valerian on human sleep. *Psychopharmacologia Berl* 897 (1985): 406–409.

Cavadas, C., Aráujo, I., Cotrim, M. D., et al. In vitro study on the interaction of Valeriana officinalis L. extracts and their amino acids on GABA receptor in rat brain. *Arzneimittel-orschung* 45 (1995): 753–755.

Chan, T. Y., Tang, C. H., and Critchley, J. A. Poisoning due to an over-the-counter hypnotic, Sleep-Qik (hyoscine, cyproheptadine, valerian). *Postgraduate Medical Journal* 71 (1995): 227–228.

Gerhard, U., Linnenbrink, N., Georghiadou, C., and Hobi, V. Vigilance-decreasing effects of 2 plant-derived sedatives. *Schweizerische Rundschau Medizin Praxis* 85 (1996): 473–481.

Kohnen, R., and Oswald, W. D. The effects of valerian, propranolol, and their combination on activation, performance, and mood of healthy volunteers under social stress conditions. *Pharmacopsychiatry* 21 (1988): 447–448.

Leathwood, P. D., and Chauffard, F. Aqueous extract of valerian reduces latency to fall asleep in man. *Planta Medica* 2 (1985): 144–148.

Leathwood, P. D., Chauffard, F., Heck, E., and Munoz Box, R. Aqueous extract of valerian root (Valeriana officinalis L.) improves sleep quality in man. *Pharmacology, Biochemistry and Behavior* 17 (1982): 65–71.

Lindahl, O., and Lindwall, L. Double blind study of a valerian preparation. *Pharmacology, Biochemistry and Behavior* 32 (1989): 1065–1066.

Santos, M. S., Ferreira, F., Cunha, A. P., Carvalho, A. P., Ribeiro, C. F., and Maçedo, T. Synaptosomal GABA release as influenced by valerian root extract—involvement of the GABA carrier. *Archives Internationales de Pharmacodynamie et de Therapie* 327 (1994): 220–231.

Santos, M. S., Ferreira, F., Faro, C., et al. The amount of GABA present in aqueous extracts of valerian is sufficient to account for [3H]GABA release in synaptosomes. *Planta Medica* 60 (1994): 475–476.

Schulz, H., Stolz, C., and Muller, J. The effect of valerian extract on sleep polygraphy in poor sleepers: A pilot study. *Pharmacopsychiatry* 27 (1994): 147–151.

Willey, L. B., Mady, S. P., Cobaugh, D. J., and Wax, P. M. Valerian overdose: A case report. *Veterinary and Human Toxicology* 37 (1995): 364–365.

Vitamin A

Butler, J. C., Havens, P. L., Sowell, A. L., et al. Measles severity and serum retinol (vitamin A) concentration among children in the United States. *Pediatrics* 91 (1993): 1176–1181.

Fawzi, W. W., Chalmers, T. C., Herrera, M. G., and Mosteller, F. Vitamin A supplementation and child mortality: A meta-analysis.

Journal of the American Medical Association 269 (1993): 898–903.

Kowalski, T. E., Falestiny, M., Furth, E., and Malet, P. F. Vitamin A hepatotoxicity: A cautionary note regarding 25,000 IU supplements. *American Journal of Medicine* 97 (1994): 523–528.

Rothman, K. J., Moore, L. L., Singer, M. R., Nguyen, U.S., Mannino, S., and Milunsky, A. Teratogenicity of high vitamin A intake. *New England Journal of Medicine* 333 (1995): 1369–1373.

Sharieff, G. Q., and Hanten, K. Psuedotumor cerebri and hypercalcemia resulting from vitamin A toxicity. *Annals of Emergency Medicine* 27 (1996): 518–521.

Silverman, A. K., Ellis, C. N., and Voorhees, J. J. Hypervitaminosis A syndrome: A paradigm of retinoid side effects. *Journal of the American Academy of Dermatology* 16 (1987): 27–39.

Sommer, A. Xerophthalmia, keratomalacia and nutritional blindness. *International Ophthalmology* 14 (1990): 195–199.

Underwood, B. A. The role of vitamin A in child growth, development and survival. *Advances in Experimental Medicine and Biology* 352 (1994): 201–208.

Underwood, B. A., and Arthur, P. The contribution of vitamin A to public health. *FASEB Journal* 10 (1996): 1040–1048.

van Poppel, G., and van den Berg, H. Vitamins and cancer. *Cancer Letters* 114 (1997): 195–202.

Vitamin B₁ (Thiamin)

Fernhoff, P. M., Lubitz, D., Danner, D. J., et al. Thiamine response in maple syrup urine disease. *Pediatric Research* 19 (1985): 1011–1016.

Khan, A. A., Maibach, H. I., Strauss, W. G., and Fenley, W. R. Vitamin B₁ is not a systemic mosquito repellent in man. *Transactions of the St. Johns Hospital Dermatological Society* 55 (1969): 99–102.

Sacks, W., Esser, A. H., Feitel, B., and Abbott, K. Acetazolamide and thiamine: An ancillary therapy for chronic mental illness. *Psychiatry Research* 28 (1989): 279–288.

Sacks, W., Esser, A. H., and Sacks, S. Inhibition of pyruvate dehydrogenase complex (PDHC) by antipsychotic drugs. *Biological Psychiatry* 29 (1991): 176–182.

Strauss, W. G., Maibach, H. I., and Khan, A. A. Drugs and disease as mosquito repellents in man. *American Journal of Tropical Medicine and Hygiene* 17 (1968): 461–464.

Vitamin B_2 (Riboflavin)

Benton, D., Haller, J., and Fordy, J. The vitamin status of young British adults. *International Journal for Vitamin and Nutrition Research* 67 (1997): 34–40.

Dawsey, S. M., Wang, G. Q., Taylor, P. R., et al. Effects of vitamin/mineral supplementation on the prevalence of histological dysplasia and early cancer of the esophagus and stomach: Results from the Dysplasia Trial in Linxian, China. *Cancer Epidemiology, Biomarkers and Prevention* 3 (1994): 167–172.

Fogelholm, M., Ruokonen, I., Laakso, J. T., Vuorimaa, T., and Himberg, J. J. Lack of association between indices of vitamin B_1, B_2, and B_6 status and exercise-induced blood lactate in young adults. *International Journal of Sport Nutrition* 3 (1993): 165–176.

Folkers, K., and Ellis, J. Successful therapy with vitamin B_6 and vitamin B_2 of the carpal tunnel syndrome and need for determination of the RDAs for vitamins B_6 and B_2 for disease states. *Annals of the New York Academy of Sciences* 585 (1990): 295–301.

Mulherin, D. M., Thurnham, D. I., and Situnayake, R. D. Glutathione reductase activity, riboflavin status, and disease activity in rheumatoid arthritis. *Annals of the Rheumatic Diseases* 55 (1996): 837–840.

van der Beek, E. J., van Dokkum, W., Wedel, M., Schrijver, J., and van den Berg, H. Thiamin, riboflavin and vitamin B_6: Impact of restricted intake on physical performance in man. *Journal of the American College of Nutrition* 13 (1994): 629–640.

Vitamin B₃ (Niacin)

Alderman, J. D., Pasternak, R. C., Sacks, F. M., Smith, H. S., Monrad, E. S., and Grossman, W. Effect of a modified, well-tolerated niacin regimen on serum total cholesterol, high density lipoprotein cholesterol and the cholesterol to high density lipoprotein ratio. *American Journal of Cardiology* 64 (1989): 725–729.

Berge, K. G., and Canner, P. L. Coronary drug project: Experience with niacin. Coronary Drug Project Research Group. *European Journal of Clinical Pharmacology* 40 suppl. (1991): S49–S51.

Blankenhorn, D. H., Nessim, S. A., Johnson, R. L., Sanmarco, M. E., Azen, S. P., and Cashin Hemphill, L. Beneficial effects of combined colestipol-niacin therapy on coronary atherosclerosis and coronary venous bypass grafts. *Journal of the American Medical Association* 257 (1987): 3233–3240.

Canner, P. L., Berge, K. G., Wenger, N. K., et al. Fifteen-year mortality in Coronary Drug Project patients: Long-term benefit with niacin. *Journal of the American College of Cardiology* 8 (1986): 1245–1255.

Farmer, J. A., and Gotto, A. M., Jr. Currently available hypolipidaemic drugs and future therapeutic developments. *Baillieres Clinical Endocrinology and Metabolism* 9 (1995): 825–847.

Gibbons, L. W., Gonzalez, V., Gordon, N., and Grundy, S. The prevalence of side effects with regular and sustained-release nicotinic acid. *American Journal of Medicine* 99 (1995): 378–385.

Jacobson, T. A., Chin, M. M., Fromell, G. J., Jokubaitis, L. A., and Amorosa, L. F. Fluvastatin with and without niacin for hypercholesterolemia. *American Journal of Cardiology* 74 (1994): 149–154.

Kleijnen, J., and Knipschild, P. Niacin and vitamin B₆ in mental functioning: A review of controlled trials in humans. *Biological Psychiatry* 29 (1991): 931–941.

McKenney, J. M., Proctor, J. D., Harris, S., and Chinchili, V. M. A comparison of the efficacy and toxic effects of sustained- vs. immediate-release niacin in hypercholesterolemic patients. *Journal of the American Medical Association* 271 (1994): 672–677.

Schulman, K. A., Kinosian, B., Jacobson, T. A., et al. Reducing high blood cholesterol level with drugs: Cost-effectiveness of pharmacologic management. *Journal of the American Medical Association* 264 (1990): 3025–3033.

Whelan, A. M., Price, S. O., Fowler, S. F., and Hainer, B. L. The effect of aspirin on niacin-induced cutaneous reactions. *Journal of Family Practice* 34 (1992): 165–168.

Vitamin B₅ (Pantothenic Acid)

Hosemann, W., Wigand, M. E., Gode, U., Langer, F., and Dunker, I. Normal wound healing of the paranasal sinuses: Clinical and experimental investigations. *European Archives of Oto-rhino-laryngology* 248 (1991): 390–394.

Leung, L. H. Pantothenic acid as a weight-reducing agent: Fasting without hunger, weakness and ketosis. *Medical Hypotheses* 44 (1995): 403–405.

Leung, L. H. Pantothenic acid deficiency as the pathogenesis of acne vulgaris. *Medical Hypotheses* 44 (1995): 490–492.

Tahiliani, A. G., and Beinlich, C. J. Pantothenic acid in health and disease. *Vitamins and Hormones* 46 (1991): 165–228.

Vitamin B₆ (Pyridoxine)

Adams, P. W., Wynn, V., Rose, D. P., et al. Effect of pyridoxine (vitamin B_6) upon depression associated with oral contraceptives. *Lancet* 1, 809 (1973): 899–904.

Berman, M. K., Taylor, M. L., and Freeman, E. Vitamin B-6 in premenstrual syndrome. *Journal of the American Dietetic Association* 90 (1990): 859–861.

Coleman, M., Sobel, S., Bhagavan, H. N., et al. A double blind study of vitamin B_6 in Down's syndrome infants. Part 1— Clinical and biochemical results. *Journal of Mental Deficiency Research* 40 (1985): 233–240.

Folkers, K., and Ellis, J. Successful therapy with vitamin B_6 and vitamin B_2 of the carpal tunnel syndrome and need for determination of the RDAs for vitamins B_6 and B_2 for disease states. *Annals of the New York Academy of Sciences* 301 (1990): 295–301.

Gunn, A. D. Vitamin B_6 and the premenstrual syndrome (PMS). *International Journal for Vitamin and Nutrition Research Supplement* 24 (1985): 213–224.

Hagen, I., Nesheim, B. I., and Tuntland, T. No effect of vitamin B-6 against premenstrual tension: A controlled clinical study. *Acta Obstetricia et Gynecologica Scandinavica* 64 (1985): 667–670.

Joosten, E., van den Berg, A., Riezler, R., et al. Metabolic evidence that deficiencies of vitamin B-12 (cobalamin), folate, and vitamin B-6 occur commonly in elderly people. *American Journal of Clinical Nutrition* 58 (1993): 468–476.

Kendall, K. E., and Schnurr, P. P. The effects of vitamin B_6 supplementation on premenstrual symptoms. *Obstetrics and Gynecology* 70 (1987): 145–149.

Kleijnen, J., and Knipschild, P. Niacin and vitamin B_6 in mental functioning: A review of controlled trials in humans. *Biological Psychiatry* 29 (1991): 931–941.

Malmgren, R., Collins, A., and Nilsson, C. G. Platelet serotonin uptake and effects of vitamin B_6 treatment in premenstrual tension. *Neuropsychobiology* 18 (1987): 83–86.

Martineau, J., Barthelemy, C., Garreau, B., and Lelord, G. Vitamin B_6, magnesium, and combined B_6-Mg: Therapeutic effects in childhood autism. *Biological Psychiatry* 20 (1985): 467–478.

Smallwood, J., Ah Kye, D., and Taylor, I. Vitamin B_6 in the treatment of premenstrual mastalgia. *British Journal of Clinical Practice* 40 (1986): 532–533.

Steegers-Theunissen, R. P., Boers, G. H., Steegers, E. A., et al. Effects of sub-50 oral contraceptives on homocysteine metabolism: A preliminary study. *Contraception* 45 (1992): 129–139.

Williams, M. J., Harris, R. I., and Dean, B. C. Controlled trial of pyridoxine in the premenstrual syndrome. *Journal of International Medical Research* 13 (1985): 174–179.

Vitamin B₁₂ (Cyanocobalamin)

Dalery, K., Lussier Cacan, S., Selhub, J., Davignon, J., Latour, Y., and Genest, J., Jr. Homocysteine and coronary artery disease in French Canadian subjects: Relation with vitamins B_{12}, B_6, pyridoxal phosphate, and folate. *American Journal of Cardiology* 75 (1995): 1107–1111.

Force, R. W., and Nahata, M. C. Effect of histamine H2-receptor antagonists on vitamin B_{12} absorption. *Annals of Pharmacotherapy* 26 (1992): 1283–1286.

Pancharuniti, N., Lewis, C. A., Sauberlich, H. E., et al. Plasma homocyst(e)ine, folate, and vitamin B-12 concentrations and risk for early-onset coronary artery disease. *American Journal of Clinical Nutrition* 59 (1994): 940–948.

Requejo, A. M., Ortega, R. M., Navia, B., Gaspar, M. J., Quintas, E., and López Sobaler, A. Folate and vitamin B_{12} status in a group of preschool children. *International Journal for Vitamin and Nutrition Research* 67 (1997): 171–175.

Shimakawa, T., Nieto, F. J., Malinow, M. R., Chambless, L. E., Schreiner, P. J., and Szklo, M. Vitamin intake: A possible determinant of plasma homocyst(e)ine among middle-aged adults. *Annals of Epidemiology* 7 (1997): 285–293.

Slot, W. B., Merkus, F. W., Van Deventer, S. J., and Tytgat, G. N. Normalization of plasma vitamin B_{12} concentration by intranasal hydroxocobalamin in vitamin B_{12}–deficient patients. *Gastroenterology* 113 (1997): 430–433.

Ubbink, J. B. Vitamin nutrition status and homocysteine: An atherogenic risk factor. *Nutrition Reviews* 52 (1994): 383–387.

Vitamin C (Ascorbic Acid)

Bendich, A., and Langseth, L. The health effects of vitamin C supplementation: A review. *Journal of the American College of Nutrition* 14 (1995): 124–136.

Charleux, J. L. Beta-carotene, vitamin C, and vitamin E: The protective micronutrients. *Nutrition Reviews* 54 (1996): 109–114.

Dylewski, D. F., and Froman, D. M. Vitamin C supplementation in the patient with burns and renal failure. *Journal of Burn Care and Rehabilitation* 13 (1992): 378–380.

Hemila, H. Vitamin C supplementation and common cold symptoms: Problems with inaccurate reviews. *Nutrition* 12 (1996): 804–809.

Mehra, M. R., Lavie, C. J., Ventura, H. O., and Milani, R. V. Prevention of atherosclerosis: The potential role of antioxidants. *Postgraduate Medicine* 98 (1995): 175–176.

Ness, A. R., Chee, D., and Elliott, P. Vitamin C and blood pressure—an overview. *Journal of Human Hypertension* 11 (1997): 343–350.

Potischman, N., and Brinton, L. A. Nutrition and cervical neoplasia. *Cancer Causes and Control* 7 (1996): 113–126.

Rimm, E. B., and Stampfer, M. J. The role of antioxidants in preventive cardiology. *Current Opinion in Cardiology* 12 (1997): 188–194.

Simon, J. A. Vitamin C and cardiovascular disease: A review. *Journal of the American College of Nutrition* 11 (1992): 107–125.

Taylor, T. V., Rimmer, S., Day, B., Butcher, J., and Dymock, I. W. Ascorbic acid supplementation in the treatment of pressure-sores. *Lancet* 2 (1974): 544–546.

Vitamin D

Chapuy, M. C., Arlot, M. E., Duboeuf, F., et al. Vitamin D_3 and calcium to prevent hip fractures in the elderly women. *New England Journal of Medicine* 327 (1992): 1637–1642.

Dabek, J. An emerging view of vitamin D. *Scandinavian Journal of Clinical and Laboratory Investigation Supplement* 201 (1990): 127–133.

Holick, M. F. McCollum Award Lecture, 1994: Vitamin D—new horizons for the 21st century. *American Journal of Clinical Nutrition* 60 (1994): 619–630.

Kim, Y. I., and Mason, J. B. Nutrition chemoprevention of gastrointestinal cancers: A critical review. *Nutrition Reviews* 54 (1996): 259–279.

Lipkin, M., and Newmark, H. Calcium and the prevention of colon cancer. *Journal of Cellular Biochemistry Supplement* 22 (1995): 65–73.

Lips, P. Prevention of hip fractures: Drug therapy. *Bone* 18 (1996): 159S–163S.

Murray, T. M. Prevention and management of osteoporosis: Consensus statements from the Scientific Advisory Board of the Osteoporosis Society of Canada. 4. Calcium nutrition and osteoporosis. *Canadian Medical Association Journal* 155 (1996): 935–939.

Reid, I. R. Therapy of osteoporosis: Calcium, vitamin D, and exercise. *American Journal of Medical Sci* 312 (1996): 278–286.

Tilyard, M. W., Spears, G. F., Thomson, J., and Dovey, S. Treatment of postmenopausal osteoporosis with calcitriol or calcium. *New England Journal of Medicine* 326 (1992): 357–362.

Vitamin E

Axford Gatley, R. A., and Wilson, G. J. Reduction of experimental myocardial infarct size by oral administration of alpha tocopherol. *Cardiovascular Research* 25 (1991): 89–92.

Calzada, C., Bruckdorfer, K. R., and Rice Evans, C. A. The influence of antioxidant nutrients on platelet function in healthy volunteers. *Atherosclerosis* 128 (1997): 97–105.

Cathcart, R. F., III. Leg cramps and vitamin E. *Journal of the American Medical Association* 219 (1972): 216–217.

Corash, L., Spielberg, S., Bartsocas, C., et al. Reduced chronic hemolysis during high-dose vitamin E administration in Mediterranean-type glucose-6-phosphate dehydrogenase deficiency. *New England Journal of Medicine* 303 (1980): 416–420.

Herold, E., Mottin, J., and Sabry, Z. Effect of vitamin E on human sexual functioning. *Archives of Sexual Behavior* 8 (1979): 397–403.

Horwitt, M. K. Data supporting supplementation of humans with vitamin E. *Journal of Nutrition* 121 (1991): 424–429.

Jacob, R. A., and Burri, B. J. Oxidative damage and defense. *American Journal of Clinical Nutrition* 63 (1996): 985S–990S.

Jenkins, M., Alexander, J. W., MacMillan, B. G., Waymack, J. P., and Kopcha, R. Failure of topical steroids and vitamin E to reduce postoperative scar formation following reconstructive surgery. *Journal of Burn Care and Rehabilitation* 7 (1986): 309–312.

Kleijnen, J., Knipschild, P., and ter Riet, G. Vitamin E and cardiovascular disease. *European Journal of Clinical Pharmacology* 37 (1989): 541–544.

London, R. S., Murphy, L., Kitlowski, K. E., and Reynolds, M. A. Efficacy of alpha-tocopherol in the treatment of the premenstrual syndrome. *Journal of Reproductive Medicine* 32 (1987): 400–404.

Meydani, S. N., Meydani, M., Rall, L. C., Morrow, F., and Blumberg, J. B. Assessment of the safety of high-dose, short-term supplementation with vitamin E in healthy older adults. *American Journal of Clinical Nutrition* 60 (1994): 704–709.

Meyer, E. C., Sommers, D. K., Reitz, C. J., and Mentis, H. Vitamin E and benign breast disease. *Surgery* 107 (1990): 549–551.

Palmieri, B., Gozzi, G., and Palmieri, G. Vitamin E added silicone gel sheets for treatment of hypertrophic scars and keloids. *International Journal of Dermatology* 34 (1995): 506–509.

Pejaver, R. K., and Watson, A. H. High-dose vitamin E therapy in glutathione synthetase deficiency. *Journal of Inherited Metabolic Disease* 17 (1994): 749–750.

Sano, M., Ernesto, C., Thomas, R. G., et al. A controlled trial of selegiline, alpha tocopherol, or both as treatment for Alzheimer's disease. *New England Journal of Medicine* 336 (1997): 1216–1222.

Seddon, J. M., Christen, W. G., Manson, J. E., et al. The use of vitamin supplements and the risk of cataract among U.S. male physicians. *American Journal of Public Health* 84 (1994): 788–792.

Simon Schnass, I. M. Nutrition at high altitude. *Journal of Nutrition* 122 (1992): 778–781.

Simon, G. A., Schmid, P., Reifenrath, W. G., van Ravenswaay, T., and Stuck, B. E. Wound healing after laser injury to skin—the effect of occlusion and vitamin E. *Journal of Pharmaceutical Sciences* 83 (1994): 1101–1106.

Traber, M. G., and Sies, H. Vitamin E in humans: Demand and delivery. *Annual Review of Nutrition* 16 (1996): 321–347.

Weber, P., Bendich, A., and Machlin, L. J. Vitamin E and human health: Rationale for determining recommended intake levels. *Nutrition* 13 (1997): 450–460.

Zidenberg Cherr, S., and Keen, C. L. Influence of dietary manganese and vitamin E on adriamycin toxicity in mice. *Toxicology Letters* 30 (1986): 79–87.

Index

About the Authors

Educated at Columbia University, **Harold M. Silverman,** Pharm.D., has worked as a hospital pharmacist, author, educator, and pharmaceutical consultant. He currently is Vice-Chairman of Interscience, a global health care communications consultancy. In addition to *The Vitamin Book,* Dr. Silverman is Editor-in-Chief of *The Pill Book* and the author of *The Pill Book Guide to Safe Drug Use, The Consumer's Guide to Poison Protection, The Women's Drug Store,* and *Travel Healthy.* Dr. Silverman has written more than seventy articles, research papers, and textbook chapters, including *The Merck Manual of Medical Information—Home Edition.* He is a member and past officer of many professional organizations, has taught pharmacology and clinical pharmacy at several universities, and has won numerous awards for his work. Dr. Silverman resides in the Washington, D.C. area with his wife, Judith Brown and their son, Joshua.

Joseph A. Romano, Pharm.D., has more than twenty-five years experience in health care as a practitioner, educator, and administrator. He is currently Vice Chairman of Nelson Communications Inc., one of the largest health care communications companies in the world. In that capacity, he serves as Chairman/Partner of two business sectors: SCIENS Worldwide Healthcare Communications and Nelson Professional Sales. Dr. Romano's past academic career includes tenure as Associate Dean and Associate Professor at the University of Washington in Seattle. He is an adjunct faculty lecturer at several institutions. He has also authored numerous professional papers and two textbooks in pharmacy and pharmacology. Dr. Romano resides in the Princeton, New Jersey, area with his wife and two children.

Gary W. Elmer, Ph.D., is an Associate Professor of Medicinal Chemistry at the University of Washington School of Pharmacy. He obtained his B.S. degree in Pharmacy and a M.S. degree in Pharmacognosy from the University of Connecticut and a Ph.D. from Rutgers University. Dr. Elmer is the coauthor of the vitamin and mineral chapter in the *Handbook of NonPrescription Drugs* and has published and lectured extensively on dietary supplements and their proper use. In his laboratories at the University of Washington, he researches herbal/drug interactions and the application of biotherapeutic agents (probiotics) in the treatment of infectious diseases.

Visit the authors' Web site at www.thevitaminbook.com